Updates in Clinical Dermatology

Series Editors:

John Berth-Jones
Chee Leok Goh
Howard I. Maibach

More information about this series at http://www.springer.com/series/13203

Ana M. Giménez-Arnau
Howard I. Maibach

Editors

Contact Urticaria Syndrome

Diagnosis and Management

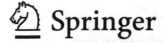 Springer

Editors
Ana M. Giménez-Arnau, MD, PhD
Hospital del Mar - Institut Mar
d'Investigacions Mediques
Universitat Autònoma de Barcelona
(UAB)
Department of Dermatology
Barcelona, Spain

Howard I. Maibach, MD
Department of Dermatology
University of California San Francisco
San Francisco, CA, USA

ISSN 2523-8884   ISSN 2523-8892   (electronic)
Updates in Clinical Dermatology
ISBN 978-3-030-07851-5   ISBN 978-3-319-89764-6   (eBook)
https://doi.org/10.1007/978-3-319-89764-6

I dedicate this book to my family, colleagues and patients –
who give me confidence in my daily work.

Ana M. Giménez-Arnau

Preface

We, as subjects who live in this world, are constantly exposed to environmental agents capable of stimulating our innate and acquired immunity. Our skin, as a complete immunological organ, recognizes such environmental agents and develops a mechanism of protection. But why does our cutaneous immune system sometimes recognize common environmental agents as foreign and develop active diseases such as eczema or urticaria? Are allergies a sign of a weak immune system?

Signs and symptoms of the contact urticaria syndrome are associated with a substantial burden in the context of health. Eczema and urticaria are prevalent disabling diseases that interfere with the quality of life and have a well-recognized occupational relevance. For this reason, early diagnosis of these diseases is recommended. From the very beginning it is crucial that the patient receive correct information. What is needed is fast identification of the disease and immediate recommendation of the patient to the correct specialist who will develop an etiological diagnosis using the proper complementary tools.

All physicians should be capable of recognizing clinically the typical signs and symptoms that define an immediate skin contact reaction, diagnostic of contact urticaria, and protein contact dermatitis. This book includes a glossary of the essential concepts necessary to understand contact urticaria syndrome. The source of exposure to potential responsible agents is broad, and wherever possible it should be verified. This book is designed to give proper general information for the correct understanding of these prevalent skin cutaneous diseases in a practical way.

Young and veteran professionals, chemists, and physicians involved in different specialties such as dermatology, allergy, or occupational medicine built the chapters of the book. We thank them all for their enthusiasm and very good work. From epidemiology to the clinical management of specific cases, pathogenic, clinical expression, and diagnostic tools are extensively reviewed and clear protocols and algorithms are provided.

Our goal was to make this book easy to read, easy to understand, and easy to apply in your daily practice. We recommend including this text in your library. It will help improve your capacity for diagnosis and consequently your relationship with your population of reference.

Barcelona, Spain   Ana M. Giménez-Arnau
San Francisco, CA, USA   Howard I. Maibach

Contents

Contributors

Jose Hernán Alfonso, MD, PhD Department of Occupational Medicine and Epidemiology, National Institute of Occupational Health, Oslo, Norway

Ricardo Cardona, MD, MSc, EAC Group of Clinical and Experimental Allergy (GACE), IPS Universitaria, University of Antioquia, Medellín, Colombia

Gustavo Deza, MD Hospital del Mar - Institut Mar d'Investigacions Mediques, Universitat Autònoma de Barcelona (UAB), Department of Dermatology, Barcelona, Spain

Ana M. Giménez-Arnau, MD, PhD Hospital del Mar - Institut Mar d'Investigacions Mediques, Universitat Autònoma de Barcelona (UAB), Department of Dermatology, Barcelona, Spain

Elena Giménez-Arnau, MD Dermatochemistry Laboratory, Institut de Chimie de Strasbourg (CNRS UMR 7177), Université de Strasbourg, Strasbourg, France

Marléne Isaksson Department of Occupational and Environmental Dermatology, Lund University, Malmö University Hospital, Malmö, Sweden

Leah Ariella Kaplan, BFA Tulane University, New Orleans, LA, USA

Emek Kocatürk, MD Okmeydanı Training and Research Hospital, Department of Dermatology, İstanbul, Turkey

Tabi A. Leslie, BSc(Hons), MBBS(Hons) Royal Free Hospital, London, UK

Howard I. Maibach, MD Department of Dermatology, University of California, San Francisco, San Francisco, CA, USA

Maria Estela Martinez Escala, MD, PhD Department of Dermatology, Northwestern University, Feinberg School of Medicine, Chicago, IL, USA

Kayria Muttardi, MBBS, BSc, MRCP (Dermatology) West Hertfordshire NHS Trust, Department of Dermatology, Hertfordshire, UK

David Orton, BSc, MSc (Allergy), MBBS, FRCP The Hillingdon Hospitals NHS Trust, Uxbridge, UK

Eduardo Rozas-Muñoz, MD Department of Dermatology, Hospital de la Santa Creu i Sant Pau, Barcelona, Spain

Jorge Sánchez, MD, MSC, Allergist Group of Clinical and Experimental Allergy, IPS Universitaria, University of Antioquia, Medellin, Colombia

Foundation for the Development of Medical and Biological Sciences (FUNDEMEB), Cartagena, Colombia

Joaquin Sastre, MD, PhD Allergy Department Fundación Jiménez Díaz, Universidad Autónoma de Madrid, and CIBER de Enfermedades Respiratorias (CIBERES, Institute Carlos III, Ministry of Economy and Competitiveness), Madrid, Spain

Esther Serra-Baldrich, MD Hospital de la Santa Creu i Sant Pau, Department of Dermatology, Barcelona, Spain

Sarah H. Wakelin, BSc, MBBS, FRCP St. Mary's Hospital, Imperial College Healthcare Trust, London, UK

Essentials and Updated Concepts

Ana M. Giménez-Arnau and Howard I. Maibach

The skin is a protective interface developed to preserve the homeostasis of the human body. A coordinated interaction between the epidermis and the dermis is responsible for the cutaneous immune response. In 1978, Streilein [1] introduced the concept of skin-associated lymphoid tissues, or "SALT," analogous to gut-, bronchial-, or conjunctival-associated lymphoid tissues. The SALT include as active principals epidermal cells—for example, keratinocytes, Langerhans cells, or resident lymphocytes—as well as migrant specific epidermotropic lymphocytes. In the dermis some tissular specialized cells such as mast cells are also involved in the response to environmental injuries. The immunological function of the skin shows a sophisticated degree of specialization as well as barrier function, melanogenesis, thermoregulation, vitamin D and B synthesis, and sensorial perception (touch, itch, pain). The skin presents a complete function of the relation between the human body and the environment. Microorganisms, toxins, physical phenomena, or chemical agents are, among others, components that exhibit a continuous interaction with the skin. Together the cells in the epidermis also serve as a vast reservoir of soluble biological response modifiers. The cytokines produced in the epidermis allow the skin to recruit and activate a wide range of inflammatory cells, providing an early signal to the host immune system that the external barrier has been disrupted.

The main objective of this chapter is to introduce the essential and updated concepts that will help the reader to understand a specific syndrome characterized by an inflammatory skin response to specific environmental agents (Table 1.1). Contact urticaria syndrome (CUS) is often misdiagnosed. It shows characteristics that break with the classical classification of hypersensitivity reactions, often exhibiting simultaneously different clinical types of immediate contact reactions. The cutaneous manifestations range from immediate wheals common in type I (IgE-mediated) to immediate eczema commonly present in type IV (cellularly mediated) hypersensitivity reactions. As a consequence of the clinical observation of isolated cases, we have learned that proteins and also chemicals with a low molecular weight can induce immediate cutaneous reactions clinically expressed with pruritus, wheals, and eczema through an immunological mechanism still not completely understood.

A. M. Giménez-Arnau (✉)
Hospital del Mar - Institut Mar d'Investigacions Mediques, Universitat Autònoma de Barcelona (UAB), Department of Dermatology,
Barcelona, Spain
e-mail: 22505aga@comb.cat

H. I. Maibach
Department of Dermatology, University of California, San Francisco, San Francisco, CA, USA

Table 1.1 Essential and updated basic concepts reviewed

Allergy
Antigen
Chronic inducible urticaria (CIndU)
Chronic spontaneous urticaria (CSU)
Contact dermatitis (CD)
Contact urticaria (CoU)
Contact urticaria syndrome (CUS)
Dermatitis
Eczema
Epitope
Hapten
Hypersensitivity
Immediate skin contact reaction (ISCR)
Immunoglobulin E
Immunological contact urticaria (ICoU)
Lymphocyte
Mast cell or mastocyte
Nonimmunological contact urticaria (NI-CoU)
Occupational dermatosis (OD)
Protein
Protein contact dermatitis (PCD)
Type I hypersensitivity
Type IV hypersensitivity
Urticaria
Work-related disease (WRD)

CUS Is Defined in Parallel and Includes Different Types of Immediate Contact Skin Reactions

CUS is a syndrome induced by environmental factors with heterogeneous clinical manifestations and a common denominator, the immediate appearance after exposure to the triggering agent. CUS shows different types of lesions that adhere to the general concept of contact dermatitis (CD). This term includes any inflammatory skin reaction, most of which are caused by direct contact with noxious agents in the environment. Although the main clinical expression of CD is eczema, contact urticaria, erythroderma, erythema multiforme, or lichenoid eruptions are also described. The history of CD in the twentieth century goes concomitantly with the history of patch testing, which is considered a useful tool for discovering the etiology of delayed cutaneous reactions. Nevertheless, for immediate CD, such as contact urticaria (CoU) or protein contact dermatitis (PCD) caused by a specific IgE, the prick test is useful as a cutaneous provocation test.

In patients suffering from CUS, immediate contact inflammatory reactions usually appear within minutes after contact with eliciting substances. Maibach and Johnson [2] defined it as an entity in 1975. Since then, new cases have been continuously reported, increasing the list of triggers, either proteins or chemicals.

The term CoU, introduced by Fisher (1973), refers to a wheal and flare reaction following external contact with a substance [3]. This phenomenon has long been recognized as usually appearing within 30 min and clearing completely within hours, without residual signs [4]. Urticarial lesions from nettles and hairy caterpillars have been reported since the nineteenth century [5]. Contact wheals and pruritus were noticed by 52.1% of 1224 adults in Spain included in a randomly designed survey, and 100% of them showed cutaneous symptoms induced by the pine processionary [6]. Naturally existing urticariogens were used therapeutically in old-style medicine as rubefacients and vesicants [7].

Protein contact dermatitis (PCD) was reported and defined by Hjorth and Roed-Petersen in 1976. It is an immediate eczematous dermatitis induced after contact with proteins [8–10]. Thirty-three food caterers suffering exacerbation of the itch, followed by erythema and vesicles immediately after contact with meat, fish, and vegetables, were described. Application of the relevant foods to the affected skin resulted in either urticaria or eczema [11]. Atopy and PCD are associated in approximately 50% of affected patients [12].

Patients suffering CUS can develop the syndrome immediately after contact with the trigger substance, CoU, and/or dermatitis/eczema. These immediate contact reactions can appear over normal or eczematous skin. Both cutaneous symptoms and entities can be induced by the same trigger factor and can be suffered by the same patient. CUS is characterized by the immediate development of contact skin reactions (ICSR), mainly consisting of wheals and/or eczema.

Basic Concepts Necessary to Understand the Contact Urticaria Syndrome

Definition of Allergy

An allergy is a condition that causes a person to become sick or develop skin or breathing problems because of an environmental trigger factor. Altered bodily reactivity (such as hypersensitivity) to an antigen occurs in response to a first exposure. A more general definition concerns any exaggerated or pathological immunological reaction (as by sneezing, difficult breathing, itching, or skin rashes) to substances, situations, or physical states that are without comparable effect on the average individual [13, 14].

Definition of Hypersensitivity

Hypersensitivity is a state of altered reactivity in which the body reacts with an exaggerated immune response to a foreign agent. Anaphylaxis and allergy are forms of hypersensitivity. The hypersensitivity states and resulting hypersensitivity reactions are usually subclassified by the Gell and Coombs classification as types I–IV [13–15].

Definition of Type I Hypersensitivity

Type I hypersensitivity is an immediate hypersensitivity that is antibody mediated, occurring within minutes when a sensitized individual is exposed to the antigen. Clinical manifestations are mostly classical IgE-mediated reactions involved in anaphylaxis and when diseases such as rhinoconjunctivitis, bronchial asthma, urticaria, or angioedema show an allergic pathomechanism. The first exposure to the antigen induces the production of IgE antibodies that bind the receptors on mast cells and basophils. Subsequent exposure to the antigen triggers production and release mediators acting on other cells responsible for the disease symptoms such as edema, bronchospasm, mucous secretion, or inflammation [13–15].

Definition of Type IV Hypersensitivity

Type IV hypersensitivity is a delayed-type hypersensitivity that takes 24–72 h or as long as 7 days to develop and is mediated by T lymphocytes rather than by antibodies. These immune reactions are not transferable by serum but through sensitized effector T lymphocytes. Cellular immunity can have a protective function, but under certain conditions may induce disease. Allergic contact dermatitis represents the classical clinical example of type IV or cellular hypersensitivity. Type IV reactions may be further subdivided into type IVa (TH1-triggered reaction, such as allergic contact dermatitis), type IVb (TH2-triggered reaction such as atopic eczema and protein contact dermatitis), or type IVc (T cyt CD8, e.g., bullous drug eruptions) [13–15].

Definition of Immunoglobulin E (IgE)

Immunoglobulin E is a type of immunoglobulin found in mammals and synthesized by plasma cells. Monomers of IgE consist of two heavy chains (ε chains) and two light chains, with the ε chain containing four Ig-like constant domains (Cε1–Cε4). It was simultaneously discovered, in 1966 and 1967, by two groups, one directed by Ishizaka and one conducted by Johansson and Bennich. The physiological function of IgE is rarely discussed in parasitic infections. IgE is involved in type I hypersensitivity. Two types of IgE receptors have been described: the high-affinity IgE receptor (type I Fcε receptor) and the low-affinity IgE receptor (type II Fcε receptor or CD63). Type I Fcε receptor is expressed on mast cells, basophils, and the antigen-presenting dendritic cells. The type II Fcε receptor is always expressed on B cells, and IL-4 can induce its expression on the surfaces of macrophages, eosinophils, platelets, and some T cells. Recently IgE and its receptors have been involved in autoimmunity based on its pathogenic role in chronic urticaria, immunotherapy, and severe atopic dermatitis [13–15].

Definition of a Lymphocyte

A lymphocyte is a type of white blood cell that is part of the immune system. There are two main types of lymphocytes: B cells and T cells. A very basic approach states that B lymphocytes recognize antigens and become plasma cells that produce antibodies. At least three types of T lymphocytes are described: cytotoxic, helper, and regulatory T cells that can become memory T cells. Helper T cells, after being stimulated by an antigen, secrete cytokines, which stimulate the differentiation of B cells into plasma cells promoting antibody production. Regulatory T cells act to control immune reactions. Cytotoxic T cells, which are activated by various cytokines, eliminate infected and cancer cells, for example. Sensitized T lymphocytes are involved in allergic contact dermatitis, protein contact dermatitis, the chronic phase of atopic dermatitis, and many drug-induced exanthematous eruptions. The tuberculin reaction as well as organ transplant rejection follow similar mechanisms. Predominantly T-helper 1 cells have a role in delayed-type hypersensitivity, whereas T-helper 2 reactions are important in the early phase of atopic eczema [13–15].

Definition of Mast Cells or Mastocytes

Mast cells or mastocytes are immune cells of the myeloid lineage that are present in connective tissues throughout the body. Paul Ehrlich first described this multidisciplinary cell in 1878. Mast cells originate from pluripotent progenitor cells of the bone narrow, and mature under the influence of the c-*kit* ligand and stem cell factor in the presence of other growth factors provided by the microenvironment of the tissue where they will reside. Under normal conditions, mature mast cells do not circulate in the bloodstream. In spite of the similarities between mast cells and basophils, the two cells seem to develop from different hematopoietic lineages and thus cannot be the same cells. Mast cells are pluripotential cells involved in many physiological functions and also in the pathomechanism of different diseases involving different vital organs. They have a central role in innate immunity (against infections) and adaptive immunity (allergy and autoimmunity) as well as in angiogenesis maintaining the immune homeostasis. One of the main receptors shown on the surface of the cutaneous mast cell is the type I Fcε IgE receptor, a cell actively involved in immunological contact urticaria [13–15].

Definition of Proteins

Proteins are large biomolecules or macromolecules in which the structure of one or more long chains of amino acid residues is present. Proteins are assembled from amino acids using information encoded in the genes. Each protein has its own unique amino acid sequence. Proteins are essential constituents in organic chemistry. Certain proteins, such as foods, can be allergens and induce an immune response. Proteins are the major responsible agents in contact urticaria and protein contact dermatitis [13–15].

Definition of Antigens

An antigen is a molecule capable of inducing an immune response to produce antibodies in the host organism. Sometimes antigens are part of the host itself. Antigenic molecules, commonly large biological polymers, usually present surface features that can act as the point of interaction for specific antibodies. Any such feature constitutes an epitope. Most antigens have the potential to be bound by multiple antibodies, each of which is specific to one antigen epitope. Antigen specificity results from the side-chain conformations of the antigen [13–15].

Definition of a Hapten

A hapten is a small molecule, not antigenic by itself, that can elicit an immune response only when is attached to a large carrier, such a protein. The carrier does not elicit the immune response by itself, but haptens combined with the carrier can induce cell-mediated hypersensitivity (type

IV) and humoral immune response hypersensitivity (type I). Commonly haptens are responsible for contact dermatitis but are also described as a cause of contact urticaria [13–15].

Immediate Contact Skin Reactions (ICSR)

An immediate contact skin reaction (ICSR) is an inflammatory cutaneous and/or mucous condition that appears within minutes of contact with various substances, including chemicals, animal products, antibiotics, cosmetics, and many other materials. Immediate contact skin reactions are manifested as itchy flares, wheals, dermatitis, or eczema. These clinical expressions characterize two defined entities, contact urticaria and protein contact dermatitis, with different mechanisms involved based on the allergen characteristics. Both diseases are included in the definition of contact urticaria syndrome [16].

Eczema

Eczema is an inflammatory dermatosis that includes a group of skin disorders exhibiting a common pattern of histological and clinical findings that vary depending on the stage of the disease. The origin of the term eczema comes from the Greek term *ekzeim*, "to boil over," which relates to the spongiotic vesiculation of the epidermis characteristic of some stages of the disorder. The clinical sequence of eczema is erythema, vesicles, and exudation (acute stage), followed by excoriation, lichenification, and fissures (chronic stage). It is characterized by a strong itchy sensation. The terms eczema and dermatitis (inflammation of the skin) are often thought of being synonymous, but not all forms of dermatitis are eczematous [13–15].

Dermatitis

Dermatitis is a general term used to describe inflammation of the skin. Most types of dermatitis are characterized by an itchy pink or red rash.

The term dermatitis includes a group of skin conditions such as atopic dermatitis, allergic contact dermatitis, irritant dermatitis, stasis dermatitis, and also protein contact dermatitis. Dermatitis does not necessarily show an eczematous clinical and pathological expression [13–15].

Urticaria

Urticaria is a disease characterized by the development of wheals (hives), angioedema, or both. Urticaria should be differentiated from other medical conditions in which wheals, angioedema, or both can occur as a symptom, such as auto-inflammatory syndromes or kinin-mediated angioedema. Three features characterize the wheal: a central swelling of variable size, almost invariably surrounded by reflex erythema, an itching or sometimes burning sensation, and a fleeting nature. The skin returns to its normal appearance, usually within 1–24 h. Angioedema involves the lower dermis and subcutis: it is sometimes painful rather than itching and can take up to 72 h to resolve [17].

Work-Related Disease

Work-related diseases (WRD) are those with solid scientific evidence concerning a possible occupational origin, which may, however, not fulfill all given criteria for recognition of an occupational disease (OD) according to the official list of ODs. Therefore, when making the diagnosis of an OD or WRD, it is necessary to establish a causal link between exposure to a risk factor and development of the disease, because definitions for both conditions are based on the notion of occupational risk. The contact urticaria syndrome frequently is caused by work exposure to environmental agents responsible for cutaneous signs and symptoms [18].

Occupational Dermatoses (OD)

The World Health Organization (WHO) defines occupational dermatoses (OD) as "any disease contracted primarily as a result of an exposure to risk factors arising from work activity." The International Labour Organization (ILO) defines the two main element requirements of an OD as follows: the causal relationship between exposure in a specific working environment or work activity and a specific disease, and the fact that the disease occurs among a group of exposed persons with a frequency above the average morbidity of the rest of the population. Based on the ILO recommendation, the evaluation of occupational causation should take into consideration the following criteria: association, consistency, specificity, time course, biological dose effects, biological plausibility, and coherence [18].

Burden of the Contact Urticaria Syndrome

ICSR are common in dermatological practice although there is a lack of general epidemiological information about CUS, CoU, or PCD [10, 19–23]. A prevalence of 5% to 10% for latex CoU has been published [12]. Only isolated cases or short series of patients are described when we consider other triggers. Because many cases show an occupational relevance, an accurate and complete reporting of such CUS that are WRD or OD is important for monitoring and allocation of resources. Current registries are incomplete [24]. A good reporting system would include a consequent reduction of cost related to medical care, retraining, and compensation.

In a few countries, as in Finland since 1989, CoU was classified as a separate occupational skin disease. The "Finnish Register of Occupational Diseases" (1990–1994) showed that CoU was the second most frequent cause of occupational dermatosis (29.5%), after contact allergic dermatitis (70.5%) [25, 26]. The most common trigger agents reported were at that time cow dander (44.4%), natural rubber latex (23.7%), and flour, grains, and feed (11.3%) [27]. Recently, the same group reviewed retrospectively a series of 291 cases of occupational CoU or PCD registered between 1995 and 2011. Concomitant occupational asthma caused by the same agent as the skin disease was detected in 60

patients (21%), and occupational rhinitis was detected in 111 patients (38%). The acid anhydrides are added to the traditional responsible agents. Because at least 46% of the patients with occupational CoU and PCD had concomitant occupational airway disease, specific questions and exploration should be considered [28]. Less prevalence of occupational CoU, about 8.3%, was found in a retrospective study done in a referral center for occupational dermatology in Melbourne, Australia [27]. Obviously hands, arms, and face were the most frequently involved body areas. Atopy was a significant risk factor for natural rubber latex, foodstuffs, or ammonium persulfate CoU. Health workers, food handlers, and hairdressers were the most commonly affected. In Singapore, in the assessment of 335 restaurant, catering, and fast-food employees, the most common occupational dermatosis was irritant contact dermatitis (10%), and CoU urticaria was sporadically reported just in 2 patients caused by lobster and prawn [29]. Exposure conditions indicate the percentage of CoU risk.

Some useful data are available for some risky occupations as such as healthcare workers. In Europe the prevalence of occupational CoU in this pool of employees was 5% to 10%, compared with the 1% and 3% described in the general population. Other occupations with high risk are as food handlers or workers in agriculture, farming, floriculture, plastics, or pharmaceutical and other laboratories, as well as hunters, veterinarians, biologists, or hairdressers. As we mentioned, when proteins are involved as triggers of CUS, atopy is a well-demonstrated risk factor [30].

The new proposed classification of occupational dermatosis for the "International Code of Diseases (ICD)-11" includes contact dermatitis (CD) joined with contact urticaria (CoU). The implementation of the proposed ICD-11 classification of WRSD/OSD is recommended by the COST Action StanDerm (TD 1206) [18]. The long version of the Nordic Occupational Skin Questionnaire (NOSQ-2002), which was developed to detect occupational hand dermatitis, includes at least nine questions about urticaria symptoms. NOSQ-2002 is a useful tool for the screening of hand eczema and CoU [31]. Very few standardized methods have been developed to evaluate easily the occupational relevance of CUS. Although the validated Mathias' criteria are available [32], only a limited number of physicians use them. An accurate and easy methodology useful to establish the occupational relevance in each case would be desirable.

Basic Pathogenic Concepts of Chronic Urticaria Syndrome

The mechanisms underlying immediate contact skin reactions are partially understood and show differences in CoU from PCD. The chemistry and the type of exposure to the trigger are important in the clinical appearance of the ISCR developed. The mechanism involved in ISCR may or may not be immunological. Nonimmunological CoU (NICoU) is caused by such vasogenic mediators as histamine, acetylcholine, leukotrienes, prostaglandins, and others without involvement of immunological processes. Damage of the blood vessels, making them leaky and inducing mast cell degranulation, is caused by dimethyl sulfoxide (DMSO) [33]. Because of the good therapeutic response to acetylsalicylic acid and nonsteroidal anti-inflammatory drugs (orally and topically); a role for prostaglandins was suggested [34–36]. Prostaglandin D2 without concomitant histamine release has been demonstrated following topical application of sorbic acid and benzoic acid [37, 38]. Capsaicin pretreatment (which depletes substance P) inhibits the allergen prick test flare of immunological CoU (ICoU) but not NICoU [39]. Nonspecific tachyphylaxis of variable duration has been associated with various urticariogens [40]. Irritant chemicals or proinflammatory mediators causing NICoU can be delivered by harp hairs from animals or spines from plants [41]. Immunological CoU (ICoU) reflects a type I hypersensitivity reaction, mediated by allergen-specific immunoglobulin E (IgE) in a previously sensitized individual [42]. IgE binding on mast cells induces its degranulation and subsequent release of histamine and other vasoactive substances such as prostaglan-

dins, leukotrienes, and kinins. The OAS is generally caused by an IgE-mediated type I allergic response involving birch pollinosis that shows cross-reactivity because of its structural homology with Rosaceae fruits such as apple or peach [43–45] and by some other foods such as peanuts (Ara h1 and 2) or other fruits. A combination of type I and type IV allergic skin reactions, the latter supported by positive delayed patch tests, has been suggested as PCD pathogenesis [46, 47]. PCD is an eczematous IgE-mediated reaction through proteins similar to the aeroallergen-induced atopic dermatitis [48].

Contact Urticaria Syndrome Chemistry

Cutaneous and systemic signs and symptoms of CUS can be induced by protein (molecular weight 10,000 to several hundred thousand daltons) and also chemicals (molecular weights less than 1000) [49]. The list of published substances responsible for CoU or PCD is very long. Not always has the agent involved in the ISCR been correctly studied according a detailed diagnostic protocol. There is, in general, a lack of studies including a control group. Nevertheless, different sources of responsible agents were described: animal and plant derivatives, foods and food additives [50], fragrances [51] and cosmetics, drugs, preservatives, rubber, metals, etc. Assessment of each occupational relevance is crucial [52, 53].

The stinging nettles wheals, induced by *Urtica dioica* for example, give the name to the disease, urticaria. Its mechanism is nonimmunological. Other responsible agents of NICoU are preservatives, fragrances, and flavorings in cosmetics, toiletries, topical medications, or in foodstuffs as benzoic and sorbic acid [54]. Household, industrial, insecticide, and laboratory chemicals can also induce NICoU. Proteins of plants, raw fruits, and vegetables, or animal proteins, chemicals such as drugs and preservatives, or more diverse substances such as metals and industrial chemicals can induce ICoU. The main risk factors for latex sensitization include atopy constitution and

Table 1.2 Substances responsible for ISCR in CSU

Animal derivatives
Plant derivatives
Foods
Food additives
Fragrances
Cosmetics
Drugs
Preservatives
Rubber
Metals

Reference numbers of isolated cases or series of cases of CUS (CoU and PCD) published in the literature are included [61–140]

prolonged exposure via damaged epidermis, such as glove wearers with hand eczema. Low molecular weight materials normally act as haptens and induce a cellular immunological response; nevertheless, for some of these IgE antibodies have been also demonstrated, such as platinum and nickel–serum albumin complexes [55, 56]. Few substances elicit mixed features of NICoU and ICoU through an unestablished mechanism. Other than IgE is involved in ammonium persulfate-induced CoU, where specific IgG and IgM activate the complement cascade through the classical pathway [57, 58]. Immediate reactions to formaldehyde seem not to be mediated by IgE, a prostaglandin role being suspected because of thromboxane B_2 and prostaglandin PGF_2 increased levels [59, 60]. For many of the trigger factors involved, the mechanism of the reaction is not fully understood. Table 1.2 includes the most common groups of substances responsible for ISCR in CSU. The references of isolated cases or series of cases of CUS (CoU and PCD) published in the literature are included [61–140].

Key Notes Messages

This book is designed as a useful tool to give to dermatologists and general practitioners the basic concepts related to the CUS. Maibach and Johnson defined PCD as an entity in 1975. Since then new cases have been continuously reported, increasing the list of triggers, either proteins or chemicals. Patients suffering from CUS can develop wheals/hives and/or dermatitis/eczema immediately after contact with the trigger substance. These immediate contact reactions can appear over normal or eczematous skin. Both cutaneous symptoms and entities can be induced by the same trigger factor and can be suffered by the same patient. CUS is characterized by the immediate development of contact skin reactions, ICSR, mainly consisting of wheals or eczema. ISCD are common in dermatological practice although there is a lack of general epidemiological information about CUS, CoU, or PCD. Because many cases show an occupational relevance, an accurate and complete reporting of such CUS that are WRD or OD is important. The ICD-11 includes both cutaneous diseases CD and CoU. The mechanism involved in ISCR may or may not be immunological. Not always has the agent involved in the ISCR been correctly studied according to a detailed diagnostic protocol. All these aspects are considered in successive chapters of this book.

References

1. Streilein JW. Chap 2: Skin-associated lymphoid tissue. In: Norris DA, editor. Immune mechanisms of cutaneous disease. New York: Marcel Dekker; 1989. p. 73–95.
2. Maibach HI, Johnson HL. Contact urticaria syndrome: contact urticaria to diethyltoluamide (immediate type hypersensitivity). Arch Dermatol. 1975;111:726–30.
3. Wakelin SH. Contact urticaria. Clin Exp Dermatol. 2001;26:132–6.
4. Fisher AA. Contact dermatitis. 2nd ed. Philadelphia: Lea & Febiger; 1973. p. 283–6.
5. Lesser E. Lehrbuch der Haut-und Teschlechtskrankheiten fur studirende und arzte (in German). Leipzig: Verlag von FCW Vogel; 1894.
6. Vega JM, Moneo I, Garcia Ortiz JC, Sánchez Palla P, Sanchis ME, Vega J, Gonzalez-Muñoz M, Battisti A, Roques A. Prevalence of cutaneous reactions to pine processionary moth (*Thaumetopoea pityocampa*) in an adult population. Contact Dermatitis. 2011;64:220–8.
7. Burdick AE, Mathias T. The contact urticaria syndrome. Dermatol Clin. 1985;3:71–84.
8. Maibach HI. Immediate hypersensitivity in hand dermatitis: role of food contact dermatitis. Arch Dermatol. 1976;112:1289–91.

9. Hannuksela M. Atopic contact dermatitis. Contact Dermatitis. 1980;6:30.

10. Veien NK, Hattel T, Justesen O, Norholm A. Dietary restrictions in the treatment of adult patients with eczema. Contact Dermatitis. 1987;17:223–8.

11. Hjorth N, Roed-Petersen J. Occupational protein contact dermatitis in food handlers. Contact Dermatitis. 1976;2:28–42.

12. Doutre M-S. Occupational contact urticaria and protein contact dermatitis. Eur J Dermatol. 2005;15(6):419–24.

13. Ring J, editor. Allergy in practice. ISBN 3-540-00219-7. New York: Springer; 2005.

14. Eric Gershwin M, Naguwa SM, editors. Allergy & Immunology Secrets. 2nd ed. Philadelphia: Elsevier Mosby; 2005.

15. The Free Dictionary by Farlex. http://medical-dictionary.thefreedictionary.com.

16. Gimenez-Arnau A, Maurer M, De La Cuadra J, Maibach H. Immediate contact skin reactions, an update of contact urticaria, contact urticaria syndrome and protein contact dermatitis "a never ending story". Eur J Dermatol. 2010;20(5):552–62.

17. Zuberbier T, Aberer W, Asero R, Bindslev-Jensen C, Brzoza Z, Canonica GW, Church MK, Ensina LF, Giménez-Arnau A, Godse K, Gonçalo M, Grattan C, Hebert J, Hide M, Kaplan A, Kapp A, Abdul Latiff AH, Mathelier-Fusade P, Metz M, Nast A, Saini SS, Sánchez-Borges M, Schmid-Grendelmeier P, Simons FE, Staubach P, Sussman G, Toubi E, Vena GA, Wedi B, Zhu XJ, Maurer M, European Academy of Allergy and Clinical Immunology, Global Allergy and Asthma European Network, European Dermatology Forum, World Allergy Organization. The EAACI/GA²LEN/EDF/WAO guideline for the definition, classification, diagnosis and management of urticaria: the 2013 revision and update. Allergy. 2014;69(7):868–87.

18. Alfonso JH, Bauer A, Bensefa-Colas L, Boman A, Bubas M, Constandt L, Crepy MN, Goncalo M, Macan J, Mahler V, Mijakoski D, Ramada Rodilla JM, Rustemeyer T, Spring P, John SM, Uter W, Wilkinson M, Giménez-Arnau AM. Minimum standards on prevention, diagnosis and treatment of occupational and work-related skin diseases in Europe-position paper of the COST action StanDerm (TD 1206). J Eur Acad Dermatol Venereol. 2017;31(suppl 4):31–43.

19. Elpern DJ. The syndrome of immediate reactivities (contact urticaria syndrome). An historical study from a dermatology practice. I. Age, sex, race and putative substances. Hawaii Med J. 1985;44:426–39.

20. Rudzki E, Rebanel P. Occupational contact urticaria from penicillin. Contact Dermatitis. 1985;13:192.

21. Nilsson E. Contact sensitivity and urticaria in "wet" work. Contact Dermatitis. 1985;13:321–8.

22. Turjanmaa K. Incidence of immediate allergy to latex gloves in hospital personnel. Contact Dermatitis. 1987;17:270–5.

23. Weissenbach T, Wutrich B, Weihe WH. Allergies to laboratory animals. An epidemiological, allergological study in persons exposed to laboratory animals. Schweiz Med Wochenschr. 1988;118:930–8.

24. Kanerva L, Jolanki R, Toikkanen J. Frequencies of occupational allergic diseases and gender differences in Finland. Int Arch Occup Environ Health. 1994;66:111–6.

25. Kanerva L, Toikkanen J, Jolanki R, Estlander T. Statistical data on occupational contact urticaria. Contact Dermatitis. 1996;35:229–33.

26. Kanerva L, Jolanki R, Toikkanen J, Estlander T. Statistics on occupational contact urticaria. In: Amin S, Lahti A, Maibach HI, editors. Contact urticaria syndrome. Boca Raton: CRC Press; 1997. p. 57–69.

27. Williams JD, Lee AY, Matheson MC, Frowen KE, Noonan AM, Nixon RL. Occupational contact urticaria: Australian data. Br J Dermatol. 2008;159:125–31.

28. Helaskoski E, Suojalehto H, Kuuliala O, Aalto-Korte K. Occupational contact urticaria and protein contact dermatitis: causes and concomitant airway diseases. Contact Dermatitis. 2017. https://doi.org/10.1111/cod.12856.

29. Teo S, Teik-Jin Goon A, Siang LH, Lin GS, Koh D. Occupational dermatoses in restaurant, catering and fast-food outlets in Singapore. Occup Med (Lond). 2009;59:466–71.

30. Bourrain JL. Occupational contact urticaria. Clin Rev Allergy Immunol. 2006;30:39–46.

31. Susitaival P, Flyvholm MA, Meding B, Kanerva L, Lindberg M, Svensson A, Olafsson JH. Nordic occupational skin questionnaire (NOSQ-2002): a new tool for surveying occupational skin diseases and exposure. Contact Dermatitis. 2003;49:70–6.

32. Mathias CG. Contact dermatitis and workers' compensation: criteria for establishing occupational causation and aggravation. J Am Acad Dermatol. 1989;20:842–8.

33. Von Krogh C, Maibach HI. The contact urticaria syndrome. An update review. J Am Acad Dermatol. 1981;5:328–42.

34. Kligman AM. Dimethyl sulphoxide I and II. J Am Med Assoc. 1965;193:796–804. 923–928

35. Lahti A, Oikarinen A, Viinikka L, Ylikorkala O, Hannuksela M. Prostaglandins in contact urticaria induced by benzoic acid. Acta Derm Venereol (Stockh). 1983;63:425–7.

36. Lahti A, Vaananen A, Kokkonen E-L, Hannuksela M. Acetylsalicylic acid inhibits non-immunologic contact urticaria. Contact Dermatitis. 1987;16:133–5.

37. Johansson J, Lahti A. Topical non-steroidal anti-inflammatory drugs inhibit non-immunological immediate contact reactions. Contact Dermatitis. 1988;19:161–5.

38. Morrow JD, Minton TA, Awad JA, Roberts LJ. Release of markedly increased quantities of prostaglandin D2 from the skin in vivo in humans

following the application of sorbic acid. Arch Dermatol. 1994;130:1408–12.

39. Downard CD, Roberts LJ, Morrow JD. Topical benzoic acid induces the increased synthesis of prostaglandin D2 in humans skin in vivo. Clin Pharmacol Ther. 1995;74:441–5.

40. Lundblad L, Lundberg JM, Anggard A, Zetterstrom O. Capsaicin sensitive nerves and the cutaneous allergy reaction in man. Possible involvement of sensory neuropeptides in the flare reaction. Allergy. 1987;42:20–5.

41. Lahti A, Maibach HI. Long refractory period after application of one nonimmunologic contact urticaria agents to the guinea pig ear. J Am Acad Dermatol. 1985;13:585–9.

42. Lovell CR. Urticaria due to plants. In: Lovell CR, editor. Plants and the skin. 1st ed. Oxford, UK: Blackwell Science; 1993. p. 29–41.

43. Amaro C, Goossens A. Immunological occupational contact urticaria and contact dermatitis from proteins: a review. Contact Dermatitis. 2008;58:67–75.

44. Lahti A, Björksten F, Hannuksela M. Allergy to birch pollen and apple, and cross-reactivity of the allergens studied with RAST. Allergy. 1980;35:297.

45. Löwenstein H, Eriksson NE. Hypersensitivity to foods among birch pollen-allergic patients. Allergy. 1983;38:577.

46. Dreborg S, Foucard T. Allergy to apple, carrot and potato in children with birch pollen allergy. Allergy. 1983;38:167.

47. Kanerva L, Estlander T. Immediate and delayed skin allergy from cow dander. Am J Contact Dermat. 1997;8:167–9.

48. Conde-Salazar L, Gonzalez MA, Guimaraens D. Type I and type IV sensitization to *Anisakis simplex* in 2 patients with hand eczema. Contact Dermatitis. 2002;46:361.

49. Tupasela O, Kanerva L. Chapter 4: Skin tests and specific IgE determinations in the diagnostics of contact urticaria caused by low-molecular-weight chemicals. In: Amin S, Lahti A, Maibach HI, editors. Contact urticaria syndrome. Boca Raton: CRC Press; 1997. p. 33–44.

50. Lukacs J, Schliemann S, Elsner P. Occupational contact urticaria caused by food: a systemic clinical review. Contact Dermatitis. 2016;75:195–204.

51. Verhulst L, Goossens A. Cosmetic components causing contact urticaria: a review and update. Contact Dermatitis. 2016;75:333–44.

52. Giménez-Arnau A, Maibach HI. Contact urticaria syndrome: definition, history, etiology and relevance. In: Gimenez-Arnau A, Maibach HI, editors. Contact urticaria syndrome. Boca Raton: CRC Press Taylor & Francis Group; 2015. p. 1–11.

53. Giménez-Arnau A. Contact Urticaria Syndrome. In: Dermatotoxicology. Eighth Edition Eds Klaus-Peter Wilhelm, Hongbo Zhai, Howrad Maibach. CRC Press Taylor & Francis Group an Informa Business. Boca Raton FL 33487-2742; 2013. p. 125–32.

54. Clemmenson O, Hjorth N. Perioral contact urticaria from sorbic acid and benzoic acid in a salad dressing. Contact Dermatitis. 1982;8:1–6.

55. Cromwell O, Pepys J, Parish WE, Hughes EG. Specific IgE antibodies to platinum salts in sensitized workers. Clin Allergy. 1979;9:109.

56. Estlander T, Kanerva L, Tupasela O, Heskinen H, Jolanki R. Immediate and delayed allergy to nickel with contact urticaria, rhinitis, asthma and contact dermatitis. Clin Exp Allergy. 1993;23:306.

57. Lahti A. Non-immunologic contact urticaria. Acta Derm Venereol (Stockh). 1980;60(Suppl):3–49.

58. Babilas P, Landthaler M, Szeimies RM. Anaphylactic reaction following hair bleaching. Hautarzt. 2005;56:1152–5.

59. Kligman AM. The spectrum of contact urticaria: wheals, erythema and pruritus. Dermatol Clin. 1990;8:57–60.

60. Barbaud A. Urticarires de contact. Ann Dermatol Venereol. 2002;128:1161–5.

61. Von Krogh G, Maibach HI. Contact urticaria. In: Adam RM, editor. Occupational skin disease. New York: Grune & Stratton; 1983. p. 58–69.

62. Bonnevie P. Occupational allergy in bakery. In: European Academy of Allergy, editor. Occupational allergy. Springfield: Thomas; 1958. p. 161–8.

63. Herxheimer H. Skin sensitivity to flour in baker's apprentices. Lancet. 1967;1:83–4.

64. Herxheimer H. The skin sensitivity to flour of baker's apprentices: a final report of long term investigation. Acta Allergol. 1967;28:42–9.

65. Nutter AF. Contact urticaria to rubber. Br J Dermatol. 1979;101:597–8.

66. Hjorth N. Occupational dermatitis in the catering industry. Br J Dermatol. 1981;105:37.

67. Sutton R, Skerritt JH, Baldo BA, Wrigley CW. The diversity of allergens involved in bakers' asthma. Clin Allergy. 1984;14:93–107.

68. Jagtman BA. Urticaria and contact urticaria due to basic blue 99 in a hair dye. Contact Dermatitis. 1996;35:52.

69. Torresani C, Periti I, Beski L. Contact urticaria syndrome from formaldehyde with multiple physical urticarias. Contact Dermatitis. 1996;35:174–5.

70. Escribano M, Muñoz-Bellido FJ, Velazquez E, Delgado E, Serrano P, Guardia J, Conde J. Contact urticaria due to aescin. Contact Dermatitis. 1997;37:233–53.

71. Gutierrez D, Conde A, Duran S, Delgado J, Guardia P, Martinez R, Garcia-Cubillana A, Gonzalez J, Conde J. Contact urticaria from lupin. Contact Dermatitis. 1997;36:311.

72. Brehler R, Sedlmayr S. Contact urticaria due to rubber chemicals? Contact Dermatitis. 1997;37:125–7.

73. Geyer E, Kränke B, Derhaschnig J, Aberer W. Contact urticaria from roe deer meet and hair. Contact Dermatitis. 1998;39:34.

74. Cancian M, Fortina AB, Peserico A. Contact urticaria syndrome from constituents of balsam of Peru

and fragrance mix in a patient with chronic urticaria. Contact Dermatitis. 1999;41:3000.

75. Kalogeromitros D, Armenaka M, Katsarou A. Contact urticaria and systemic anaphylaxis from codfish. Contact Dermatitis. 1999;41:170.

76. Schalock PC, Storrs FJ, Morrison L. Contact urticaria from panthenol in a hair conditioner. Contact Dermatitis. 2000;43:223.

77. Foti C, Nettis E, Panebianco R, Cassano N, Diaferio A, Porzia Pia D. Contact urticaria from *Matricaria chamomilla*. Contact Dermatitis. 2000;42:360–1.

78. Le Coz CJ, Ball C. Contact urticaria syndrome from mustard in anchovy fillet mustard sauce. Contact Dermatitis. 2000;42:114–5.

79. Guin JD, Goodman J. Contact urticaria from benzyl alcohol presenting as intolerance to saline soaks. Contact Dermatitis. 2001;45:182–3.

80. Yamakawa Y, Ohsuna H, Aihara M, Tsubaki K, Ikezawa Z. Contact urticaria from rice. Contact Dermatitis. 2001;44:91–3.

81. Porcel S, León F, Cumplido J, Cuevas M, Guimaraens D, Conde-Salazar L. Contact urticaria caused by heat-sensitive raw fish allergens. Contact Dermatitis. 2001;45:139–42.

82. Conde-salazar L, Guimaraens D, Gonzalez MA, Mancebo E. Occupational allergic contact urticaria from amoxicillin. Contact Dermatitis. 2001;45:109.

83. Kanerva L, Vanhanen M. Occupational allergic contact urticaria and rhinoconjunctivitis from a detergent protease. Contact Urticaria. 2001;45:49–51.

84. Hernández B, Ortiz-Frutos FJ, Garcia M, Palencia S, Garcia MC, Iglesias L. Contact urticaria from 2-phenoxyethanol. Contact Dermatitis. 2002;47:54.

85. Narayan S, Sanson JE. Contact urticaria from runner bean (*Phaseolus coccineus*). Contact Dermatitis. 2002;47:243.

86. Sugiura K, Sugiura M, Shiraki R, Hayakawa R, Shamoto M, Sasaki K, Itoh A. Contact urticaria to polyethylene gloves. Contact Dermatitis. 2002;46:262–6.

87. Sugiura K, Sugiura M, Hayakawa R, Shamoto M, Sasaki K. A case of contact urticaria syndrome due to di(2-ethylhexyl)phthalate (DOP) in work clothes. Contact Dermatitis. 2002;46:13–6.

88. Hannuksela M. Mechanisms in contact urticaria. Clin Dermatol. 1997;15:619–22.

89. Suzuki T, Kawada A, Yashimoto Y, Isogai R, Aragane Y, Tezuka T. Contact urticaria to ketoprofen. Contact Dermatitis. 2003;48:284–5.

90. Diva VC, Statham BN. Contact urticaria from cinnamal leading to anaphylaxis. Contact Dermatitis. 2003;48:119.

91. Bourrain JL, Amblard P, Béani JC. Contact urticaria photoinduced by benzophenones. Contact Dermatitis. 2003;48:45–6.

92. Monteseirín J, Pérez-Formoso JL, Hérnandez M, Sánchez-Hernández MC, Camacho MJ, Bonilla I, Chaparro A, Conde J. Contact urticaria from dill. Contact Dermatitis. 2003;48:275.

93. Yung A, Papworth-Smith J, Wilkinson SM. Occupational contact urticaria from solid-phase peptide synthesis coupling agents HATU and HBTU. Contact Dermatitis. 2003;49:108–9.

94. Rudzki E, Rapiejko P, Rebandel P. Occupational contact dermatitis, with asthma and rhinitis, from camomile in a cosmetician also with contact urticaria from both camomile and lime flowers. Contact Dermatitis. 2003;49:162.

95. Torresani C, Zendri E, Vescovi V, De Panfilis G. Contact urticaria syndrome from occupational triphenyl phosphite exposure. Contact Dermatitis. 2003;48:237–8.

96. Waton J, Boulanger A, Trechot PH, Schumtz JL, Barbaud A. Contact urticaria from Emla® cream. Contact Dermatitis. 2004;51:284–7.

97. Walker SL, Chalmers RJG, Beck MH. Contact urticaria due to *p*-chloro-*m*-cresol. Br J Dermatol. 2004;151:936–7.

98. Lin-Feng L, Sujan SA, Li QX. Contact urticaria syndrome from occupational benzonitrile exposure. Contact Dermatitis. 2004;50:377–8.

99. Baron SE, Moss C. Contact urticaria to play dough: a possible sign of dietary allergy. Br J Dermatol. 2004;151:945–7.

100. Krakowiak A, Kowalczyk M, Palczyñski C. Occupational contact urticaria and rhinoconjunctivitis in a veterinarian from bull terrier's seminal fluid. Contact Dermatitis. 2005;51:34.

101. Jovanovic M, Karadaglic D, Brkic S. Contact urticaria and allergic contact dermatitis to lidocaine in a patient sensitive to benzocaine and propolis. Contact Dermatitis. 2006;54:124–6.

102. Birnie AJ, English JS. 2-Phenoxyethanol-induced contact urticaria. Contact Dermatitis. 2006;54:349.

103. Quiñones Estevez MD. Occupational contact urticaria-dermatitis by *Tyrophagus putrescentiae*. Contact Dermatitis. 2006;55:308–9.

104. Majmudar V, Azam NAM, Finch T. Contact urticaria to *Cannabis sativa*. Contact Dermatitis. 2006;54:127.

105. Co-Minh HB, Demoly P, Guillot B, Raison-Peyron N. Anaphylactic shock after oral intake and contact urticaria due to polyethyleneglycols. Allergy. 2007;62:92–3.

106. Pérez-Calderon R, Gonzalo-Garijo A, Bartolomé-Zavala B, Lamilla-Yerga A, Moreno-Gastón I. Occupational contact urticaria due to pennyroyal (*Mentha pulegium*). Contact Dermatitis. 2007;57:285–6.

107. Williams JD, Moyle M, Nixon RL. Occupational contact urticaria from parmesan cheese. Contact Dermatitis. 2007;56:113–4.

108. Liu W, Nixon RL. Corn contact urticaria in a nurse. Australas. J Dermatol. 2007;48:130–1.

109. Foti C, Antelmi A, Mistrello G, Guarneri F, Filotico R. Occupational contact urticaria and rhinoconjunctivitis from dog's milk in a veterinarian. Contact Dermatitis. 2007;56:169–71.

110. Crippa M, Balbiani L, Baruffini A, Belleri L, Draicchio F, Feltrin G, Larese F, Maaggio GM, Marcer G, Micheloni GP, Montomoli L, Moscato G, Previdi M, Sartorelli P, Sossai D, Spatari G, Zanetti C. Consensus document. Update on latex exposure and use of gloves in Italian health care settings. Med Lav. 2008;99:387–99.

111. Williams C, Thompstone J, Wilkinson M. Work-related contact urticaria to *Cannabis sativa*. Contact Dermatitis. 2008;58:62–3.

112. Houtappel M, Bruijnzeel-Koomen CAFM, Röckmann H. Immediate-type allergy by occupational exposure to didecyl dimethyl ammonium chloride. Contact Dermatitis. 2008;59:116–1.

113. Willi R, Pfab F, Huss-Marp J, Buters JTM, Zilker T, Behrendt H, Ring J, Darsow U. Contact anaphylaxis and protein contact dermatitis in a cook handling chicory leaves. Contact Dermatitis. 2009;60:226–7.

114. Davies E, Orton D. Contact urticaria and protein contact dermatitis to chapatti flour. Contact Dermatitis. 2009;60:113–4.

115. Valsecchi R, Santini M, Leghissa P. Contact urticaria and asthma from *Sarcophaga carnaria*. Contact Dermatitis. 2009;61:186–7.

116. Galvez Lozano JM, Alcantara M, Saenz de San Pedro B, Quiralte J, Caba I. Occupational contact urticaria caused by donepezil. Contact Dermatitis. 2009;61:176.

117. Olaiwan A, Pecquet C, Mathelier-Fusade P, Francès C. Urticaire de contact aux hydrolysats de proteins de blé contenudans es cosmétiques. Ann Dermatol Venereol. 2010;137:281–4.

118. Spoerl D, Scherer K, Bircher AJ. Contact urticaria with systemic symptoms due to hexylene glycol in a topical corticosteroid: case report and review of hypersensitivity to glycols. Dermatology. 2010;220:238–42.

119. Foti C, Cassano N, Mistrello G, Amato S, Romita P, Vena GA. Contact urticaria due to raw arugula and parsley. Ann Allergy Asthma Immunol. 2011;106:447–8.

120. Erkek E, Sahin S, Ince Ü, Özkut K. Mucosal contact urticaria to sesame seeds. J Eur Acad Dermatol Venereol. 2011;26:790–1.

121. Viinanen A, Salokannell M, Lammintausta K. Gum Arabic as a a cause of occupational allergy. J Allergy. 2011; 2011:841508.

122. Ruiz Oropeza A, Fischer Friis U, Duus Johanssen J. Occupational contact urticaria caused by didecyl dimethyl ammonium chloride. Contact Dermatitis. 2011;64:289–302.

123. Hansson C, Bergendorff O, Wallengren J. Contact urticaria caused by carvone in toothpaste. Contact Dermatitis. 2011;65:362–4.

124. Seitz CS, Trautmann A. Cosmetic facial peel-induced contact anaphylaxis: chestnut allergy without latex-fruit syndrome. J Invest Allergol Clin Immunol. 2011;21:494–5.

125. Doukaki S, Pistone G, Arico M, Bongiorno MR. Allergic contact dermatitis with contact urticaria to colophony from an alternative remedy. Dermatitis. 2012;23:298–9.

126. Vanstreels L, Merk HF. Protein contact dermatitis in a butcher. Hautarzt. 2012;63:926–8.

127. Nishida K, Tateishi C, Tsuruta D, Shimauchi T, Ito T, Hirakawa S, Tokura Y. Contact urticaria caused by a fish-derived elastin-containing cosmetic cream. Contact Dermatitis. 2012;67:171–2.

128. Barrientos N, Vazquez S, Dominguez JD. Contact urticaria induced by hydrolyzed wheat protein in cosmetic cream. Actas Dermosifiliogr. 2012;103:750–2.

129. Vishal B, Rao SS, Pavithra S, Shenoy MM. Contact urticaria to glycolic acid peel. J Cutan Aesthet Surg. 2012;5:58–9.

130. Pala G, Pignatti P, Perfetti L, Gentile E, Moscato G. Occupational allergic contact urticaria to crustacean in a cook. J Invest Allergol Clin Immunol. 2012;22:142–3.

131. Doyen V, Leduc V, Corazza F, Mairesse M, Ledent C, Michel O. Protein contact dermatitis and food allergy to mare milk. Ann Allergy Asthma Immunol. 2013;110:390–1.

132. Valsecchi R, Leghissa P. Contact allergy due to lychee. Acta Dermato-Venereol. 2013;93:90–1.

133. Saito M, Nakada T. Contact urticaria syndrome from eye drops levofloxacin hydrate ophthalmic solution. J Dermatol. 2013;40:130–1.

134. Shutty B, Swender D, Chernin L, Tcheurekdjian H, Hostoffer R. Insect repellents and contact urticaria: differential response to DEET and picaridin. Cutis. 2013;91:280–2.

135. Leheron C, Bourrier T, Albertini M, Giovannini-Chami L. Immediate contact urticaria caused by hydrolysed wheat proteins in a child via maternal skin contact sensitization. Contact Dermatitis. 2013;68:379–80.

136. Park MR, Kim DS, Kim J, Ahn K. Anaphylaxis to topically applied sodium fusidate. Allergy Asthma Immunol Res. 2013;5:110–2.

137. Ozkaya E, Kavlak Bozkurt P. An unusual case of triclosan-induced immunological contact urticaria. Contact Dermatitis. 2013;68:121–3.

138. Chinuki Y, Takahashi H, Dekio I, Kaneko S, Tokuda R, Nagao M, Fujisawa T, Morita E. Higher allergenicity of high molecular weight hydrolysed wheat protein in cosmetics for percutaneous sensitization. Contact Dermatitis. 2013;68:86–93.

139. Gomulka K. Panaszek contact urticaria syndrome caused by haptens. Postepy Dermatol Alergol. 2014;31:108–12.

140. Suzuki R, Fukuyama K, Miyazaki Y, Namiki T. Contact urticaria and protein contact dermatitis caused by glycerin enema. JAAD Case Rep. 2016;2:108–10.

Basic Epidemiology Concepts Relevant in Contact Urticaria

2

Jose Hernán Alfonso

List of Abbreviations

95% UI	95% uncertainty intervals
DALYs	Disability-adjusted life-years
GBD 2016	Global Burden of Disease 2016 Project
YLDs	Years lived with disability

Epidemiology: A Necessary Approach for Dermatology

Epidemiology is directly concerned with public health and the prevention of disease, and it has been defined by Last [1] as

"the study of the distribution and determinants of health-related states or events in specific populations, and the application of this study to control of health problems."

For instance, skin diseases are associated with a substantial burden in the context of health: they are both widespread and among the most prevalent and disabling diseases, representing a source of considerable loss of quality of life [2]. Collectively, skin diseases were the fourth leading cause of nonfatal burden expressed as years lost because of disability in 2010 [2]. As an example, work-related and occupational skin diseases, most of them preventable by reduction of occupational exposures and early diagnosis, impose a significant burden to society. According to the World Health Organization, they represent a challenge for all workers, and the EU Commission has defined insufficient prevention as a top priority problem [3].

In this context, contact urticaria is the most frequent work-related and occupational skin disease after contact dermatitis. An epidemiological approach, therefore, intends to identify risk subgroups within a population and to examine associations that may explain such excess risks in order to define effective prevention strategies. For clinical dermatology, prevention is often linked to early diagnosis (secondary prevention) as well as to effective treatment and rehabilitation (tertiary prevention).

Nevertheless, epidemiology and clinical dermatology should not be regarded as completely different disciplines. In fact, there is a great need to gather approaches from both disciplines together with occupational medicine for the purposes of comprehensive prevention of work-related and occupational skin affections. By knowing about the epidemiology of contact urticaria, we not only understand more about its distribution and causes in a population, but also know more about creating a basis for its prevention.

J. H. Alfonso (✉)
Department of Occupational Medicine and Epidemiology, National Institute of Occupational Health, Oslo, Norway
e-mail: jose.alfonso@stami.no

© Springer International Publishing AG, part of Springer Nature 2018
A. M. Giménez-Arnau, H. I. Maibach (eds.), *Contact Urticaria Syndrome*, Updates in Clinical Dermatology, https://doi.org/10.1007/978-3-319-89764-6_2

This chapter does not attempt to review methods used in epidemiology to assess the occurrence and causes of diseases; however, it does provide a systematic summary of the evidence available on the epidemiology of contact urticaria. For readers interested in more complex and sophisticated issues of epidemiology, we refer to basic texts on epidemiology [4]. Chapters 3 and 12, focusing on occupational relevance of immediate-contact reactions and preventive measures, are complementary to this chapter.

Urticaria in the Context of the Global Burden of Disease

The Global Burden of Diseases, Injuries, and Risk Factors (GBD 2016) provides a comprehensive assessment of prevalence, incidence, years lived with disability (YLDs), and disability-adjusted life-years (DALYs) for 333 diseases and injuries in 195 countries and territories from 1990 to 2016 (GBD 2016 Disease and Injury Incidence and Prevalence Collaborators 2016) [5]. Concepts of prevalence, incidence, YLDs, and DALYs are defined in this chapter before specific data are presented.

In the Global Burden of Diseases Project, all accessible information on disease occurrence, natural history, and severity that passes minimum inclusion criteria is included. It must be highlighted that the availability and quality of epidemiological data gathered vary among diseases and by location. For example, survey data can be biased by low response frequency, as well as register data from official health statistics that usually include people seeking and receiving healthcare, leading to selection bias [5]. Overall, these sources of bias may lead to an underestimation of the real occurrence of contact urticaria.

However, the GBD attempts to identify and adjust for known sources of measurement error by advanced and sophisticated statistical methods.[1] For more details regarding data sources and methods, please refer to the original publication from *Lancet* [5].

Prevalence

The term prevalence denotes the number of cases of the disease at a particular time [6]. It can be defined as follows:

- Point prevalence: estimates the number of cases of disease at one point in time. (*Do you have contact urticaria now?*)
- Period prevalence: denotes the number of cases of disease during some time interval, e.g., 1 year. (*Have you had contact urticaria in the last year?*)
- Lifetime prevalence: denotes the number of cases of disease during a lifetime. (*Have you ever had contact urticaria?*)

Prevalence as a measure of burden of disease is good for planning the allocation of resources in health services. For example, it is useful to compare disease prevalence in or within a specific population (e.g., prevalence of contact urticaria among cooks versus prevalence of contact urticaria among cleaners in a population of kitchen workers), communities, or countries (e.g., high-income countries vs. middle-income countries vs. low-income countries). When estimating the prevalence of a disease, the hypothesis can be tested by comparing prevalence in subgroups of people who have or not have been exposed to a particular risk factor (e.g., food proteins in the same population of kitchen workers). Prevalence is not an appropriate measure to assess temporal associations between a specific exposure (e.g., food proteins) and the occurrence of disease.

---

[1]Bayesian metaregression tool DisMod-MR 2.1 was used to combine all available sources of information for a specific disease.

Table 2.1 Global prevalence of skin and subcutaneous diseases for both sexes

	Prevalence in thousands (95% UI)
Skin and subcutaneous diseases	2,266,315 (2,242,994–2,285,332)
1. Fungal skin diseases	626,700 (568,967–690,267)
2. Acne vulgaris	614,771 (560,634–672,878)
3. Dermatitis	306,359 (290,041–324,193)
4. Viral skin diseases	193,171 (184,773–201,619)
5. Scabies	146,785 (127,773–170,009)
6. Urticaria	**67,060 (59,299–77,018)**
7. Pruritus	66,780 (59,262–74,868)
8. Psoriasis	65,135 (62,708–67,812)
9. Pyoderma	21,020 (20,491–21,564)
10. Cellulitis	3018 (2842–3210)

Adapted from table of global prevalence, incidence, and years lived with disability (YLDs) for 2016, percentage change of YLD counts, and percentage change of age-standardized YLD rates between 2006 and 2016 for all causes and nine impairments [5]
GBD (2016) [5]
UI uncertainty intervals: both sexes and all ages are included

Estimates for the worldwide prevalence of urticaria were not available before the publication of the study Global Burden of Diseases, Injuries, and Risk Factors (GBD 2016) [5]. However, occupational relevance of contact urticaria has been documented by register-based studies, case-reports, and case-series (Chap. 3). Although the current worldwide estimates on urticaria may also include cases of chronic urticaria, contact urticaria is frequent in everyday practice.

Table 2.1 shows that contact urticaria was in sixth place among the ten most prevalent skin and subcutaneous diseases in 2016 [approximately 67 million cases, 95% UI (uncertainty intervals[2]) (59.3–77 million)]. The worldwide distribution

of prevalent cases by sex is shown for males in Fig. 2.1 and for females in Fig. 2.2.

Incidence

Incidence can be defined as new cases of disease in a defined time period, divided by the number of persons at risk for the disease in the same period [4]. The resulting proportion can be multiplied by 1000 to obtain the number of cases per 1000 inhabitants. What is critical for incidence is that every person in the denominator must have the potential to become a part in the numerator. The transition from disease-free (denominator) to diseased (numerator) is a measure of events, and therefore incidence is a measure of risk. We can say that every single person in the denominator (disease-free) must have the potential to be a part of the numerator (diseased).

Estimates for the worldwide incidence of urticaria were not available before the publication of the Global Burden of Disease 2016 Study. In fact, as Table 2.2 shows, urticaria is placed number seven among the ten leading skin diseases with highest incidence in 2016 [119,403 million cases, 95% UI (105,497 million to 135,993 million cases)] [5].

Table 2.3 shows the temporal trends for global incidence for urticaria for the period 1990–2016 in three ways:

1. Mean percentage change in number of incidence cases, which reflects the combined effects of population growth, population aging, and epidemiological change.
2. Mean percentage change in all-age incidence rate, which explains the effects of population aging and epidemiological change.
3. Mean percentage change in age-standardized reflects epidemiological change that is not explained by aging or population growth.

Urticaria is placed number 29 among the 30 diseases with highest incidence between 1990 and 2016 in the Global Burden of Diseases 2016 Project. For the periods 1990–2006 and 2006–2016, there has been an increasing trend in the

[2]95% Uncertainty intervals (95% UI): it is derived from 1000 draws from the posterior distribution of each step in the estimation process, capturing uncertainty from multiple modeling steps, as well as from sources such as model estimation and model specification, rather than from sampling error alone. For estimation of prevalence, incidence, and YLDs, UIs incorporated variability from sample sizes within data sources, adjustments to data to account for non-reference definitions, parameter uncertainty in model estimation, and uncertainty associated with establishment of disability weights.

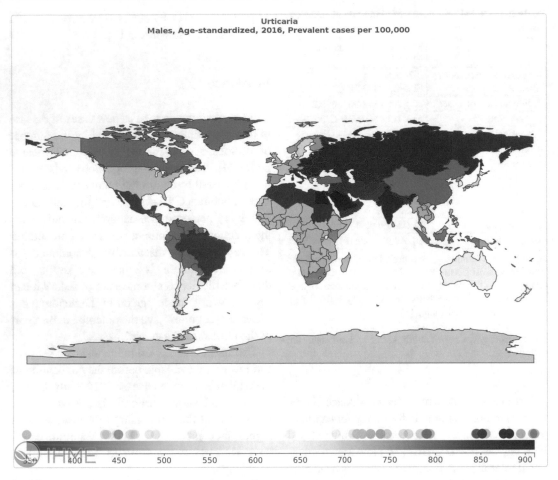

Fig. 2.1 Urticaria: age-standardized prevalent cases among males, 2016 (GBD 2016) [7]. (With permission from Institute for Health Metrics and Evaluation (IHME) [7])

global incidence of urticaria (Table 2.3). The worldwide distribution for incidence is shown for males in Fig. 2.3 and for females in Fig. 2.4.

Years Lived with Disability

Years lived with disability (YLDs) refer to the number of years that a subject lives with some disease, and it is closely related to the severity of the disability that the disease causes to the affected individual [5]. This measure is obtained by multiplying the prevalence of a disorder by the short- or long-term loss of health associated with that disability (the disability weight) [5].

Urticaria is number five among the ten leading skin and subcutaneous diseases with high-est YLDs (Table 2.4). This figure is not surprising, as patients with a diagnosis of allergic contact dermatitis and urticaria reported the most extensive disturbances in physical and psychosocial functioning, with the highest levels of somatic symptoms, anxiety, insomnia, and symptoms of depression. Urticaria was associated with the highest level of tension, hostility, and fatigue [8].

Table 2.4 shows the change in global YLDs over time in three different ways:

1. YLDs counts for 2016.
2. Percentage change in counts between 2006 and 2016, which reflects the combined effects of population growth, population aging, and epidemiological change.

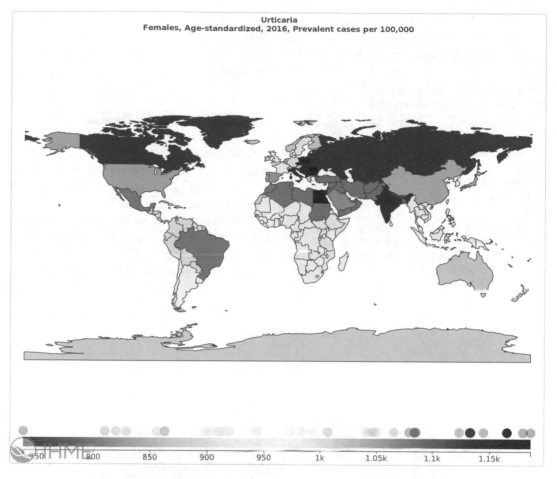

Fig. 2.2 Urticaria: age-standardized prevalent cases among females, 2016 (GBD 2016) [7]. (With permission from Institute for Health Metrics and Evaluation (IHME) [7])

Table 2.2 Global incidence of skin and subcutaneous diseases for both sexes, 2016

	Incidence in thousands (95% UI)
Skin and subcutaneous diseases	5,074,605 (4,838,566–5,335,844)
1. Fungal skin diseases	2,098,743 (1,884,346–2,337,325)
2. Pyoderma	474,384 (461,024–488,662)
3. Scabies	454,671 (392,690–529,184)
4. Dermatitis	430,376 (398,274–462,932)
5. Acne vulgaris	429,822 (361,790–521,114)
6. Viral skin diseases	276,755 (263,471–290,189)
7. Urticaria	**119,403 (105,497–135,993)**
8. Cellulitis	61,333 (58,280–64,556)
9. Pruritus	53,046 (47,751–59,503)
10. Psoriasis	8170 (7861–8478)

Adapted from table of global prevalence, incidence, and YLDs for 2016, percentage change of YLDs counts, and percentage change of age-standardized YLDs rates between 2006 and 2016 for all causes and nine impairments [5] GBD (2016) [5]

UI uncertainty intervals: both sexes and all ages are included

3. Percent change in age-standardized YLDs, which reflects epidemiological change that is not explained by aging or population growth.

Table 2.3 Temporal trends for global incidence of urticaria for both sexes from 1990 to 2016

Urticaria (mean % change)	1990–2006 (%)	2006–2016 (%)
Number of incidence (cases)	16.6	9.2
All-age incidence rates	−6.7	−2.8
Standardized incidence rate	−0.3	−0.3

Adapted from table of global prevalence, incidence, and YLDs for 2016, percentage change of YLDs counts, and percentage change of age-standardized YLD rates between 2006 and 2016 for all causes and nine impairments [5] GBD (2016) [5]

An increasing trend is observed from 2006 to 2016 (data not shown); however, little variation is observed in age-standardized rates between 2006 and 2016.

Disability-Adjusted Life-Years

Disability-adjusted life-years (DALYs), a summary measurement of the overall burden of disease, refers to health loss from both fatal and nonfatal disease burden [9].

DALYs consists of the sum of the years of life lost because of premature mortality and years of life lived with disability (YLDs). One DALY represents one year of healthy life lost [9].

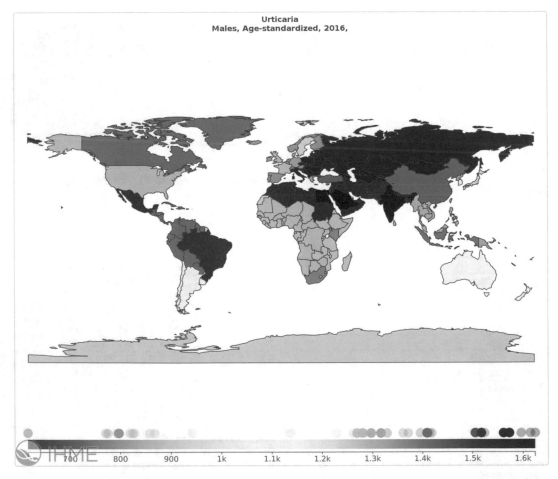

Fig. 2.3 Urticaria: age-standardized incidence among males, 2016 (GBD 2016) [7]. (With permission from Institute for Health Metrics and Evaluation (IHME) [7])

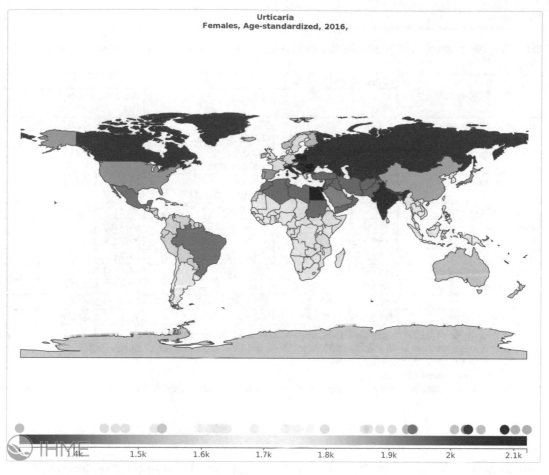

Fig. 2.4 Urticaria: age-standardized incidence among females, 2016 (GBD 2016) [7]. (With permission from Institute for Health Metrics and Evaluation (IHME) [7])

Table 2.4 Global YLDs for 2016, percentage change of YLDs counts, and percentage change of age-standardized YLDs rates between 2006 and 2016 for skin and subcutaneous diseases

	Years lived with disability (YLDs), 95% (UI)	
	2016 counts	Percentage change in age-standardized rates between 2006 and 2016
Skin and subcutaneous diseases	54,635 (36,830–79,320)	1.2 (0.9–1.5)[a]
1. Acne vulgaris	15,836 (10,644–22,843)	2.1 (1.5–2.6)[a]
2. Dermatitis	11,210 (6714–18,218)	1.1 (0.3–1.8)[a]
3. Viral skin diseases	5915 (3674–8828)	−0.1 (−0.5–0.2)
4. Psoriasis	5643 (4040–7377)	4.2 (3.6–5.0)[a]
5. Urticaria	**4030 (2576–5745)**	**−0.3 (−0.8–0.3)**
6. Scabies	3788 (2104–6029)	−5.4 (−6.2–4.8)[a]
7. Fungal skin diseases	3509 (1403–7271)	2.5 (2.2–2.9)[a]
8. Pruritus	709 (330–1299)	1.3 (0.8–1.8)[a]
9. Alopecia areata	504 (323–760)	−1.3 (−2.2 to −0.5)[a]
10. Decubitus ulcer	290 (203–388)	−0·8 (−2.8–1.0)

Adapted from table of global prevalence, incidence, and YLDs for 2016, percentage change of YLD counts, and percentage change of age-standardized YLD rates between 2006 and 2016 for all causes and nine impairments [5]
GBD (2016) [5]
UI uncertainty intervals
[a]Percentage changes that are statistically significant

Table 2.5 Global all-age DALYs rates for skin and subcutaneous diseases in 1990 and 2016 with mean percentage changes [10]

	Global all-age DALYs		
	1990	2016	Percentage change, 1990–2016
Skin and subcutaneous diseases	41366.2 (28152.7–59346.6)	57394.0 (39334.2–81653.4)	38.8 (37.0–41.0)[a]
1. Acne vulgaris	12086.8 (8150.7–17552.7)	15836.0 (10643.5–22842.6)	31.0 (29.7–32.4)[a]
2. Dermatitis	8427.2 (5021.7–13797.8)	11210.2 (6714.5–18218.1)	33.0 (31.2–35.0)[a]
3. Viral skin diseases	4543.4 (2823.8–6780.1)	5915.2 (3674.3–8828.1)	30.2 (29.2–3.2)[a]
4. Psoriasis	3321.0 (2384.1–4347.4)	5643.4 (4039.7–7377.2)	69.9 (68.4–71.5)[a]
5. Urticaria	**3155.2 (2020.3–4556.7)**	**4029.9 (2575.9–5745.3)**	**27.7 (24.9–31.0)[a]**
6. Scabies	3332.5 (1844.4–5364.2)	3787.8 (2103.6–6029.0)	13.7 (10.8–16.7)[a]
7. Fungal skin diseases	2267.4 (900.2–4720.9)	3508.8 (1403.0–7271.0)	54.8 (51.8–57.7)[a]
8. Pyoderma	1094.9 (615.2–1411.5)	1944.8 (1249.8–2603.1)	77.6 (42.6–123.0)[a]
9. Pruritus	452.1 (211.1–825.5)	709.1 (329.7–1298.7)	56.8 (52.5–61.0)[a]
10. Decubitus ulcer	377.1 (291.5–475.3)	670.4 (513.0–836.1)	77.8 (65.5–86.8)[a]

Adapted from table of global all-age DALYs and age-standardized DALY rates in 1990, 2006, and 2016 with mean percentage changes between 1990 and 2016, 2006 and 2016, and 1990 and 2016, for all causes [10]

Data in parentheses are 95% uncertainty intervals

DALYs disability-adjusted life-years

[a]Percentage changes that are statistically significant; skin cancer is not included among skin and subcutaneous diseases

Examination of the levels and trends of DALYs facilitates quicker comparison between different diseases and injuries.

Worldwide, urticaria is placed number five among the ten leading skin and subcutaneous diseases with highest DALYs (Table 2.5). All-age DALYs count for urticaria increased by 27.7% (95% UI 24.9–31.0%) between 2000 and 2016; however, age-standardized DALYs rates showed little variation between 1990 and 2016 (Table 2.6). The increasing trend in the all-age DALYs rates for urticaria as well as for the other skin and subcutaneous diseases can be explained by population growth and higher life expectancy, which has resulted in a significant increase in total DALYs from noncommunicable diseases [10]. As life expectancy becomes higher across a population, the absolute amount of functional health loss increases [10]. Health systems should consider the increasing need for expertise and improvements within dermatology as the global population is still growing.

The worldwide distribution for DALYs for males is shown in Fig. 2.5 and for females in Fig. 2.6.

Overall, the total burden of contact urticaria is probably greatly underestimated in the Global Burden of Diseases 2016 project, because data sources for severity are mostly from high-income countries. Moreover, many immediate-contact reactions are often not registered. Late diagnosis, underdiagnosis, and deficiencies in health registry systems not only in low-income and middle-income countries, but also in high-income countries, should be addressed to achieve completeness of registries and accuracy of the estimates.

Unmet Needs to Be Addressed in Future Epidemiological Studies

Most of the available studies on contact urticaria consist of case reports, case series, retrospective register-based studies, and reviews of such cases.

Table 2.6 Age-standardized DALYs rate for skin and subcutaneous diseases [10]

	Age-standardized DALYs (per 100,000)		
	1990	2016	Percentage change 1990–2016
Skin and subcutaneous diseases	756.7 (518.9–1081.9)	781.3 (535.8–1110.4)	3.2 (2.5–4.4)[a]
1. Acne vulgaris	202.3 (136.5–292.9)	212.1 (143–306.4)	4.9 (4.2–5.6)[a]
2. Dermatitis	151.8 (91–246.4)	153.0 (91.6–248.4)	0.7 (−0.3–1.8)
3. Viral skin diseases	80.2 (49.9–119.5)	79.9 (49.6–119.3)	−0.4 (−0.8–0.0)
4. Psoriasis	69.7 (50–91.2)	76.6 (54.9–100)	9.8 (9.1–10·6)[a]
5. Urticaria	**55.1 (35.3–78.7)**	**54·9 (35.1–78.6)**	**−0.5 (−1.1–0.1)**
6. Scabies	58.6 (32.4–93.0)	51 (28.3–81)	−13.0 (−13.9–12.2)[a]
7. Fungal skin diseases	46.1 (18.3–95.7)	48.9 (19.5–101.4)	6.0 (5.3–6.8)[a]
8. Pyoderma	22.1 (12.9–27.9)	27.7 (17.8–37.0)	25.1 (3.6–51.2)[a]
9. Pruritus	9.4 (4.4–17.2)	9.7 (4.5–17.8)	2.9 (2.4–3.5)[a]
10. Decubitus ulcer	10.7 (8.2–13.6)	10.2 (7.8–12.6)	−5.1(−11.6–0.4)

Adapted from table in global all-age DALYs and age-standardized DALYs rates in 1990, 2006, and 2016 with mean percentage changes between 1990 and 2016, 2006 and 2016, and 1990 and 2016 for all causes. [10]

Data in parentheses are 95% uncertainty intervals

Skin cancer is not included among skin and subcutaneous diseases

DALYs disability-adjusted life-years

[a]Percentage changes that are statistically significant

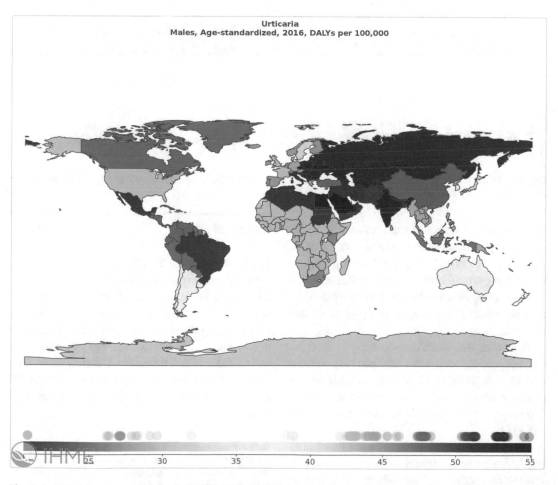

Fig. 2.5 Urticaria: age-standardized disability-adjusted life-years (DALYs) among males per 100,000, 2016 (GBD 2016) [7]. (With permission from Institute for Health Metrics and Evaluation (IHME) [7])

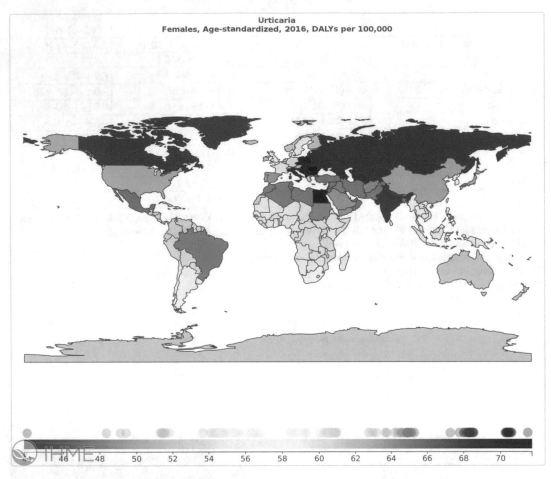

Fig. 2.6 Urticaria: age-standardized DALYs among females per 100,000, 2016 (GBD 2016) [7]. (With permission from Institute for Health Metrics and Evaluation (IHME) [7])

Population-based studies and prospective studies on contact urticaria are scarce. Stratification according to sex, age, temporal trends, occupational category, adjustment for population at risk, and potential confounders would be most desirable to assess the true epidemiology of contact urticaria.

Accurate and complete reporting is essential for preventing chronic and relapsing disease course. Registries should be improved by enhancement of reporting procedures, which should be transparent, simple, and easily accessible [11].

Continuous surveillance of substances leading to immediate-contact reactions is also necessary for primary, secondary, and tertiary prevention.

Conclusion

Worldwide, the burden of urticaria is substantial, being among the ten leading skin and subcutaneous diseases with the highest prevalence and incidence. Urticaria leads to considerable health loss, being among the ten leading skin and subcutaneous diseases with highest number of years lived with disability and disability-adjusted years. The total burden of urticaria may be highly underestimated as the result of late diagnosis, underdiagnosis, and subregistration.

Acknowledgments The author is grateful to the Global Burden of Disease 2016 Project and [7] Institute for Health Metrics and Evaluation (IHME), University of Washington, for providing the permission to reproduce the figures presented in this chapter.

References

1. Last JM, Spasoff RA, Harris SS, editors. Dictionary of epidemiology. 4th ed. New York: Oxford University Press; 2001. p. 224.
2. Hay RJ, Johns NE, Williams HC, Bolliger IW, Dellavalle RP, Margolis DJ, et al. The global burden of skin disease in 2010: an analysis of the prevalence and impact of skin conditions. J Invest Dermatol. 2014;134:1527–34.
3. Occupational skin diseases and dermal exposure in the European Union (EU-25): Policy and practice review [homepage on the Internet]. European Agency for Safety and Health at Work; 2008 [cited 2017 Oct 20]; Available from: https://osha.europa.eu/en/publications/reports/TE7007049ENC_skin_diseases.
4. Rothman K, Greenland S, editors. Modern epidemiology. 3rd ed. Philadelphia: Lippincott Williams & Wilkins; 2008. p. 757.
5. GBD 2016 Disease and Injury Incidence and Prevalence Collaborators. Global, regional, and national incidence, prevalence, and years lived with disability for 328 diseases and injuries for 195 countries, 1990–2016: a systematic analysis for the Global Burden of Disease Study 2016. Lancet. 2017;390(10100):1211–59.
6. Pearce N. Prevalence studies. In: Pearce N, editor. A short introduction to epidemiology. 2nd ed. Wellington: Centre for Public Health Research; 2005. p. 33–41.
7. Institute for Health Metrics and Evaluation (IHME). GBD compare. Seattle: IHME, University of Washington; 2017. Available from http://vizhub.healthdata.org/gbd-compare. Accessed 02 Nov 2017.
8. Kiec-Swierczynska M, Krecisz B, Potocka A, Swierczynska-Machura D, Dudek W, Palczynski C. Psychological factors in allergic skin diseases. Med Pract. 2008;59:279–85.
9. Murray CJ. Quantifying the burden of disease: the technical basis for disability-adjusted life-years. Bull World Health Org. 1994;72:429–45.
10. GBD Disease and Injury Incidence and Prevalence Collaborators. Global, regional, and national disability-adjusted life-years (DALYs) for 333 diseases and injuries and healthy life expectancy (HALE) for 195 countries and territories, 1990–2016: a systematic analysis for the Global Burden of Disease Study 2016. Lancet. 2017;390(10100):1260–344.
11. Alfonso JH, Bauer A, Bensefa-Colas L, Boman A, Bubas M, Constandt L, et al. Minimum standards on prevention, diagnosis and treatment of occupational and work-related skin diseases in Europe. Position paper of the COST Action StanDerm (TD 1206). J Eur Acad Dermatol Venereol. 2017;31(Suppl 4):31–43.

Occupational Relevance of Contact Urticaria Syndrome

Jose Hernán Alfonso

"...Now and then I have noticed that bakers have swollen, aching hands. Everyone in this trade -gets rough hands by kneuding the dough. A baker just has to show his hands to reveal this trade. No other tradesman has similar hands."

"De Morbis Artificum Diatriba" [1]
Bernardino Ramazzini (1633–1714)

Work-Related Skin Disease and Occupational Skin Disease

In 1700 Bernard Ramazzini, the father of modern occupational medicine, described cases of work-related skin diseases among bakers in *De Morbis Artificum Diatriba* (*Diseases of Workers*), which is the first comprehensive book on occupational diseases [1]. The first recorded observation of occupational disease is even older and dates back to Hippocrates (ca. 460–377 BC); however, as of 2018 it is still challenging to define work-related and occupational skin disease.

Therefore, to understand the occupational relevance of immediate contact skin reactions, we should start by defining work-related and occupational skin diseases. Although these concepts are often used as synonyms, they are not.

The American Medical Association defined, in 1930, occupational dermatoses as

"all dermatologic conditions where it can be demonstrated that the work is its fundamental cause or a contributing factor to it" [2, 3]

The Tenth Ibero-Latin American Congress of Dermatology, in 1983, defined occupational dermatoses as

"any affection of the skin, mucous or skin adnexa directly or indirectly caused, conditioned, maintained or worsened by anything that is used in professional activity or exists in the work environment" [4, 5].

The common pattern in both definitions is that the development or worsening of the skin disease has to be related directly or indirectly to chemical, physical, biological, mechanical, or psychosocial exposures in the work environment.

Work-related Skin Disease: A Preventive Context

"Work-related diseases" are diseases with multiple causes for development in which factors of the work environment may be involved together with other risk factors, such as atopic predisposition. For instance, work-related

J. H. Alfonso (✉)
Department of Occupational Medicine and Epidemiology, National Institute of Occupational Health, Oslo, Norway
e-mail: jose.alfonso@stami.no

diseases include diseases with solid scientific evidence of a possible occupational origin, which may not fulfill all given criteria to recognize an occupational disease according to the official list of occupational diseases, which differs among countries [4, 5]. For example, when establishing a diagnosis of work-related or occupational contact urticaria, it is necessary to identify a causal link between exposure to a risk factor at work and the development or worsening of the disease [6].

The Health & Safety Executive (United Kingdom) defines three patterns of a work–illness relationship [7]:

- *Causation:* the illness would not have occurred without the work effect.
- *Contributory causation:* work is one of several factors directly affecting the disease process; absence of the work effect could influence the onset and course of the illness but not remove the disease altogether.
- *Symptom exacerbation:* the illness is worsened by work, but work does not contribute to the underlying disease process.

If our aim is to prevent disease, the definition should be sufficiently broad and include a scientific (medical) approach [8, 9]; in this case the term "work-related urticaria/protein contact dermatitis" may be preferable to prevent illness as much as possible.

Occupational Skin Disease: A Compensatory Context

For compensation, the definition of occupational skin disease is used differently in each country because of the different legal and political systems [10].

The World Health Organization (WHO) defines the term occupational disease as

"any disease contracted primarily as a result of an exposure to risk factors arising from work activity" [11, 12].

According to The International Labour Organization, an occupational disease comprises two main elements:

1. A causal relationship between exposure in a specific working environment or work activity and a specific disease.
2. The fact that the disease occurs among a group of exposed persons with a frequency above the average morbidity of the rest of the population [13].

Generally, criteria for recognition and compensation of an occupational disease are the following:

- The disease has to be listed in the official national list of occupational diseases.
- The occupational risk factor should stem from the patient's job.
- The worker's exposure to an occupational risk factor must be documented [14].

In a few words, the "causal relationship" should be established based on clinical, pathological data, and epidemiological evidence [14].

Sometimes it can be challenging and time-demanding to assess whether an immediate skin contact reaction is related to work because evaluation of occupational and non -occupational risk factors should be considered, for example, in the case of a patient with previous respiratory atopy developing contact urticaria at work, or a patient suffering from chronic urticaria that worsens in response to a mechanical or physical stimulus at work. In all cases is essential to document in detail the association between exposures at work and development or worsening of symptoms, as well as improvement of skin symptoms during free time, weekends, holidays, or sick leave periods.

Toward a Common Definition

It is apparent that definitions are conditioned by the context, purposes, locations, and time [8, 9]. For instance, no international official agreement exists on the best reliable and applicable definition. However, a European Consensus (Minimum Standards on Prevention, Diagnosis, and Treatment of Occupational and Work-related Skin Diseases, STANDERM) has recently suggested the following definition: "both work-related and occupational skin diseases comprise entities/conditions with an occupational contribution. Occupational skin diseases *sensu stricto* are additionally defined by diverging national legal requirements, with an impact on registration, prevention, management, and compensation" [15].

Immediate Contact Reactions in the Classification of Work-Related and Occupational Skin Diseases

Lachapelle et al. [16] suggested a classification of skin conditions according to different types of occupational exposure (Table 3.1). Immediate contact reactions can be related to chemical exposures (contact urticaria, contact urticaria syndrome, and protein contact dermatitis), physical and mechanical exposures (worsening of chronic urticaria), and biological agents (contact urticaria and protein contact dermatitis).

Contact dermatitis of the hands constitutes the majority of the cases (between 90% and 95%) of work-related and occupational skin diseases. As immediate contact reactions are common in dermatological practice, and may be frequent in occupational settings [18], it is important to always ask for the patient's occupation and consider potential work-related or occupational immediate contact reaction as a potential diagnosis.

The draft of the next International Code Diseases (ICD)-11 proposes a comprehensive classification of work-related skin diseases, which includes protein contact dermatitis, occupational allergic contact urticaria, occupational nonallergic contact urticaria, and in addition, exacerbation of constitutional dermatitis. The implementation of the proposed ICD-11 classification of work-related skin diseases and occupational skin diseases has been recommended by a consensus of European experts because it will enable a comprehensive identification of work-related skin diseases and occupational skin diseases, and thereby valid surveillance [15].

Table 3.1 Classification of work-related and occupational skin diseases

Occupational exposure	Skin disease
Chemical agents	Chemical skin injury
	Irritant contact dermatitis
	Allergic contact dermatitis
	Protein contact dermatitis
	Phototoxic dermatitis
	Urticaria
	Acne (e.g., oil acne, chloracne)
	Leucoderma/vitiligo-like skin diseases (phenols, catechol, and hydroquinone causing death of melanocytes and subsequent depigmentation)
	Scleroderma-like diseases (vinyl chloride monomer, silica dust, organic solvents, and epoxy resins have all been reported as associated with scleroderma-like conditions)
	Cutaneous squamous cell carcinoma Melanoma skin cancer
Physical agents	Irritant contact dermatitis caused by physical agents (heat, cold, dry air)
	Physical urticaria (cold urticaria, delayed pressure urticaria, solar urticaria, heat urticaria, vibratory angioedema) [17]
	Cutaneous squamous cell carcinoma (UVB radiation, ionizing radiation)
	Melanoma skin cancer (UVB radiation)
	Raynaud phenomenon (vibration)
Biological agents	*Protein contact dermatitis* Bacteria (e.g., erysipeloid, quarry fever, borreliosis)
	Virus (e.g., orf, contagious pustular dermatitis)
	Fungi (e.g., tinea pedis)
	Parasites, algal (prototheccosis)

Adapted from Lachapelle et al. [16]

Occurrence of Occupational Contact Urticaria and Protein Contact Dermatitis

Although the worldwide burden of urticaria is substantial (Chap. 2), little is known about the real occurrence of occupational contact urticaria and protein contact dermatitis in the general population [18].

A systematic literature search aimed to identify epidemiological studies focusing on occupa-

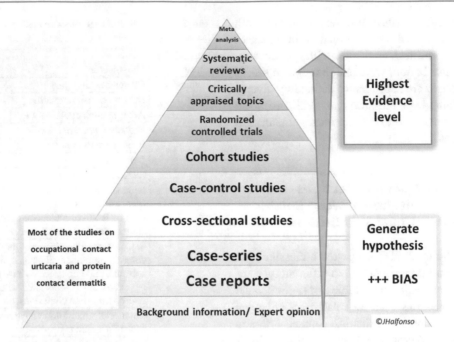

Fig. 3.1 Type of epidemiological studies most commonly used for occupational contact urticaria and protein contact dermatitis

tional urticaria and protein contact dermatitis for the period 1974–2017[1] identified mostly case reports, case series, and register-based studies with a retrospective design.

As Fig. 3.1 shows, case reports and case series provide the lowest level of epidemiological evidence; however, they contribute to identifying environmental and occupational exposures leading to immediate contact skin reactions and to initiate local preventive actions. Therefore, the publication of clinical cases is highly encouraged.

According to available register-based studies (Table 3.2), occupational contact urticaria accounts for about 1–29.5% of the reported cases of occupational skin disease. The annual population incidence of occupational contact urticaria ranges from an estimated 0.3 to 6.2 cases per 100,000 workers per year [27].

Most of the available studies stem from official registers whereof underreporting may undermine findings from register-based studies. Current registries are usually incomplete as work-related and occupational skin diseases are highly underdiagnosed, underreported, and undertreated [15]. These studies have usually a retrospective design, which is inexpensive, but cannot show temporal associations and determine the incidence of a disease. Thus, these provide a low level of evidence, but are useful to generate hypotheses. In some cases when registries are almost complete, such studies may be useful to follow the trends of a disease in a population and to evaluate the impact of preventive interventions [27, 28].

Although protein contact dermatitis in an occupational setting (food handlers) was described for the first time in 1976 [29], most of the available studies consist of case reports and case series, which are not suitable to draw statistical conclusions. In fact, protein contact dermatitis is still a little-known disease.

---

[1]The systematic literature search was conducted in the database Embase, Medline with the last search on 8 august 2017. The search strategy included a combination of free text terms indexed by a hierarchical controlled vocabulary (MeSH and Emtree adapted for OVID Medline).

Table 3.2 Overview of selected register-based studies with data on occupational contact urticaria (OCU)

Region	Study design	Population	Main findings
France (Bensefa-Colas et al. 2015) [19]	Retrospective, register-based study	Reports to the French National Network for Occupational Disease Vigilance and Prevention (RNV3P) for the period 2001–2010	251 cases of OCU were reported in RNV3P, half of which were caused by natural rubber latex, in particular in the health and social work activity sector. The number of these cases declined significantly over the study period (19% per year), and particularly after 2006. Conversely, the other causes of OCU did not decrease.
Norway (Alfonso et al. 2015) [20]	Retrospective, register-based study	Reports to the Norwegian Labour Inspectorate's Registry for work-related diseases for the period 2000–2013	3% of cases of 3142 cases of work-related skin diseases consisted of contact urticaria. Occupational exposures most commonly notified consisted of gloves, plants, animals, and animal products, fish and shellfish, and medicines.
Australia (Williams et al. 2008) [21]	Retrospective, register-based study	Cases of occupational contact urticaria diagnosed at an occupational dermatology clinic in Melbourne between 1 January 1993 and 31 December 2004.	8.3% of 1720 patients with occupational skin disease were diagnosed with occupational contact urticaria. *Exposures most frequently reported*: Natural rubber latex, foodstuffs, and ammonium persulfate. *Sites most commonly affected*: hands, followed by the arms and face. *Occupations*: healthcare workers, food handlers, and hairdressers. *Significant risk factor*: Atopy
United Kingdom (Mc Donald et al. 2006) [22]	Retrospective, register-based study	Cases reported in 1996–2001 to the EPIDERM and OPRA national surveillance schemes	*Exposures most frequently reported for OCU*: Rubber chemicals and materials, foods and flour, aldehydes, fragrance, and cosmetics. *Types of industry*: Food and organic material manufacturing, health and social services, metallic and automotive product manufacturing. Rates for urticaria in women where twice those in men. Incidence rates were six to eight times higher when based on reports from occupational physicians than from dermatologists.
Scotland (Chen et al. 2005) [23]	Retrospective, register-based study	Cases of work-related diseases reported to The Health and Occupation network (THOR) for Scotland in 2002–2003.	Contact urticaria accounted for 6% of all reported cases of skin diseases (16% of all cases of notified work-related diseases).
Pakistan (Arif, and Haroon 2001) [24]	Prospective study with 2-year follow-up	One hundred consecutive patients (97 males and 3 females), aged between 13 and 65 years with suspected occupational contact dermatitis were patch tested with the European Standard Series and with material samples from the workplace, during 1997–1998.	Occupational contact urticaria accounted for 1% of all reported cases. More common among males. Many of the workers did not use any protective equipment.

(continued)

Table 3.2 (continued)

Region	Study design	Population	Main findings
Finland (Kanerva et al. 1996) [25]	Retrospective, register-based study	Reports on occupational dermatoses to the Finnish Register of Occupational Diseases for the period 1990–1994	815 cases (29.5%) of contact urticaria (protein contact dermatitis included) were reported to the Finnish Register of Occupational Diseases. Occupations mostly affected: farmers, domestic animal attendants, bakers, nurses, chefs, dental assistants, veterinary surgeons, domestic animal attendants, farmers and silviculturists, chefs, cooks, and cold buffet managers.
Norway (Bakke et al. 1990) [26]	Cross-sectional, population-based study	Self-administered questionnaire to a random sample of 4992 subjects of the general population aged 15–70 years of the Hordaland county. Response frequency: 90%	The lifetime prevalence of eczema and urticaria was of 25% and 9%. More frequent among women. The lifetime prevalence of eczema and urticaria were associated with occupational dust or gas exposure after adjusting for sex, age, smoking habits, and area of residence.

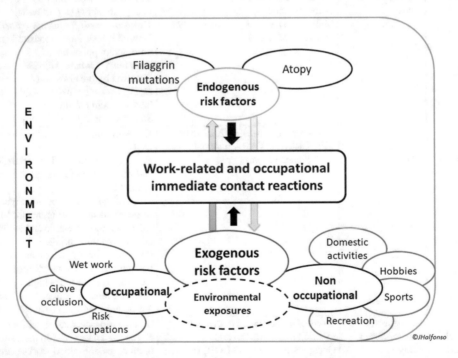

Fig. 3.2 Risk factors for work-related and occupational immediate contact reactions

Risk Factors for Work-Related and Occupational Immediate Contact Reactions

The development of work-related immediate contact reactions is influenced by a combination of endogenous risk factors (individual susceptibility) and exogenous risk factors (environmental exposures) (Fig. 3.2). Environmental exposures can occur either at the workplace, during leisure time, or a combination of both.

Occupational skin exposure to hazardous substances such as chemical, biological, and physical factors is a *sine qua non* condition of work-related and occupational immediate contact reactions.

Moreover, individual susceptibility character-istics may influence the development of these conditions, and make some individuals more prone to develop such diseases, for example, atopic predisposition [21]. Skin barrier disrup-tion and irritant contact dermatitis predispose to the penetration of allergens that may cause con-tact urticaria, or proteins which may lead to pro-tein contact dermatitis [18].

Endogenous Risk Factors

Atopy

Atopy is a significant risk factor for the develop-ment of immediate contact reactions [18, 21]. Atopy can be defined as

> "A personal or family tendency to produce IgE antibodies in response to low doses of allergens, usually proteins, and to develop typical symptoms such as asthma, rhinoconjunctivitis, or eczema/dermatitis" [30].

Atopic predisposition includes food allergy, eczema, asthma, and seasonal and persistent rhi-nitis and urticaria. Atopic dermatitis, a chronic skin disease, generally starts in infancy and affects between 5% and 20% of individuals worldwide [31]. A history of atopic dermatitis in childhood is associated with an increased risk of hand eczema in adulthood, up to a threefold risk [32–34]. For instance, atopic dermatitis is associ-ated with persistent and incident hand eczema, according to a Danish population-based cohort study with 5-year follow-up [35].

People with specific food allergies to banana, mangos, figs, papayas, and pineapple may react to natural rubber latex protein because of IgE cross-reactivity [36].

Filaggrin Mutations

Filaggrin, a structural protein, influences integ-rity in the stratum corneum. Filaggrin loss-of-function mutations are associated with an elevated risk of developing atopic dermatitis and irritant contact dermatitis [37, 38]. Filaggrin mutations affect between 8% and 10% of adults from the general population, but the frequency is even higher in individuals with atopic dermatitis

[37, 39]. The identification of individual suscep-tibility markers such as loss of filaggrin muta-tions is a fascinating research area because of their potential preventive implications. Consequently, workers with elevated individual susceptibility can be identified and theoretically prevented from developing work-related and occupational contact dermatitis eczema. For instance, an association between filaggrin and irritant contact dermatitis was reported among high-risk occupations such as healthcare, metal-work and construction, hairdressing, food and catering, and cleaning [40–42].

Future epidemiological studies focusing on immediate contact reactions should address whether filaggrin mutations are an independent risk factor for contact urticaria and protein con-tact dermatitis.

Ethnicity

Some immediate contact reactions such as alco-hol urticaria syndrome are reported to be more common among persons of East Asian descent who have aldehyde dehydrogenase deficiency, leading to increased serum aldehyde levels in alcohol breakdown [43–45]. For example, alco-hol urticaria syndrome presenting after a reaction to hand sanitizer has been described [46].

Exogenous Risk Factors

Wet Work

Wet work is defined as activities in which work-ers have to immerse their hands in liquids, wear waterproof (occlusive) gloves for more than 2 hours per shift, or wash their hands more than 20 times per shift [47]. Frequent exposure to water causes swelling and shrinking of the stra-tum corneum and subsequent epidermal barrier disruption, leading to the development of irritant contact dermatitis. In addition, wet work with the simultaneous effect of cleaning products, disin-fectants, solvents, alkalis, and acids leads to addi-tional damage that facilitates the penetration of allergens, which may lead to contact urticaria and proteins that may lead to protein contact dermati-tis. For instance, wet work is a well-known risk factor for hand eczema in hairdressing, nursing, cleaning, food handling, metal working, manufacturing, construction, machine tool operation, food preparation, printing, metal plating, leather work, engine servicing, and floristry [48].

Glove Occlusion

Gloves provide workers with protection, but extensive and prolonged glove occlusion may lead to skin barrier disruption and subsequent development of irritant contact dermatitis, which again is a prerequisite for the development of contact urticaria and protein contact dermatitis. Glove occlusion significantly enhances skin barrier damage following exposure to cleaning products in a dose–response manner [49]. Use of gloves may take place at the workplace, but also during domestic activities such as cleaning and leisure time activities such as gardening, painting, sports, recreation, or other hobbies. It is important, therefore, to document the number of hours using gloves at both occupational and non-occupational activities, the type of gloves in use, and the presence of skin symptoms while using gloves.

In addition to the negative effects following glove occlusion, immediate contact reactions can follow exposure to rubber gloves and, more rarely, to plastic gloves [50].

Skin Exposure to Chemical Products

Cleaning products enhance skin barrier disruption leading to an easier penetration of allergens such as fragrances and preservatives. Skin contact with *organic solvents*, in addition to systemic adverse effects, can lead to skin dryness, whitening, sensory irritation, contact urticaria, cumulative irritant contact dermatitis, skin chemical injuries, and scleroderma [51]. The effects vary according to the chemical structure, concentration, and duration of exposure.

Metallic coatings containing nickel can lead to immediate contact reactions in addition to delayed allergy [52, 53]. Direct or airborne contact with specific polymers from *plastic resins* and paint coatings can also induce irritant contact dermatitis, allergic contact dermatitis, contact urticaria, mucosal irritation, allergy, and sclero-

derma [54, 55]. For example, low molecular weight chemicals such as the epoxy resin hardener methyl tetrahydrophthalic anhydride (MTHPA) may lead to immunological contact urticaria [56]. Severe reactions after exposure to epoxy and hardeners have also been described [57]. Skin contact and airborne exposure to medicaments and cosmetics are also reported as exposures leading to immediate contact reactions [18, 58, 59]. Table 3.3 shows an overview of selected reviews summarizing the agents leading to immediate contact reactions. In addition, Chap. 8 focuses on immediate contact reactions induced by chemicals.

Skin Exposure to Biological Agents

Vegetables, fruits, plants, flowers, flower extracts, and contact with animals may lead to immediate contact reactions [60–68].

Skin Exposure to Physical and Mechanical Stimuli

This book focuses on immediate contact reactions, but it needs to be highlighted that physical and mechanical stimuli at work may trigger and worsen inducible urticaria (approximately half the cases of chronic urticaria in the general population are caused by inducible urticaria). In addition, physical urticaria can have occupational consequences. Table 3.4 shows some case reports of work-related physical urticaria. Atopic predisposition and occupations with frequent and repetitive mechanical stimuli are a common feature.

High-Risk Occupations for Urticaria and Protein Contact Dermatitis

Contact Urticaria

At the weakest end of the contact urticaria syndrome, patients may experience itching, tingling, or burning accompanied by erythema (wheal and flare). At the more extreme end of the spectrum, extracutaneous symptoms may accompany the local urticarial response, ranging from rhinoconjunctivitis to anaphylactic shock. The typical pri-

Table 3.3 Some selected studies on agents leading to immediate contact reactions

Author, year and type of study	Main findings
Helaskoski et al., 2017[60] Retrospective, register-based study	*Occupational contact urticaria and protein contact dermatitis: causes and concomitant airway diseases* Between 1995 and 2011, 291 cases of occupational contact urticaria or protein contact dermatitis were diagnosed in the Finnish Institute of Occupational Health. The most common causes were flour, cow dander, natural rubber latex, and acid anhydrides. Concomitant occupational airway disease was detected in 46% of patients with skin disease (occupational asthma or rhinitis)
Verhulst and Goossens, 2016 [59] Non-systematic review	*Cosmetics component causing contact urticaria: a review and update* Hair dyes and bleaches, preservatives, fragrance and aroma chemicals, sunscreens, hair glues, plant-derived and animal-derived components, permanent makeup and tattoos, glycolic acid peel, lip plumper, and alcohols. Many of the reported cases lack appropriate controls and detailed investigation. Contact urticaria may include life-threating systemic manifestations.
Lukacs et al., 2016 [61] Systematic clinical review	*Occupational contact urticaria caused by food* Food handlers are at increased risk for occupational contact urticaria and protein contact dermatitis. Individuals handling seafood, meat, vegetables, and fruits, such as chefs, cooks, bakers, butchers, slaughterhouse workers, and fish-factory workers. Foodstuffs that commonly induce occupational protein contact dermatitis include fish, seafood, meats, vegetables, and fruits.
Paulsen and Andersen, 2016 [62] Non-systematic review	*Lettuce contact allergy* Concomitant or isolated immediate lettuce reactions in patients who presented with dermatitis. In cases of concomitant immediate and delayed sensitization, the patients often had clinical features of both dermatitis and contact urticaria.
Barbaud, et al., 2015 [63] Retrospective, register-based study	*Protein contact dermatitis in France* Of 7560 patients tested, 22 had occupational protein contact dermatitis. Most of them were among food handlers, but also in gardeners, grocer, hairdresser, florists, veterinary worker, and nurses. 59% of cases were in females. A history of atopy was found in 56–68% of cases.
Wang and Maibach, 2013 [64] Non-systematic review	*High-risk occupations for occupational immediate contact reactions* Review of high- risk occupations for occupational contact urticaria and new technologies that may lead to development of occupational immediate contact reactions.
Vester et al., 2012 [65] Retrospective, case-series	*Protein contact dermatitis among food handlers* Of 372 food handlers diagnosed with occupational skin disease in a period of 10 years, 57.0% had irritant contact dermatitis, 22.0% had protein contact dermatitis, 2.4% had contact urticaria, and 1.8% had allergic contact dermatitis. Frequent risk occupations were cooking in restaurants, baking, and kitchen work. Substantially more patients reacted in skin prick testing with fresh foods than with food extracts
Davari and Maibach, 2011 [66] Non-systematic review	*Contact urticaria to cosmetic and industrial dyes* Widespread use of dyes in textiles, cosmetics, and foods. Hair dyes, basic blue 99 dye, patent blue dyes, henna, red dyes, curcumin, and reactive dyes can potentially cause contact urticaria. Hair-dye constituents such as preservatives and intensifiers may be important as causative agents of CU.
Gimenez-Arnau et al., 2010 [18] Non-systematic review	*Update of contact urticaria, contact urticaria syndrome, and protein contact dermatitis* Overview of substances leading to immediate contact reactions such as animal, plants, derivatives, food and food additives, fragrances and cosmetics, drugs, preservatives, and miscellaneous chemicals and metals.

(continued)

Table 3.3 (continued)

Author, year and type of study	Main findings
Amaro and Goossens, 2008 [67] Non-systematic review	*Immunological occupational contact urticaria and contact dermatitis from proteins* Comprehensive overview of proteins leading to immunological contact urticarial and/or protein contact dermatitis, i.e., fruits, vegetables, spices, plants, and woods; animal proteins; grains and enzymes, all affecting a wide variety of jobs.
Santos and Goossens, 2007 [68] Non-systematic review	*An update on airborne contact dermatitis: 2001–2006* *Contact urticaria:* amoxicillin, curcumin, epoxy resin HATU and HBTU, hyacinth, pine processionary caterpillar (*Thaumetopoea pityocampa*), *Spathiphyllum wallisii* flower, weeping fig (*Ficus benjamina*), yucca (*Yucca aloifolia*). *Contact urticaria syndrome: Anisakis simplex*, Compositae, diphenylmethane-4,49-diisocyanate, ferns, goat dander, protease, lupine flour, triphenyl phosphate *Protein contact dermatitis:* flour, sapele wood
Valsecchi et al., 2003 [69] Cross-sectional study	*Occupational contact dermatitis and contact urticaria in veterinarians* Contact urticaria due to latex, cow dander and obstetric fluids. Cross-sectional study with low response frequency, but the specific exposures linked to contact urticaria are in line with reports from both Europe and USA
Warner et al., 1997 [70] Non-systematic review	*Agents causing contact urticaria* *Immunological:* seafood, fruits, animals, plants, honey, nuts, spices, plants substances, medicaments, germicides, hair-care products, beans, meats, industrial chemicals, and others. *Nonimmunological:* foods, fragrance and flavoring, medicaments, animals, plants, preservatives.

mary lesion (erythema, or wheal and flare) with or without secondary organ involvement resolves in hours, but atypical recurrent episodes via unknown mechanisms may convert into dermatitis (eczema) [76].

Workers at risk of suffering from work-related and occupational urticaria include those in all kinds of food, health, chemical, and biological occupations such as cooks, bakers, butchers, restaurant personnel [63, 65, 67, 77–81], surgeons, nurses [82–84], dental nurses [85], veterinarians [69, 86], laboratory technicians handling laboratory animals [87], biologists, pharmaceutical industry workers [88], hairdressers [89–91], agriculture, farming, floriculture, and industry workers [88], and construction. Population-based and prospective studies addressing occupational contact urticaria are available for healthcare workers [28, 84, 92, 93], hairdressers [90, 91], and hairdressing apprentices [91].

Healthcare Workers

The prevalence of contact urticaria in healthcare workers in Europe varies between 5% and 10%, whereas in the general population it varies between 1% and 3% [18]. Natural rubber latex was responsible for an epidemic of occupational contact urticaria among health workers during the 1990s from extensive glove use. In studies of hospital personnel, latex sensitivity was found to be three to five times higher among nurses and doctors than among workers not involved in patient care [82–84, 93].

The decreasing prevalence of occupational contact urticaria as a result of the use of low-allergen/low-protein non-powdered protective gloves is a successful example of the prevention of occupational contact urticaria [28, 92]. In countries without such legislation, occupational contact urticaria from natural rubber latex may still be a problem [94].

Hairdressing

The prevalence of contact urticaria in hairdressing apprentices has been reported to be 7.3%, compared to 4.2% in controls from the general population. In addition, it increased with increasing level of apprenticeship [90]. Among hairdressers, the prevalence is about 16% [90, 95].

Table 3.4 Occupational exposures and physical urticaria

Occupational exposure	Type of physical urticaria
Heavy work	Cholinergic and delayed-pressure urticaria [71]
An atopic 29-year-old man presented with 3-year-duration recurrent edematous lesions and itch to the palm of the hands owing to the use of a planing machine and during journeys on a motorbike.	Nonfamiliar vibratory angioedema [72]
Backs of truck drivers and in professional football players from the pressure of the shoulder pads.	Pressure urticaria owing to repetitive mechanical trauma [73]
A 42-year-old nurse working in a surgical department for 11 years developed urticaria, rhinitis and bronchospasm in contact with formaldchyde. In addition, she developed demographic, aquagenic, cholinergic, and delayed pressure urticaria in exposed areas.	Contact urticaria syndrome from formaldehyde with multiple physical urticaria [74]
A 40-year-old women with atopic rhinitis, presented with pruriginous wheals, occurring only in areas in contact with hot objects while making churros (Spanish sweet food)	Heat urticaria [75]

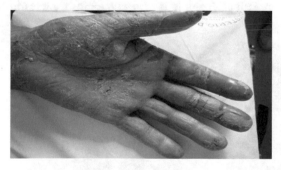

Fig. 3.3 Protein contact dermatitis in the context of chronic hand eczema in a greengrocer

Protein Contact Dermatitis

Protein contact dermatitis, an underdiagnosed skin disease, is characterized by chronic and recurrent dermatitis of the hands and forearms

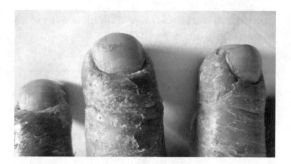

Fig. 3.4 Finger dermatitis in the same greengrocer

occurring a few minutes after contact with allergens (Fig. 3.3). It may also be manifested as just a fingertip dermatitis (Fig. 3.4) The lesions are at first urticarial; and then, as Figs. 3.3 and 3.4 show, they develop the eczematous type, with erythema, scaling, and fissures [63, 96]. Some cases of chronic paronychia were considered a variety of protein contact dermatitis, with redness and swelling of the proximal nail fold, for example, after handling food, and natural rubber latex [67].

Protein contact dermatitis affects occupations with frequent wet work, glove occlusion, and skin contact with irritants such as food handling, such as bakers, pastry cooks, fishmongers, cooks, greengrocers, cheese producers, florists, and veterinary workers. For example, in a 10-year retrospective study among 373 food handlers with occupational dermatoses in Denmark, 22% had protein contact dermatitis and 2.4% of the patients had contact urticaria. In this case series, substantially more patients reacted in skin prick testing with fresh foods than with food extracts [65]. Figure 3.4 shows results after prick-by-prick with fresh vegetables in a greengrocer with protein contact dermatitis in the context of chronic hand eczema. Patch testing was negative.

In the seafood industry, the reported prevalence of occupational protein contact dermatitis is between 3% and 11% [77–81], but these estimates arise from old studies. A newer French study revealed that chefs who have to cook seafood are more at risk for occupational protein contact dermatitis than fishermen. The authors hypothesized that skin protection is better implemented in the fishing sector than in the catering profession, where it is more difficult to use gloves to perform work tasks [97].

Assessment of Occupational Relevance in a Clinical Context

The diagnosis of work-related and occupational immediate contact reactions is essential for effective prevention and treatment. Such a diagnosis is based on medical history, physical examination, skin testing, and assessment of occupational relevance. The gold standard for diagnosing immediate contact reactions such as contact urticaria and protein contact dermatitis is the prick test and the prick-by-prick test (Fig. 3.5) [6, 15]. Chapters 4 and 10 give more details about diagnostic methods.

It should be highlighted that even when contact urticaria or protein contact dermatitis are the sole suspected diagnoses, patch testing should also be performed to not miss a diagnosis of delayed-type reactions. This provision is particularly important in patients with occupational hand dermatitis, chronic hand eczema, or atopic eczema and when latex rubber allergy is suspected [98]. Given that repeated episodes of contact urticaria may cause dermatitis, differential diagnosis may be difficult. Moreover, the same agent can originate different clinical pictures from distinct mechanisms. For example, curcumin, a potential cause of immediate and delayed allergic reactions, has also been reported as a cause of non-immunological contact urticaria in a woman exposed to this spice powder at work [99]. Therefore, atopic, allergic, and irritant contact dermatitis have to be considered in the differential diagnosis.

The apparition of immediate contact reactions in relationship to the workplace and improvement during sick leave periods and holidays raises suspicion on a work-related problem [6, 15]. For instance, the use of a symptom diary on work and non-work days is useful to investigate work-related urticaria and to identify allergens in the workplace that lead to urticaria [100]. Photographic documentation provided by the patients and by the attending physician is also useful to assess disease evolution.

The clinical manifestations are heterogeneous, varying from localized or generalized urticaria to concurrent involvement of other organs, mainly the respiratory and gastrointestinal tracts. For instance, occupational airway disease and occupational contact urticaria may occur [60]. Occupational airway, conjunctival, and skin allergy has also been reported among seafood workers handling squid [101]. Another practical example is airborne exposure to gum

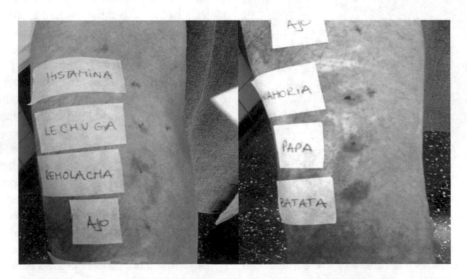

Fig. 3.5 Prick-by-prick test positives to carrots, potato, and sweet potato (picture on the right)

arabic in the food industry leading to allergic rhinitis, asthma, and urticaria [102]. Airborne exposure leading to urticaria associated with angioedema, conjunctivitis, and anaphylaxis has also been reported among pine processionary caterpillars [103, 104]. Therefore, it is important to ask for previous or concomitant nasal, conjunctival, or respiratory symptoms related to the occupational exposure. Patients often recall that contact with urticariogens elicited immediate pruritic wheals and swelling in the contact area, symptoms that may subside spontaneously after a few hours without further exposure and after taking antihistamines.

To document respiratory symptoms, peak flow at workdays and periods off can demonstrate airflow obstruction and greater variability in peak expiratory flow rates on workdays compared to rest days. When the clinical picture includes a combination of cutaneous and respiratory symptoms, they should be regarded as a third-stage contact urticaria [105]. Nevertheless, it must be highlighted that the diagnosis of contact urticaria should be restricted to situations in which patients develop a skin reaction after direct skin contact [106].

Occupational Exposure Assessment

Table 3.5 summarizes requirements for workplace exposure assessment that may be useful in the diagnosis of work-related and occupational immediate skin contact reactions.

The occupational history, assessment of occupational exposure, exploration of product labels, and a Material Safety Data Sheet (MSDS) will additionally help to establish the occupational relevance of immediate contact reactions [15]. History taking and occupational exposure assessment is time-demanding, but is always the most cost-effective part of the assessment because of the implications for diagnosis and prevention. For example, in more than 80% of cases with occupational allergic contact dermatitis, work exposure assessment in terms of medical history,

assessment of product labels, and the MSDS has been contributory to a correct diagnosis [107]. Dermatologists and occupational physicians, and other health professionals handling the management of work-related and occupational skin diseases may find challenges when assessing MSDS, as they are often incomplete. The most frequent shortcoming is "Missing H317" (labels for skin sensitizers) although a known contact allergen was present [108]. Often, the allergen is not listed because its concentration is less than the mandatory labeling concentration, which may be too high in relation to common elicitation concentration levels. Thus, if the composition of the implicated product still remains (partially) unknown or is not fully known as in the case of commercial products and complex mixtures, the manufacturer should be contacted to provide a detailed description of a product in question [107]. Unfortunately, information by manufacturers or importers is voluntary and a legal basis is lacking to support full diagnostic workup.

A workplace visit is often necessary to correctly identify relevant exposure and perform a complete assessment. For example, a workplace visit is useful to confirm the exposure source and allow patients to be cured of occupational contact urticaria and continue working [109]. Conducting a workplace visit is a challenge as in many countries there is no legal basis for who is going to perform a workplace visit and how it has to be performed [15].

Prognosis

Occupational immediate contact reactions such as contact urticaria and protein contact dermatitis may have quite disabling consequences and lead to significant social consequences such as sick leave, job loss, job change, and early retirement. A Finnish 6-month follow-up study in which 15.50% of 1048 patients were diagnosed with occupational contact urticaria, reported that contact urticaria was healed in 35% of the patients, 23% were on sick leave, 17% had changed work tasks, and 14% reported job loss [110]. However, duration of sick leave was not specified, and a

Table 3.5 Workplace exposure assessment in the diagnosis of work-related and occupational immediate skin contact reactions

Tool	Information to be collected
Worker's medical and occupational history	Profession, industrial sector
	Former and current workplaces, and work tasks (type and duration, skin hazards, collective and personal protective equipment)
	Current skin problems (time of appearance, relation to workplace and nonoccupational exposures such as leisure and domestic activities)
	Symptom diary on work and nonwork days
	Glove use, type, hours, change of gloves
	If respiratory symptoms, peak flow at workdays and periods off to demonstrate airflow obstruction and greater variability in peak expiratory flow rates on workdays compared to rest days
	Concomitant airway disease in relation to occupational or nonoccupational exposures
	Other previous or current skin problems or airway disease
	Leisure and domestic activities including skin hazards.
Clinical examination	Skin findings: localizations correlated with exposure Photographic documentation
Product labels and material safety data sheets	Objective data about chemicals with relevant work-related epidermal and dermal contact as well as exposure scenarios.
Workplace visit	
Spot tests	Spot tests for detection of cobalt, nickel, chrome, and formaldehyde
Skin testing	Prick test, prick by prick test

Adapted from [15]

6-month follow-up is too short to assess the long-term consequences of occupational contact urticaria. In general, predictors for continuation of occupational skin disease consisted of continuing in the job that caused the occupational skin disease, age over 45 years, food-related occupation, male sex, and respiratory atopy [110]. In this study, patients with occupational contact urticaria had the best outcome as compared to occupational allergic and irritant contact dermatitis.

On the other hand, a Danish study reported that occupational contact urticaria was associated with a risk of long-term sick leave [111].

A Danish cohort included 2703 employees with recognized occupational hand eczema and contact urticaria in 2010 were followed up for 4 to 5 years, with a response frequency of 58%. Approximately 6% of this population was diagnosed with occupational contact urticaria, whereof 54.2% remained in the same profession and 45.8% changed jobs by the end of the follow-up [112]. Important predictors for job change in patients with occupational hand eczema and/or

contact urticaria were a positive patch test reaction, severe symptoms, and working in the cleaning sector. Demographic factors, such as young age and low educational level, were also of importance, whereas factors such as atopic dermatitis and diagnosis (allergic versus irritant dermatitis) did not show any marked association with change of profession [112].

Differences in the factors predicting prognosis of occupational contact urticaria should be explained in the light of different legal definitions of work-related and occupational contact urticaria, study design, health systems, industry, length of follow-up, and social differences. Nevertheless, studies are consistent regarding the negative socioeconomic consequences.

Occupational protein contact dermatitis has a very negative impact on the working life of food handlers compared to other occupational skin diseases in the same field. For example, among 175 food handlers with occupational hand dermatitis, 30% suffered from protein contact dermatitis and all reported negative consequences on their work [65].

The negative consequences of work-related and occupational contact urticaria and protein contact dermatitis can be effectively avoided by preventive strategies that are presented in Chap. 12.

Further Needs and Available Standardized Questionnaires

More population-based and follow-up studies on work-related and occupational contact urticaria and protein contact dermatitis are needed to understand the real occurrence in emergent risk groups and the general working population, the interplay between risk factors and modifying and confounding factors. Future register-based studies should include adjustments for populations at risk, as well present results stratified by sex and age when possible.

As most of the available studies arise from Western Europe and Scandinavian countries, more research activity in other latitudes of the globe will contribute to enhance our current knowledge on work-related and occupational immediate contact reactions.

Future studies should use standardized and validated questionnaires to assess the occurrence and consequences of work-related and occupational immediate reactions.

The Nordic Occupational Skin Questionnaire–2002 short and long form (NOSQ-2002), a standardized questionnaire, includes nine specific questions on urticaria including intensity, risk factors, work activities, occupational exposures, and non-occupational exposures [113]. NOSQ-2002 is available in English, Swedish, Finnish, Norwegian, Icelandic, Danish, Spanish, Catalan, Turkish, and Italian [114–116].

Useful and standardized questionnaires to define the impact of contact urticaria on patients include the urticaria activity score (UAS), the angioedema activity score (AAS), the CU quality of life questionnaire (CU-Q2oL), the angioedema quality of life questionnaire (AE QoL), and the urticaria control test (UCT) [117].

Conclusion

Work-related and occupational urticaria are different definitions, but both are related to exposures at work. In a compensatory context, the term "occupational urticaria" is used most, wherein legal requirements for recognition are different among countries. If the aim is prevention, a wide definition such as "work-related urticaria" is preferable to prevent as much illness as possible. In all cases is essential to document the association between exposures at work and development of immediate contact reactions or worsening of symptoms. Occupational urticaria accounts for 1% to 29.5% of notified work-related and occupational skin diseases, but these are probably underdiagnosed and underreported.

The development of work-related and occupational immediate contact reactions is influenced by a combination of endogenous risk factors (individual susceptibility) and exogenous risk factors (environmental exposures). Environmental exposures can occur at the workplace, or during leisure time, or at a combination of both. Occupational and non-occupational exposures include chemical and biological agents. Mechanical and physical exposures at work may trigger or worsen physical urticaria. Risk professions include food industry workers, healthcare workers, hairdressers, industrial workers, and workers handling animals, fruits, plants, and vegetables. Wet work and irritant contact dermatitis may be prerequisites to develop contact urticaria and protein contact dermatitis. Concomitant occupational airway disease may occur.

Assessment of occupational relevance is an exhaustive, but essential, process for diagnosis and prevention that includes the worker's medical and occupational history, clinical examination, exposure information from product labels and material safety data sheets, workplace visits, spot tests, and skin testing with prick testing or prick-by-prick test. Differential diagnosis with atopic, allergic, or irritant contact dermatitis should be included. These work-related skin affections are associated with negative socioeconomic consequences.

More population-based and follow-up studies are necessary. Standardized questionnaires to assess both the occurrence and the consequences of immediate contact reactions are available and should be used in future studies.

Acknowledgments The author is grateful to Dr. Juan Pedro Russo, Hospital San Martín de La Plata, Argentina for providing the pictures of the patient with protein contact dermatitis.

References

1. Ramazzini B. De morbis artificum diatriba. Mutinae: Typis Antonii Capponi; 1700.
2. Wise F, Sulzberger MB. Industrial dermatoses. Am Med. 1933;28:4–7.
3. Sulzberger MB, Finnerud CW. Industrial dermatitis definitions and criteria of diagnosis. JAMA. 1938;111:1528–32.
4. Ortiz de Frutos FJ, Conde Salazar L. Eczemas y dermatosis profesionales. In:Tratado de dermatología. Madrid: LUZÁN 5; 1994. p. 351–401.
5. Ruíz-Frutos C, Benavides FG, Delclós J, García AM. Salud Laboral. Conceptos y Técnicas Para la Prevención de Riesgos Laborales. 3rd ed. Masson: ELSE-VIER; 2007. ISBN13: 978844581712.
6. Adisesh A, Robinson E, Nicholson PJ, Sen D, Wilkinson M, Standards of Care Working Group. U.K. standards of care for occupational contact dermatitis and occupational contact urticaria. Br J Dermatol. 2013;168:1167–75.
7. Jones JR, Hodgson JT, Clegg TA, Elliot RC. Self-reported work related illness in 1995: results from a household survey. Norwich (UK): Her Majesty´s Stationary Office; 1998. p. 282.
8. World Health Organization. Epidemiology of work-related diseases and accidents: tenth report of the Joint ILO/WHO Committee on Occupational Health. Geneve (Switzerland): WHO; 1989. Technical Report Series No. 777.
9. Clayton A, Johnstone R, Sceats S. The legal concept of work-related injury and disease in australian OHS and Workers´ Compensation Systems. Aust J Labour Law. 2002;15:105–53.
10. Mahler V, Aalto-Korte K, Alfonso JH, Bakker JG, Bauer A, Bensefa-Colas L, et al. Occupational skin diseases: actual state analysis of patient management pathways in 28 European countries. J Eur Acad Dermatol Venereol. 2017;31(Suppl. 4):12–30. El
11. Batawi MA. Work-related diseases. A new program of the World Health Organization. Scand J Work Environ Health. 1984;10:341–6.
12. World Health Organization (WHO). Occupational Health. Occupational and work-related diseases. http://www.who.int/occupational_health/activities/ occupational_work_diseases/en/. Last accessed 19 Nov 2017.
13. International Labour Organization (ILO). Encyclopaedia of occupational health and safety. http://www.iloencyclopaedia.org/. Last accessed 19 Nov 2017.
14. International Labour Organization (ILO). Recommendation No. 194 onthe List of Occupational Diseases. http://www.ilo.org/safework/info/publications/WCMS_125137/lang–en/index.htm. Last accessed 19 Nov 2017.
15. Alfonso JH, Bauer A, Bensefa-Colas L, Boman A, Bubas M, Constandt L, et al. Minimum standards on prevention, diagnosis and treatment of occupational and work-related skin diseases in Europe – position paper of the COST Action StanDerm (TD 1206). J Eur Acad Dermatol Venereol. 2017;31(Suppl. 4):31–43.
16. Lachapelle JM, Frimat P, Tennstedt D, Ducombs G. Dermatologie professionnelle et de l'environnement. Paris: Masson; 1992. p. 372.
17. Zuberbier T, Aberer W, Asero R, Bindslev-Jensen C, Brzoza Z, Canonica GW, et al. The EAACI/GA(2) LEN/EDF/WAO guideline for the definition, classification, diagnosis, and management of urticaria: the 2013 revision and update. Allergy. 2014;69:868–87.
18. Gimenez-Arnau A, Maurer M, De La Cuadra J, Maibach H. Immediate contact skin reactions, an update of contact Urticaria, contact Urticaria syndrome and protein contact dermatitis – "a never ending story". Eur J Dermatol. 2010;20:552–62.
19. Bensefa-Colas L, Telle-Lamberton M, Faye S, Bourrain J-L, Crépy M-N, Lasfargues G, Choudat D, RNV3P members, Momas I. Occupational contact urticaria: lessons from the French National Network for occupational disease vigilance and prevention (RNV3P). Br J Dermatol. 2015;173:1453–61. https://doi.org/10.1111/bjd.14050.
20. Alfonso JH, Løvseth EK, Samant Y, Holm JØ. Work-related skin diseases in Norway may be underreported: data from 2000 to 2013. Contact Dermatitis. 2015;72:409–12.
21. Williams JDL, Lee AYL, Matheson MC, Frowen KE, Noonan AM, Nixon RL. Occupational contact urticaria: Australian data. Br J Dermatol. 2008;159:125–31.
22. McDonald JC, Beck MH, Chen Y, Cherry NM. Incidence by occupation and industry of work-related skin diseases in the United Kingdom, 1996-2001. Occup Med. 2006;56:398–405.
23. Chen Y, Turner S, McNamee R, Ramsay CN, Agius RM. The reported incidence of work-related ill-health in Scotland (2002 & 2003). Occup Med. 2005;55:252–61.
24. Arif M, Haroon TS. Occupational contact dermatitis in Lahore, Pakistan. J Pak Assoc Dermatol. 2001;11:20–6.
25. Kanerva L, Toikkanen J, Jolanki R, Estlander T. Statistical data on occupational contact urticaria. Contact Dermatitis. 1996;35:229–33.

26. Bakke P, Gulsvik A, Eide GE. Hay fever, eczema and urticaria in Southwest Norway. Lifetime prevalences and association with sex, age, smoking habits, occupational airborne exposures and respiratory symptoms. Allergy. 1990;45:515–22.

27. Turner S, McNamee R, Agius R, Wilkinson SM, Carder M, Stocks SJ. Evaluating interventions aimed at reducing occupational exposure to latex and rubber glove allergens. Occup Environ Med. 2012;69:925–31.

28. Allmers H, Schmengler J, John SM. Decreasing incidence of occupational contact urticaria caused by natural rubber latex allergy in German health care workers. J Allergy Clin Immunol. 2004;114(2):347–51.

29. Hjorth N, Roed-Petersen J. Occupational protein contact dermatitis in food handlers. Contact Dermatitis. 1976;2:28–42.

30. Johansson SGO, Bieber T, Dahl R, Friedmann PS, Lanier BQ, Lockey RF, et al. Revised nomenclature for allergy for global use: report of the nomenclature review Committee of the World Allergy Organization. J Allergy Clin Immunol. 2004;113:832–6.

31. Beasley R. Worldwide variation in prevalence of symptoms of asthma, allergic rhinoconjunctivitis, and atopic eczema: ISAAC. Lancet. 1998;351:1225–32.

32. Johannisson A, Pontén A, Svensson Å. Prevalence, incidence and predictive factors for hand eczema in young adults – a follow-up study. BMC Dermatol. 2013;13:14.

33. Nyren M, Lindberg M, Stenberg B, Svensson M, Svensson Å, Meding B. Influence of childhood atopic dermatitis on future worklife. Scand J Work Environ Health. 2005;31:474–8.

34. Thyssen JP, Johansen JD, Linneberg A, Mennê T. The epidemiology of hand eczema in the general population-prevalence and main findings. Contact Dermatitis. 2010;62:75–87.

35. Heede NG, Thyssen JP, Thuesen BH, Linneberg A, Johansen JD. Predictive factors of self-reported hand eczema in adult Danes – a population based cohort study with 5-year follow-up. Br J Dermatol. 2016;175:287–95.

36. Sussman GL, Beezhold DH. Allergy to latex rubber. Ann Intern Med. 1995;122:43–6.

37. Palmer CN, Irvine AD, Terron-Kwiatkowski A, Zhao Y, Liao H, Lee SP. Common loss-of-function variants of the epidermal barrier protein are a major predisposing factor for atopic dermatitis. Nat Genet. 2006;38:441–6.

38. Visser MJ, Landeck L, Campbell LE, McLean WH, Weidinger S, et al. Impact of atopic dermatitis and loss-of-function mutations in the gene on the development of occupational irritant contact dermatitis. Br J Dermatol. 2013;168:326–32.

39. Henderson J, Northstone K, Lee SP, Liao H, Zhao Y, Pembrey M, et al. The burden of disease associated with mutations: a population-based, longitudinal birth cohort study. J Allergy Clin Immunol. 2008;121:872–877.e879.

40. Visser MJ, Verberk MM, Campbell LE, McLean WH, Calkoen F, Bakker JG, et al. Filaggrin loss-of-function mutations and atopic dermatitis as risk factors for hand eczema in apprentice nurses: part II of a prospective cohort study. Contact Dermatitis. 2014;70:139–50.

41. Kezic S, Visser MJ, Verberk MM. Individual susceptibility to occupational contact dermatitis. Ind Health. 2009;47:469–78.

42. Timmerman JG, Heederik D, Spee T, van Rooy FG, Krop EJ, Koppelman GH, et al. Contact dermatitis in the construction industry: the role of loss-of-function mutations. Br J Dermatol. 2016;174:348–55.

43. Rilliet A, Hunziker N, Brun R. Alcohol contact urticaria syndrome (immediate type hypersensitivity). Dermatologica. 1980;161:361–4.

44. Matuse H, Shimoda T, Fukushima C, , Mitsuta K, Kawano T, Tomari S,et al. Screening for acetaldehyde dehy-drogenase 2 genotype in alcohol-induced asthma by using the ethanol patch test. Fukushima J Allergy Clin Immunol 2001; 108:715–719.

45. Tsutaya S, Shoji M, Saito Y, Kitaya H, Nakata S, Takamatsu H, Yasujima M. Analysis of aldehyde dehydrogenase 2 gene polymorphism and ethanol patch test as a screening method for alcohol sensitivity. Tohoku J Exp Med. 1999;187:305–10.

46. Wong JW, Harris K, Powell D. Alcohol urticaria syndrome. Dermatitis. 2011;22:350–4.

47. Bundesanstalt für Arbeitsschutz und Arbeitsmedizin. [TRGS 401: risks resulting from skin contact – determination, evaluation, measures]; 2008. Available at: http://www.baua.de/cln_135/en/Topicsfrom-A-to-Z/Hazardous-Substances/TRGS/TRGS.html.

48. Behroozy A, Keegel TG. Wet-work exposure: a main risk factor for occupational hand dermatitis. Saf Health Work. 2014;5:175–80.

49. Tiedemann D, Clausen ML, John SM, Angelova-Fischer I, Kezic S, Agner T. Effect of glove occlusion on the skin barrier. Contact Dermatitis. 2016;74:2–10.

50. Estlander T, Jolanki R, Kanerva L. Dermatitis and urticaria from rubber and plastic gloves. Contact Dermatitis. 1986;14:20–5.

51. Schliemann S, Boman A, Wahlberg J. Organic solvents. In: Rustemeyer T, Elsner P, John SM, Maibach H, editors. Kanerva's occupational dermatology, vol. 2. Second ed. Berlin: Springer; 2012. p. 701–15.

52. Estlander T, Kanerva L, Tupasela O, Keskinen H, Jolanki R. Immediate and delayed allergy to nickel with contact urticaria, rhinitis, asthma and contact dermatitis. Clin Exp Allergy. 1993;23:306–10.

53. Hostynek JJ. Sensitization to nickel: etiology, epidemiology, immune reactions, prevention, and therapy. Rev Environ Health. 2006;21:253–80.

54. Salavastru C, Bucur L, Bucur G, Sorin Tiplica G. Coatings. In: Rustemeyer Elsner TP T, John SM, Maibach H, editors. Kanerva's occupational derma-

tology, vol. 2. Second ed. Berlin: Springer; 2012. p. 691–701.

55. Tosti A, Guerra L, Vincenzi C, Peluso AM. Occupational skin hazards from synthetic plastics. Toxicol Ind Health. 1993;9:493–502.

56. Jolanki R, Kanerva L, Estlander T, Tarvainen K. Epoxy dermatitis. Occup Med. 1999;9:97–112.

57. Woyton A, Wasik F, Blizanowska A. An uncommon anaphylactic and eczematous reaction after contact with epoxide resins [polish]. Przegl Dermatol. 1974;61:303–8.

58. KwoHJ KMY, Kim HO, Park YM. The simultaneous occurrence of contact urticaria from sulbactam and allergic contact dermatitis from ampicillin in a nurse. Contact Dermatitis. 2006;54:176–8.

59. Verhulst L, Goossens A. Cosmetics component causing contact urticaria: a re-view and update. Contact Dermatitis. 2016;75:333–44.

60. Helaskoski E, Suojalehto H, Kuuliala O, Aalto-Korte K. Occupational contact urticaria and protein contact dermatitis: causes and concomitant airway diseases. Contact Dermatitis. 2017. https://doi.org/10.1111/cod.12856. [Epub ahead of print]

61. Lukacs J, Schliemann S, Elsner P. Occupational contact urticaria caused by food – a systematic clinical review. Contact Dermatitis. 2016;75:195–204.

62. Paulsen E, Andersen KE. Lettuce contact allergy. Contact Dermatitis. 2016;74:67–75.

63. Barbaud A, Poreaux C, Penven E, Waton J. Occupational protein contact dermatitis. Eur J Dermatol. 2015;25:527–34.

64. Wang CY, Maibach H. Immunologic contact urticaria—the human touch. Cutan Ocul Toxicol. 2013;32:154–60.

65. Vester L, Thyssen JP, Menne T, Johansen JD. Occupational food-related hand dermatoses seen over a 10-year period. Contact Dermatitis. 2012;66:264–70.

66. Davari P, Maibach H. Contact urticaria to cosmetic and industrial dyes. Clin Exp Dermatol. 2011;36:1–5.

67. Amaro C, Goossens A. Immunological occupational contact urticaria and contact dermatitis from proteins: a review. Contact Dermatitis. 2008;58:67–75.

68. Santos R, Goossens A. An update on airborne contact dermatitis: 2001–2006. Contact Dermatitis. 2007;57:353–60.

69. Valsecchi R, Leghissa P, Cortinovis R. Occupational contact dermatitis and contact urticaria in veterinarians. Contact Dermatitis. 2003;49:167–8.

70. Warner MR, Taylor JS, Leow YH. Agents causing contact urticaria. Clin Dermatol. 1997;15:623–35.

71. Thawer-Esmail F. Physical urticaria presenting as cholinergic urticaria with dermatographism. Curr Allergy Clin Immunol. 2008;4:187–8.

72. Ricci L, Francalanci S, Giorgini S, Fabbri P, Sertoli A. A case of vibratory angioedema. [Italian]. Annali Italiani di Dermatologia Allergologica Clinica e Sper-imentale. 2001;55:40–2.

73. Samitz MH. Repeated mechanical trauma to the skin: occupational aspects. Am J Ind Med. 1985;2011:265–71.

74. Torresani C, Periti I, Beski L. Contact urticaria syndrome from formaldehyde with multiple physical urticarias. Contact Dermatitis. 1996;35:174–5.

75. Miranda-Romero A, Navarro L, Pérez-Oliva N, González-López A, García-Muñoz M. Occupational heat contact urticaria. Contact Dermatitis. 1998;38:358–9.

76. Maibach HI, Johnson HL. Contact urticaria syndrome: contact urticaria to diethyltoluamide (immediate- type hypersensitivity). Arch Dermatol. 1975;111:726–30.

77. Peltonen L, Wickstrom G, Vaahtoranta M. Occupational dermatoses in the food industry. Dermatosen. 1985;33:166–9.

78. Fisher AA. Allergic contact urticaria of the hands due to seafood in food handlers. Cutis. 1988;42:388–9.

79. Cronin E. Dermatitis in food handlers. Adv Dermatol. 1989;4:113–23.

80. Cronin E. Dermatitis of the hands in caterers. Contact Dermatitis. 1987;17:265–9.

81. Tosti A, Fanti PA, Guerra L, Piancastelli E, Poggi S, Pileri S. Morphological and immunohistochemical study of immediate contact dermatitis of the hands due to foods. Contact Dermatitis. 1990;22:81–5.

82. Turijanma K. Incidence of immediate latex allergy to latex gloves in hospital personnel. Contact Dermatitis. 1987;17:270–5.

83. Yassin MS, Lierl MB, Fischer TJ, O'Brien K, Cross J, Steinmetz C. Latex allergy in hospital employees. Ann Allergy. 1994;72:245–9.

84. Garabrant DH, Roth HD, Parsad R, Gui-Shuang Y, Weiss J. Latex sensitization in health care workers and in the US general population. Am J Epidemiol. 2001;153:515–22.

85. Alanko K, Susitaival P, Jolanki R, Kanerva L. Occupational skin diseases among dental nurses. Contact Dermatitis. 2004;50:77–82.

86. Bulcke DM, Devos SA. Hand and forearm dermatoses among veterinarians. J Eur Acad Dermatol Venereol. 2007;21:360–3.

87. Agrup G, Sjostedt L. Contact urticaria in laboratory technicians working with animals. Acta Derm Venereol. 1985;65:111–5.

88. Le Coz CH. Urticaria. In: Rustemeyer T, Elsner P, John SM, Maibach H, editors. Kanerva's occupational dermatology, vol. 1. Second ed. Berlin: Springer; 2012. p. 217–30.

89. Lyons G, Roberts H, Palmer A, et al. Hairdressers presenting to an occupational dermatology clinic in Melbourne, Australia. Contact Dermatitis. 2013;68:300–6.

90. Foss-Skiftesvik MHL, Winther CR, Johnsen CZ, Johansen JD. Incidence of skin and respiratory diseases among Danish hairdressing apprentices. Contact Dermatitis. 2017;76:160–6.

91. Hougaard MG, Winther L, Søsted H, Zachariae C, Johansen JD. Occupational skin diseases in

hairdressing apprentices – has anything changed? Contact Dermatitis. 2015;72:40–6.
92. Larese Filon F, Bochdanovits L, Capuzzo C, Cerchi R, Rui F. Ten years incidence of natural rubber latex sensitization and symptoms in a prospective cohort of health care workers using non-powdered latex gloves 2000-2009. Int Arch Occup Environ Health. 2017;87:463–9.
93. Liss GM, Sussman GL. Latex sensitization: occupational versus general population prevalence rates. Am J Ind Med. 1999;35:196–200.
94. Pradeep Kumar R. Latex allergy in clinical practice. Indian J Dermatol. 2012;57:66–70.
95. Zorba E, Karpouzis A, Zorbas A, Bazas T, Zorbas S, Alexopoulos E, et al. Occupational dermatoses by type of work in Greece. Saf Health Work. 2013;4:142–8.
96. Romita P, Mistrello G, Antelmi A, Foti C. Occupational protein contact dermatitis in a bakcr. 'Case'. Annali Italiani di Dermatologia Allergologica Clinica e Sperimentale. 2011;65:96–8.
97. Lodde B, Cros P, Roguedas-Contios AM, Pougnet R, Lucas D, Dewitte JD, Misery L. Occupational contact dermatitis from protein in sea products: who is the most affected the fisherman or the chef? J of Occup Med Toxicol. 2017;10:12–4. E- collection 2017
98. Usmani N, Wilkinson SM. Allergic skin disease: investigation of both immediate- and delayed-type hypersensitivity is essential. Clin Exp Allergy. 2007;37:1541–6.
99. Liddle M, Hull C, Liu C, Powell D. Contact urticaria from curcumin. Dermatitis. 2006;17:196–7.
100. Waclawski ER, Beach J. Using a symptom diary to investigate work-related urticaria. Occup Med. 2013;63:160–1.
101. Wiszniewska M, Tymoszuk D, Pas-Wyroślak A, Nowakowska-Świrta E, Chomiczewska-Skóra D, Pałczyński C, Walusiak-Skorupa J. Occupational allergy to squid (Loligo vulgaris). Occup Med. 2013;63:298–300.
102. Viinanen A, Salokannel M, Lammintausta K. Gum arabic as a cause of oc-cupational allergy. J Allergy. 2011;2011:841508. Epub 2011
103. Vega JM, Moneo I, Armentia A, Vega J, De la Fuente R, Fernandez A. Pine processionary caterpillar as a new cause of immunologic contact urticaria. Contact Dermatitis. 2000;43:129–32.
104. Vega J, Vega JM, Moneo I, Armentia A, Caballero ML, Miranda A. Occupational immunologic contact urticaria from pine processionary caterpillar (Thaumetopoea pityocampa): experience in 30 cases. Contact Dermatitis. 2004;50:60–4.
105. Krogh G, Maibach HI. The contact urticaria syndrome--an updated review. J Am Acad Dermatol. 1981;5:328–42.

106. Aalto-Korte K. When should the diagnosis 'contact urticaria' be used? Contact Dermatitis. 2017;77:323–4.
107. Friis UF, Menne T, Flyvholm MA, Bonde JP, Johansen JD. Occupational allergic contact dermatitis diagnosed by a systematic stepwise exposure assessment of allergens in the work environment. Contact Dermatitis. 2013;69:153–63.
108. Friis UF, Menne T, Flyvholm M-A, Bonde JPE, Johansen JD. Difficultiesin using material safety data sheets to analyse occupational exposures to contact allergens. Contact Dermatitis. 2015;72:147–53.
109. Weiss RR, Mowad C. Contact urticaria from xylene. Am J Contact Dermat. 1998;9:125–7.
110. Mälkönen T, Jolanki R, Alanko K, Luukkonen R, Aalto-korte K, Lauerma A, Susitaival P. A 6-month follow-up study of 1048 patients diagnosed with an occupational skin disease. Contact Dermatitis. 2009;61:261–8.
111. Cvetkovski RS, Zachariae R, Jensen H, Olsen J, Johansen JD, Agner T. Prognosis of occupational h and eczema: a follow-up study. Arch Dermatol. 2006;142:305–11.
112. Carøe TK, Ebbehøj NE, Bonde JP, Agner T. Occupational hand eczema and/or contact urticaria: factors associated with change of profession or not remaining in the workforce. Contact Dermatitis. 2018;1:55–63. https://doi.org/10.1111/cod.12869.
113. Susitaival P, Flyvholm MA, Meding B, Kanerva I., Lindberg M, Svensson Å, Ólafsson JH. Nordic Occupational Skin Questionnaire (NOSQ-2002): a new tool for surveying occupational skin diseases and exposure. Contact Dermatitis. 2003;49:70–6.
114. Sala-Sastre N, Herdman M, Navarro L, De La Prada M, Pujol RM, Serra C, Alonso J, et al. Principles and methodology for translation and cross-cultural adaptation of the Nordic Occupational Skin Questionnaire (NOSQ-2002) to Spanish and Catalan. Contact Dermatitis. 2009;61:109–16.
115. Aktas E, Esin MNA. Turkish translation of the Nordic Occupational Skin Questionnaire (NOSQ-2002/LONG) adapted for young workers in high-risk jobs. Int J Dermatol. 2016;55:278–88.
116. Chiesi A, Pellacani G, Di Rico R, Farnetani F, Giusti G, Pepe P, et al. Italian translation and validation of the Nordic Occupational Skin Questionnaire (NOSQ-2002). [Article in Italian]. Med Lav. 2016;107:205–12.
117. Baiardini I, Braido F, Bindslev-Jensen C, Bousquet PJ, Brzoza Z, Canonica G, et al. Recommendations for assessing patient-reported outcomes and health-related quality of life in patients with urticaria: a GA2LEN taskforce position paper. Allergy. 2011;66:840–4.

Clinical Diagnosis of Immediate Contact Skin Reactions

Ana M. Giménez-Arnau and Marléne Isaksson

The diagnosis of the contact urticaria syndrome (CUS) is mostly clinical. The CUS includes signs and symptoms that define two classical clinical pictures, contact urticaria (CoU) and also protein contact dermatitis (PCD). Both entities, initially identified as independent diseases, are characterized by the immediate development of contact skin reactions (ICSR) showing clinically different patterns of inflammation such as erythema, wheals or hives, eczema, or dermatitis. CoU shows immediate itchy hives, even painful angioedema, or both that appear immediately after contact with the culprit agent. PCD shows immediate itchy erythema, papules, and vesicles or lichenified skin unleashed by the responsible contact agent. Pruritus is the hallmark symptom. CoU and PCD can be induced by the same trigger and be manifested simultaneously or consecutively in the same patient [1]. The chemistry of the trigger factor influences the clinical expression of the immunological response. The same patient can suffer both entities simultaneously. CoU and PCD belong to the CUS.

A. M. Giménez-Arnau (✉)
Hospital del Mar - Institut Mar d'Investigacions Mediques, Universitat Autònoma de Barcelona (UAB), Department of Dermatology, Barcelona, Spain
e-mail: 22505aga@comb.cat

M. Isaksson
Department of Occupational and Environmental Dermatology, Lund University, Malmö University Hospital, Malmö, Sweden

Contact Urticaria Syndrome: Clinical Signs and Symptoms Useful for Differential Diagnosis

Contact Urticaria: Cutaneous Manifestations and Differential Diagnosis

The wheal, also called a hive, is the cutaneous elemental lesion that defines urticaria. With the term urticaria, a heterogeneous group of types were identified based on the clinical course and also the trigger factor (Table 4.1). Wheals, angioedema, or both are the clinical lesions that define any type of urticaria. Three features characterize a wheal: central swelling of variable size, almost invariably surrounded by reflex erythema; an itching or sometimes burning sensation; and a fleeting nature. The skin returns to its normal appearance, usually within 1–24 h [2, 3], Angioedema is characterized by a sudden, pronounced erythematous or skin-colored swelling of the lower dermis and subcutis with frequent involvement below the mucous membranes that sometimes is painful rather than itchy. It resolves more slowly than wheals and can take up 72 h. Table 4.1 presents a classification of chronic urticaria (CU) approved by international consensus [3]. Contact urticaria (CoU) belongs to the group of inducible urticarias (CIndU) [3] (Table 4.1).

Table 4.1 Contact urticaria is a subtype of chronic urticaria that is inducible by a contact environmental agent

Chronic urticaria	
Chronic spontaneous urticaria (CSU)	Spontaneous appearance of wheals, angioedema, or both at 6 weeks or more from known or unknown causes
Inducible urticaria (CIndU)	Symptomatic dermographism[a] Cold urticaria[b] Delayed pressure urticaria[c] Solar urticaria Heat urticaria[d] Vibratory angioedema Cholinergic urticaria *Contact urticaria* Aquagenic urticaria

[a]Also called urticaria factitia, dermographic urticaria
[b]Also called cold contact urticaria or afrigore
[c]Also called pressure urticaria (immediate and delayed)
[d]Also called heat contact urticaria

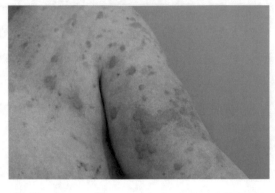

Fig. 4.1 Chronic spontaneous urticaria (CSU). Complete involvement of the skin with itchy wheals fleeting in nature; in this case the patient showed more than 50 wheals daily from more than 6 weeks. The hives spontaneously appear in any area of the body surface, and the crisis of CSU started 6 months ago

Histologically, wheals are characterized by edema of the upper and mid-dermis, with dilatation of the postcapillary venules and lymphatic vessels of the upper dermis. In angioedema, primarily the lower dermis and the subcutis are involved. A mild to moderate increase of dermal mast cell numbers is characteristic. The wheal shows upregulation of endothelial cell adhesion molecules, chemokines, neuropeptides, and growth factors and an inflammatory perivascular infiltrate, consisting mainly of neutrophils and/or eosinophils, basophils, macrophages, and T cells, but without vessel wall necrosis.

CoU was described for the first time in the Greek literature more than 2000 years ago [4]. The earliest recorded reports include one from Pliny the Younger who, in the first century AD, noticed individuals with severe itching and wheals when cutting pine trees. Wheals and sometimes even angioedema appear after the contact of the skin with the trigger agent, involving the hands, lips, or another cutaneous location. The inflammatory cutaneous swelling and redness reaction appear immediately (within a few minutes) after the contact and also can (but rarely) appear with a certain delay (after a few hours). In severe cases, generalized cutaneous reactions, systemic involvement as rhinitis or asthma, and sometimes anaphylactic reactions may be associated. The etiology and mechanisms of CoU thus differ from those of other types of urticaria primarily by the route of access by the antigen or the noxious agent to the body. It penetrates through the epidermis. Second, because it is either immunological (caused by specific IgE) or nonimmunological (from unspecified histamine releasers), the environmental character makes it different from other types of CU. Chronic spontaneous urticaria (CSU) or other CIndU types show an endogenous pathogenesis mainly caused by an autoimmune mechanism through the activation and overexpression of mast cells and basophils, the high-affinity receptors of the IgE (FcεRI) [5].

In CSU the wheals appear daily, predominantly in the evening and at night. Any part of the body can be affected, showing a variable number of lesions, from fewer than 15 to more than 50 per day (Fig. 4.1) The size of the wheal can reach a few centimeters or grow further, developing large plaques. The lesions always disappear in a few hours, however, with new ones appearing in areas of the skin that were free of symptoms at least 24 h earlier—a consequence of the continuous activation of the cutaneous mast cells by the endogenous factor. In CSU even the apparently nonlesional skin shows a distinctive genetic pathway, suggesting a global involvement of the cutaneous tegument [6]. Upregulation of adhesion molecules, infiltrating eosinophils, and altered cytokine expression are also seen in uninvolved skin.

The basic characteristic of the wheal in CoU does not differ from that of other types of urticaria: it is itchy, shows a reflex erythema, and also is fleeting in nature. The clinical aspect can change according with the type of the contact substance. The wheals are distributed linearly arranged if these are habitually caused by nettles of plants. Punctate wheals arise in the site where the stinging hairs penetrate the skin. Wheals can start in a follicular pattern if the contact agent penetrates through the hair follicles. The wheal shape changes with time. The lesions can be confluent. Tingling, itching, and sometimes burning symptoms are common. A burning sensation is often described when the lips are involved after contact with food, as a fruit and vegetable seller described it (Fig. 4.2).

The lesion starts with redness at the site of contact. The wheal appears at the same site within 10–30 min after contact. The maximal size is reached often at 45 min afterward, and within 2 h, the swelling disappears. Redness can persist, even for 6 h. Exceptionally, the hive can persist for more than 24 h. It was described that contact

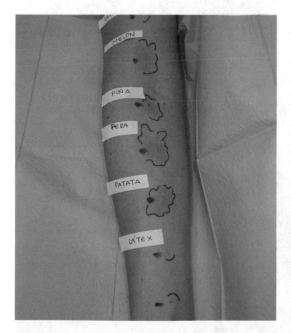

Fig. 4.2 Contact urticaria (CoU). Contact wheals induced by prick-by-prick with fruits (banana, melon, pear, potato) responsible for CoU in a fruit and vegetable seller

urticaria can reappear after 4–5 h in the same site as the previous contact with no new contact with the responsible agent. This dual wheal response has been demonstrated experimentally in the ears of BALB/mice and in humans [7]. Delayed onset of contact urticaria was also described after repeated applications of the trigger substance [8]. The time course and intensity of contact urticaria lesions differ depending on the nature of the eliciting agent. The different type of response may also be caused by the reactivity of the cells, which secrete the vasoactive amines, or the sensitivity of the target tissue to the mediators or chemical released.

CIndUs, in contrast to chronic spontaneous urticaria (CSU), are characterized by the need for specific external triggers for wheals, angioedema, or both of these symptoms to develop. CoU is classified as CIndU. An accurate differential diagnosis is required between different types of CIndUs based in the clinical expression and the trigger factor [9]. CIndU wheals are induced after contact or exposure to physical stimulus (cold, solar, heat, friction, pressure, or vibration) as well as by contact with water (aquagenic) or by increase of body temperature (sweating). The hives appear immediately (after 10 min) with the sole exception of delayed pressure urticaria, which shows hives 3–6 h after the stimulus. CIndU signs and symptoms are usually confined to skin areas that are exposed to the specific trigger. The morphology of the hives tends to be follicular in cholinergic urticaria. The lesions range from extensive erythema, papules, and extensive plaques in cold and solar urticaria. When the stimulus is friction in symptomatic dermographism, the cutaneous lesion tends to be linear, reproducing the scratching. If pressure is the responsible for the delayed reaction, commonly an erythematous and edematous itchy and painful plaque is present in the involved area. Complete exposure of the body to triggers such as cold, solar light, or sweating as a consequence of the increased body temperature in cholinergic urticaria, can induce global involvement of the body with, occasionally, systemic involvement or even anaphylaxis. Individual patients may exhibit two or more CIndUs, and in rare cases, two or more specific triggers are needed to produce urticarial signs and symptoms. It is important to accurately identify and characterize the eliciting trigger and individual elicitation thresholds and to distinguish CIndUs from spontaneous urticaria. CIndUs are diagnosed based on the patient history and the results of specific provocation testing (Table 4.2; Fig. 4.3).

Table 4.2 Recommended diagnostic tests in chronic inducible urticaria (CIndU)

Chronic inducible urticaria (CIndU)	Routine diagnostic tests (recommended)
Cold urticaria	Cold provocation and threshold test (ice cube, cold water, cold wind, TempTest)
Delayed pressure urticaria	Pressure test and threshold test
Heat urticaria	Heat provocation and threshold test
Solar urticaria	UV and visible light of different wavelengths and threshold test
Symptomatic dermographism	Elicit dermographism and threshold test (dermographometer or Fric Test)
Vibratory angioedema	Test with vortex (e.g.)
Aquagenic urticaria	Wet cloths at body temperature applied for 20 min
Cholinergic urticaria	Exercise and hot bath provocation
Contact urticaria	Cutaneous provocation test; skin tests with immediate readings, e.g., prick test

Protein Contact Dermatitis (PCD): Cutaneous Manifestations and Differential Diagnosis

Contact dermatitis is a term used to define any inflammatory skin reaction caused by direct contact with environmental noxious agents. Pruritus is the hallmark symptom of contact dermatitis. Although an eczematous reaction is the most common encountered adverse reaction to contact substances, other cutaneous clinical manifestations can also be present. Within the term contact dermatitis, different types of skin lesions can be included, such as eczema (Fig. 4.4), erosions, urticaria, lichenoid eruptions, erythroderma, lymphocytoma (Fig. 4.5), or photosensitive reactions (Table 4.3). An appropriate diagnosis of contact dermatitis requires a detailed clinical his-

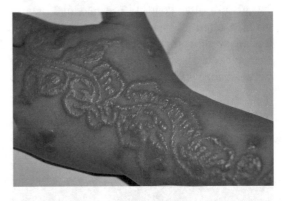

Fig. 4.4 Contact dermatitis: acute eczema with well-defined vesicles and bullae from a false henna tattoo responsible for contact sensitization to *p*-phenylenediamine

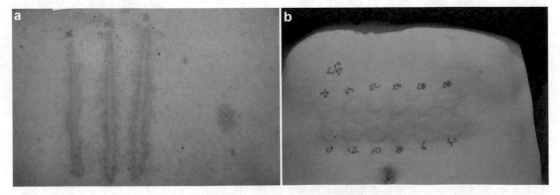

Fig. 4.3 Chronic inducible urticaria (CIndU). (**a**) Symptomatic dermographism. (**b**) Cold urticaria with a positive provocation test showing a critical temperature threshold (CTT) of 24 °C

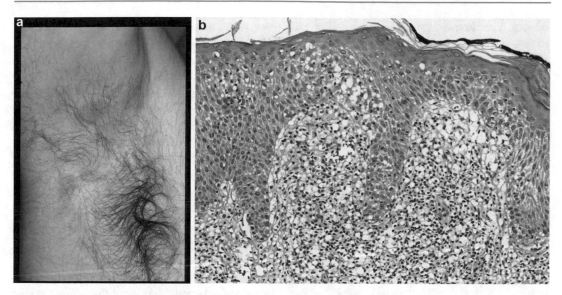

Fig. 4.5 Contact dermatitis. (**a**) Chronic dermatitis with recurrent itchy and desquamative skin caused by methyl-chloroisothiazolinone/methylisothiazolinone contact allergy. (**b**) Atypical intraepithelial lymphocytes in a lymphomatoid contact reaction

Table 4.3 Clinical manifestations caused by environmental agents that can be responsible for contact dermatitis

Patterns of immediate or delayed cutaneous reactions that can be induced by environmental skin contact triggers through an allergic or irritant mechanism
Allergic contact granuloma
Contact leukoderma
Contact urticaria may become anaphylaxis
Eczema
Erosions
Exanthemas
Erythema multiforme
Erythroderma
Generalized symptoms
Lichenoid eruptions
Lymphocytoma
Nodular lesions
Photosensitive reactions
Pigmented contact dermatitis
Purpura
Sarcoidal reactions
Toxic epidermal necrolysis
Ulcerations
Urticaria

tory (including occupational background), an accurate physical examination (sometimes the patient brings excellent pictures showing the active lesions), and an etiological study with adequate in vitro and cutaneous testing.

Histologically, spongiosis of the epidermis is the defining pathological characteristic of eczematous reactions. The confluence of spongiosis leads to the appearance of vesicles and even bullae. The vesicle is the elemental lesion of eczema. It is preceded by erythema and dermal thickening and, because of scratching, the crust appears. The vesicular response is associated with acute contact dermatitis. Once contact dermatitis becomes chronic, the skin becomes acanthotic. Macroscopically chronic eczema shows lichenified skin and characteristic painful fissures. Chronic dermatitis shows such characteristic features as pruritus, lichenification, erythema, scaling, excoriation, and fissures (Fig. 4.6).

The classification of the different types of eczema can be based on the clinical morphology but also on the different etiologies involved. At times, acute and chronic clinical forms of eczema are present simultaneously in the same patient. It is common that more than one relevant etiology can be the cause of the disease. This fact makes mandatory the etiological evaluation of each patient through the design of an accurate protocol using a useful diagnostic test based on the clinical history. The knowledge of useful in vitro and in vivo provocation tests is required. How to classify the different types of eczema is not easy. The European guidelines of hand dermatitis include useful hand dermatitis etiological classifications [10]. Proposed definitions of the different classic forms of eczema are included in Table 4.4.

The irritant and a classical allergic contact eczema can be clinically identical. In both cases,

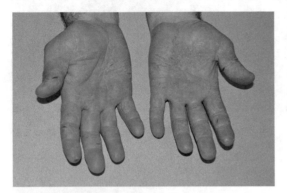

Fig. 4.6 Contact dermatitis. Chronic contact hand dermatitis, showing lichenified erythematous skin with broken skin with desquamation and fissures. In this case, the origin combines irritancy because of the wet work and a relevant contact allergy from methylisothiazolinone that was included in a hand soap

very small molecules (molecular weight less than 1000 Da) are the responsible agents. Few differences between irritant and allergic dermatitis were described based on the characteristics of the response to the occluded patch test (an in vivo provocation test). When a primary irritant is occluded in a patch test and placed on the skin, the eczematous reaction induces minimal itch. The provoked dermatitis shows erythema and slight infiltration strictly limited to the area of the patch. If the contact irritant is strong, a bullous or pustular reaction limited to the occluded area is observed. When an occlusive test is done with a substance that induces a type 4 hypersensitivity cutaneous response, a typically cellular immune reaction, eczema is pruritic, infiltrated, papular, or vesicular beyond the rim of the occluding ring or patch test [11].

Protein contact dermatitis (PCD) is considered a special type of eczema based on the nature of the trigger and the immunological pathway involved. Proteins can induce immunological CoU and also PCD. Proteins (molecular weight 10,000 to several hundred thousand Da) can be responsible for chronic and recurrent eczema. Fingertip dermatitis, hand, wrists, and arms are the more frequently

Table 4.4 Definitions of the different types of eczema according to etiology that can involve the hands and other body sites (definitions based on the European Hand Dermatitis Guidelines [10]) (patient can suffer more than one cause of eczema simultaneously)

Allergic contact dermatitis	Eczema caused by relevant contact allergens or cross-reactors identified by patch testing. Relevance means that there is a current exposure of the allergen to the hands, typically a delayed reaction immunologically defined as type 4.
Irritant contact dermatitis	Eczema with documented irritant exposure, which is quantitatively likely to cause dermatitis; no relevant contact allergy (no current exposure to allergens to which the patient has reacted positive in patch test)
Contact urticaria/ protein contact dermatitis	Eczema in patients exposed to proteins (food, latex, and other biological material) with a positive prick test, or proven specific IgE, to suspect items. Symptoms can be present combined with itchy wheals or hives. The cutaneous reactions are present immediately after the contact of the trigger. A considerable proportion of patients with contact urticaria will also have atopic symptoms. It is a typically an immediate reaction immunologically defined as type I.
Atopic eczema/ dermatitis	Eczema in a patient with a familial and personal medical history of atopy, previous or current. The main atopic diseases are dermatitis, rhinoconjunctivitis, and asthma. No documented irritant exposure and/or relevant contact allergen likely to cause eczema.
Vesicular eczema, classically dyshidrotic	Recurrent eczema with vesicular eruptions. Commonly involve the hand; specially lateral side of the fingers. No relevant contact allergy, no documented irritant exposure likely to cause dermatitis, and no personal history of atopic dermatitis.
Hyperkeratotic eczema	Chronic eczema with hyperkeratosis specially involves the palms, or pulpitis, and no vesicles or pustules. No documented irritant exposure to the involved skin areas, likely to cause irritant exposure

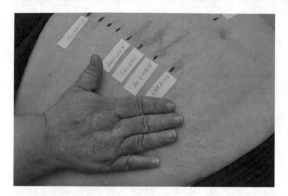

Fig. 4.7 Protein contact dermatitis showing eczema at the dorsum of the hands induced by immediate contact with fish

Table. 4.5 Stages of the contact urticaria syndrome (CUS)

Stage 1	Localized urticaria (redness, wheals/hives, angioedema) Immediate contact dermatitis (eczema–protein contact dermatitis) Itching, tingling, or burning sensation
Stage 2	Generalized urticaria
Stage 3	Bronchial asthma (wheezing) Rhinitis, conjunctivitis (runny nose, watery eyes) Orolaryngeal symptoms (lip swelling, hoarseness, difficulty swallowing) Gastrointestinal symptoms (nausea, vomiting, diarrhea, cramps)
Stage 4	Anaphylactic or anaphylactoid reaction (shock)

body sites involved (Fig. 4.7). PCD usually shows a characteristic occupational relevance involving food caterers, sellers, or handlers. Some cases of chronic paronychia were considered a variety of PCD, with redness and swelling of the proximal nail fold, for example, after handling food [12] or natural rubber latex [13]. An urticarial or vesicular exacerbation can be noted a few minutes after contact with the causal agent, especially on previously affected skin. As for CoU, extracutaneous symptoms can appear when PCD is present, as rhinoconjunctivitis or asthma and even anaphylaxis. An "oral allergy syndrome" with abdominal pain and diarrhea may occasionally develop when the allergen comes in contact with the oropharyngeal mucosa [14].

PCD belong to the first staging of the contact urticaria syndrome, as does CoU. The same protein can be responsible for both clinical entities in the same patients showing eczema and wheals. Both immediate reactions can be maintained chronically by accumulative exposure to the contact allergen.

Contact Urticaria Syndrome: Stages of Severity

Four stages characterize the contact urticaria syndrome (CUS) (Table 4.5). Cutaneous symptoms define stages 1 and 2. Stage 1 includes flare reactions, wheals, and eczema as well as symptoms such as itching, tingling, or a burning sensation. When CoU is present it shows itchy wheals that are usually strictly limited to contact areas and which disappear within a few hours without residual lesions. PCD shows eczema, typically affects the hands (especially the fingertips, wrists, and arms), lasts many days, and may lead to residual lesions (hypo- or hyperpigmentation). Wheals and eczema can be present simultaneously in the same patient, induced by the same trigger. Stage 2 refers to the development of urticaria over all the body after a local contact. Stages 3 and 4 include extracutaneous reactions or symptoms. Stage 3 may include bronchial asthma, rhinoconjunctivitis, orolaryngeal symptoms, or gastrointestinal dysfunctions. Systemic involvement depends upon the allergen or preexisting conditions such as atopic dermatitis [12, 13]. Volatile allergen can induce dermatitis, rhinoconjunctivitis, and asthma. Bakers who are in continuous contact with flour are a very useful example. Abdominal pain, diarrhea, and the oral allergy syndrome are caused by the allergen contact with the oropharyngeal mucosa [15]. Multisystemic disease implies a severe CUS [16]. Stage 4 refers to anaphylactic or anaphylactoid reactions. It is the most severe type of CUS manifestation because it is life threatening.

The oral allergy syndrome (OAS) is considered as a special form of CUS, localized in the mouth and throat. Usually its symptoms occur immediately after oral contact with the food involved and include oropharyngeal pruritus (itching of mouth, palate, and throat), angioedema of lips, tongue, and palate, and hoarseness. The oral syndrome can be accompanied by gastrointestinal reactions and systemic involvement showing urticaria, rhinitis, asthma, or even anaphylaxis.

Contact Urticaria Syndrome: Diagnostic Exploratory Tests

The diagnosis of CUS is based on a full medical history and diagnostic exploratory tests. The diagnosis protocol of study should include the suspected etiological substances, protein or chemical. In vitro techniques are available for only a few allergens. The measurement of specific IgE in serum is useful for some proteins such as latex, and vegetables or fruits. The basophil activation test analyzing CD63 expression following exposure to the allergens by flow cytometry can be useful when rare allergens are studied for which a specific IgE is not found, such as chicken meat [17].

The cutaneous provocation test should take into account if the reaction is only cutaneous or if there is also systemic involvement. Diluted allergen concentrations and serial dilutions to minimize allergen exposure are recommended. Nonsteroidal antiinflammatory drugs and antihistamines should be avoided because of the risk of false-negative results. Life-threatening reactions have been documented during skin tests; therefore, caution is advised, especially when testing certain occupational substances. Skin tests should be performed only if resuscitation equipment and trained personnel are readily available [18–20]. When poorly or nonstandardized substances are studied, testing a healthy population as control to avoid false-positive interpretations is suggested.

The "open test" is the simplest cutaneous provocation test for immediate contact reactions including immunological and nonimmunological CoU and PCD. The suspected substance is applied and gently rubbed on slightly affected skin or on a normal-looking 3 × 3 cm area of the skin, either on the upper back or the extensor side of the upper arm. Often contact urticants should be applied to skin sites suggested by the patient's history. Open testing is generally negative unless the substance is applied on damaged or eczematous skin, where it may cause a vesicular reaction. A positive result is an immediate itchy edema and/or erythema typical of CoU, or tiny intraepidermal spongiotic vesicles typical of acute eczema. An immunological and nonimmunological contact reaction usually appears within 15–20 min. The nonimmunological result lasts between 45 and 60 min instead of disappearing after a few hours as do the immunological results. Occasionally a delayed onset of ICoU is reported. The "open test" is the less invasive diagnostic test.

The "prick testing" of suspected allergens is often the method of choice to study immediate contact reactions. A skin prick test with fresh material or commercial reagents is the gold standard. The principle of the prick test relies on bringing a small volume of allergen (approximately 5–10 nl) into contact with mast cells by puncturing the skin with a lancet. When a prick-by-prick is done, with the same lancet the fresh material is pricked and immediately after the skin is punctured. A positive reaction elicited is assessed after 15–20 min compared with the positive control (histamine hydrochloride) and the negative control (sodium chloride). A flare is considered neuronally mediated and a papule is caused by histamine release (Fig. 4.8).

Sometimes a "rubbing test," gentle rubbing with the material on intact or lesional skin might be indicated, if an open test is negative. The

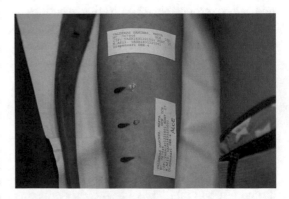

Fig. 4.8 Prick-by-prick test is the gold standard technique to demonstrate the etiology of immediate contact reactions. Contact wheals induced by contact with *Aloe vera* plant. Positive prick-by-prick with aloe vera leaf

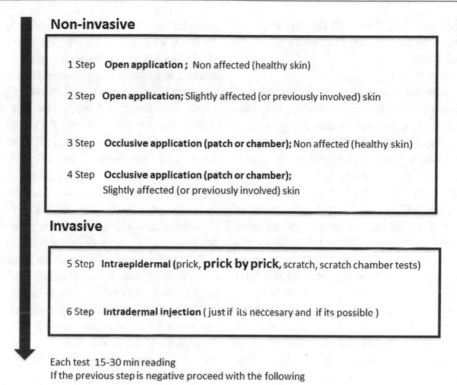

Fig. 4.9 Simple protocol proposed to study immediate contact skin reactions responsible of CUS, including typical lesions from both CoU and PCD diseases

"scratch test" and "chamber scratch test" (contact with a small aluminum chamber for 15 min) are less standardized than the prick test but are useful when a nonstandard allergen must be studied. It carries a higher risk of false-positive reactions and lacks sensitivity compared with the prick test.

A simple protocol with consecutive steps has been proposed to study immediate contact skin reactions involved in the CUS (Fig. 4.9).

Short Approach to Prevention and Treatment of the Contact Urticaria Syndrome

CUS clinical symptoms are determined by the route, duration, and extent of exposure, the inherent sensitizing properties of the allergen, and an individual's genetic and/or acquired susceptibility. Discovering the responsible agent is required to identify the correct avoidance of the eliciting trigger. Avoidance of further exposure will improve occupational contact dermatitis and CoU. Primary and secondary prevention are highly recommended as being necessary common guidelines to prevent such well-known occupational risks as latex allergy [21].

Considering their good safety profile, second-generation antihistamines must be considered the preferred first-line symptomatic treatment for most CoU. Before considering alternative treatment, higher doses of antihistamines should be used. When dermatitis is present, topical immunomodulation can be conducted using topical steroids [22, 23]. Severe cases of CUS require a short course of oral steroids or even treatment in an emergency unit.

Protein Contact Dermatitis. How to Proceed? Learning Through a Clinical Case

The 31-year-old female patient was a married office worker with three small children. She presented with a history of atopic finger eczema since childhood, which had worsened the preceding 3 months. A history of atopy in her near family included bronchial asthma in her father, sister, and brother, and allergic rhinitis in a brother. As a child she had had bronchial asthma but not as an adult. At presentation, slightly hyperkeratotic eczema with erythema, dry vesicles, and some scaling was seen on the volar surfaces of hands and fingertips and also on the proximal nail folds (Fig. 4.10).

The patient reported that she developed itchy wheals on her hands 20 min after handling wet chapatti flour, made from the mixture of wheat and rye. Being of Pakistani origin she made chapatti bread each day at home and never wore any gloves during the procedure. She had noticed that handling dry flour did not provoke any itchy wheals, and that she could also eat cooked chapattis without any symptoms.

The patient had been patch tested in another clinic 4 years before presentation with negative results, and her eczema was then diagnosed as

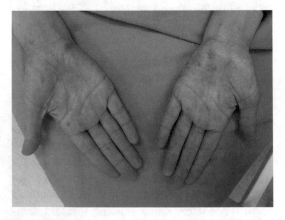

Fig. 4.10 Protein contact dermatitis. This clinical case showed at presentation slightly hyperkeratotic eczema with erythema, dry vesicles, and some scaling seen on the volar surfaces of hands and fingertips and also on the proximal nail folds

being irritant. We performed a new patch test to the Swedish baseline series with again negative results. However, prick-prick testing to the wet chapatti flour (consisting of wheat and rye, wheal diameter 7 × 7 mm), wet wheat (prick test wheal diameter 5 × 5 mm), and wet rye flour (wheal diameter 4 × 4 mm) as well as gluten (wheal diameter 5 × 5 mm) all were positive. Prick test to latex (100 IR/ml; Alyostal, Stallergenes, France) was negative. A positive histamine test (wheal diameter 7 × 7 mm) (histamine hydrochloride 10 mg/ml; Alk-Abelló, Denmark) and a negative saline control (0.9% sodium chloride) were demonstrated.

The patient was advised to avoid direct contact with both wet and dry chapatti flour by wearing nitrile gloves while preparing and cooking the bread. This regimen was successful, as the eczema had improved considerably when we saw the patient after 1 month. The patient informed us that if she occasionally forgot to wear gloves, immediate pruritus and wheals would appear on her hands while handling the flour or the dough [24].

In 1976 the Danes Hjorth and Roed-Petersen described hand and forearm eczema in several kitchen workers in whom high molecular weight proteins were suspected as allergens. They named the condition protein contact dermatitis [25]. In 1983 specific criteria were defined by Veien et al.: a chronic or recurrent dermatitis caused by contact with high molecular weight proteins in foods; an immediate, itching, urticarial eruption occurring within 30 min of contact with the offending agent; positive prick/or scratch testing with the suspected causative substance, and often negative patch-test results [26].

Flour-associated protein contact dermatitis has been reported primarily among food handlers, kitchen workers, caterers, bar staff, food vendors, food packers, gardeners, dairy farmers, housewives, and home helpers, sometimes with allergic rhinitis or asthma symptoms [27, 28].

It seems that irritant contact dermatitis with a compromised skin barrier is a prerequisite for this condition [29]. The most common culprits are wheat and rye flour [30].

Key Notes/Messages

Clinical symptoms of the immediate contact reactions in the CUS are determined by the route, duration, and extent of exposure to the contact trigger, the inherent sensitizing properties of the allergen, and an individual's genetic or acquired susceptibility. Based in the clinical history, the type of immediate contact reactions, and the substance involved (protein or chemical), a specific protocol can be designed for each patient. Discovering the responsible agent is required to identify the correct avoidance of the eliciting trigger. Avoidance of further exposure will improve CUS. Primary and secondary prevention are highly recommended [21].

References

1. Gimenez-Arnau A, Maurer M, de la Cuadra J, Maibach H. Immediate contact skin reactions, an update of contact urticaria, contact urticaria syndrome and protein contact dermatitis – "a never ending story.". Eur J Dermatol. 2010;20:1–11.
2. Czarnetzki B. Chapter 2: Basic mechanisms. In: Czarnetzki MB, editor. Urticaria. Berlin: Springer; 1986. p. 5–25.
3. Zuberbier T, Aberer W, Asero R, Baker D, Ballmer-Weber B, Bernstein JA, Bindslev-Jensen C, Brzoza Z, Buense Bedrikow R, Canonica GW, Church MK, Craig T, Damilicheva IV, Dressler C, Ensina LF, Giménez-Arnau A, Godse K, Gonçalo M, Grattan C, Hebert J, Hide M, Kaplan A, Kapp A, Katelaris C, Kocatürk Göncü E, Kulthanan K, Larenas-Linnemann D, Abdul Latiff AH, Leslie T, Magerl M, Mathelier-Fusade P, Meshkova RY, Metz M, Nast A, Oude-Elberink H, Rosumeck S, Saini SS, Sánchez-Borges M, Schmid-Grendelmeier P, Staubach P, Sussman G, Toubi E, Vena GA, Vestergaard C, Wedi B, Werner RN, Zhao Z, Maurer M. The EAACI/GA2LEN/EDF/WAO Guideline for the definition classification, diagnosis and management of Urticaria. The 2016 revision and update. Allergy. 2018 Jan 15. https://doi.org/10.1111/all.13397.
4. Czarnetzki B. Chapter 6: Basic mechanisms. In: Czarnetzki MB, e, editor. Urticaria. Berlin: Springer; 1986. p. 89–95.
5. Deza G, Bertolín-Colilla M, Pujol RM, Curto-Barredo L, Soto D, García M, Hernández P, Gimeno R, Giménez-Arnau AM. Basophil FcεRI expression in chronic spontaneous urticaria: a potential immunological predictor of response to omalizumab therapy. Acta Derm Venereol. 2017;97(6):698–704.
6. Giménez-Arnau A, Curto-Barredo L, Nonell L, Puigdecanet E, Yelamos J, Gimeno R, Rüberg S,

Santamaria-Babi L, Pujol RM. Transcriptome analysis of severely active chronic spontaneous urticaria shows an overall immunological skin involvement. Allergy. 2017. https://doi.org/10.1111/all.13183.
7. Ray MC, Tharp MD, Sullivan TJ, Tigelaar RE. Contact hypersensitivity reactions to dinitrofluorobenzene mediated by monoclonal IgE anti-DNP antibodies. J Immunol. 1983;131:1096–102.
8. Andersen KE, Maiback HI. Multiple application delayed onset urticaria. Possible relation to certain unusual formalin and textile reactions. Contact Dermatitis. 1984;10:227–34.
9. Magerl M, Altrichter S, Borzova E, Giménez-Arnau A, Grattan CE, Lawlor F, Mathelier-Fusade P, Meshkova RY, Zuberbier T, Metz M, Maurer M. The definition, diagnostic testing, and management of chronic inducible urticarias – the EAACI/GA(2) LEN/EDF/UNEV consensus recommendations 2016 update and revision. Allergy. 2016;71(6):780–802.
10. Diepgen TL, Andersen KE, Chosidow O, Coenraads PJ, Elsner P, English J, Fartasch M, Gimenez-Arnau A, Nixon R, Sasseville D, Agner T. Guidelines for diagnosis, prevention and treatment of hand eczema: short version. J Dtsch Dermatol Ges. 2015;13(1):77–85.
11. Veien NK. Chapter 15: Clinical features. In: Johanssen JD, Frosch PJ, Lepoittevin J-P, editors. Contact dermatitis. 5th ed. Heidelberg: Springer; 2011. p. 255–303.
12. Tosti A, Guerra L, Morelli R, Bardazzi F, Fanti R. Role of foods in the pathogenesis of chronic paronychia. J Am Acad Dermatol. 1992;27:706–10.
13. Kanerva L. Occupational protein contact dermatitis and paronychia from natural rubber latex. J Eur Acad Dermatol Venereol. 2000;14:504–6.
14. Goossens A, Amaro C. Chapter 21: Protein contact dermatitis. In Johanssen JD, Frosch PJ, Lepoittevin J-P, eds. Contact dermatitis 5th edn. Heidelberg: Springer; 2011, pp 407–413.
15. Crisi G, Belsito D. Contact urticaria from latex in a patient with immediate hypersensitivity to banana, avocado and peach. Contact Dermatitis. 1993;28:247–8.
16. Jeannet-Peter N, Piletta-Zanin PA, Hauser C. Facial dermatitis, contact urticaria, rhinoconjunctivitis, and asthma induced by potato. Am J Contact Dermat. 1999;10:40–2.
17. Morren M, Janssens V, Dooms-Goossens A, Van Hoeyveld E, Cornelis A, De Wolf-Peeters C, Heremans A. Alpha-amylase, a flour additive: an important cause of protein contact dermatitis in bakers. J Am Acad Dermatol. 1993;29:723–8.
18. Von Krogh C, Maibach HI. The contact urticaria syndrome. An update review. J Am Acad Dermatol. 1981;5:328–42.
19. Gonzalez-Muñoz M, Gómez M, Aldalay E, Del Castillo A, Moneo I. Occupational protein contact dermatitis to chicken meat studied by flow cytometry. Contact Dermatitis. 2007;57:62–3.

20. Haustein UF. Anaphylactic shock and contact urti-
    caria after patch test with professional allergens.
    Allerg Immunol. 1976;22:349–52.
21. Maucher OM. Anaphylaktische Reaktionen beim
    Epicutantest. Hautarzt. 1972;23:139–40.
22. Nicholson PJ. Evidence-based guidelines: occupa-
    tional contact dermatitis and urticaria. Occup Med.
    2010;60:502–6.
23. Zuberbier T, Asero R, Bindslev-Jensen C, Canonica W,
    Church MK, Giménez-arnau AM, Grattan CEH, Kapp
    A, Maurer M, Merk HF, Rogala B, Saini S, Sánchez-
    Borges M, Schmid-Grendelmeier P, Schünemann H,
    Staubach P, Vena GA, Wedi B. EAACI/GA₂LEN/
    EDF guideline: management of urticaria. Allergy.
    2009;64:1427–43.
24. Malinauskiene L, Isaksson M. Protein contact der-
    matitis caused by allergy to chapatti flour. Acta Derm
    Venereol. 2013;93:91–3.
25. Hjorth N, Roed-Petersen J. Occupational protein con-
    tact dermatitis in food handlers. Contact Dermatitis.
    1976;2:28–42.
26. Veien NK, Hattel T, Justesen O, Norholm A. Causes
    of eczema in the food industry. Derm Beruf Umwelt.
    1983;31:84–6.
27. Amaro C, Goossens A. Immunological occupational
    contact urticaria and contact dermatitis from proteins:
    a review. Contact Dermatitis. 2008;58:67–75.
28. Levin C, Warshaw E. Protein contact dermatitis: aller-
    gens, pathogenesis, and management. Dermatitis.
    2008;19:241–51.
29. Kanerva L. Occupational fingertip protein contact
    dermatitis from grain flours and natural rubber latex.
    Contact Dermatitis. 1998;38:295–6.
30. Davies E, Orton D. Contact urticaria and protein con-
    tact dermatitis to chapatti flour. Contact Dermatitis.
    2009;60:113–4.

Oral Allergy Syndrome: Rethinking Concepts

Jorge Sánchez and Ricardo Cardona

Introduction

So far, of more than 200,000 known plant species, about 50 are registered in the official allergen list of the International Union of Immunological Societies (http://www.allergen.org) as capable of inducing pollen allergy in susceptible individuals [1].

As its name implies, the oral allergy syndrome (OAS) consists of a set of symptoms that usually occur in the oral cavity after the intake of various foods, mainly fruits and vegetables, that usually have cross-reactivity with pollen. OAS has been a challenging diagnosis since it was first published in 1942 by Tuft and Blumstein, who discussed the clinical features of four adult patients who presented with itching on the soft palate and mucosal swelling after eating various raw fruits [2, 3]. This syndrome was first recognized in

patients with birch pollen allergy, suggesting a possible cross-reactivity between some of their proteins, which was later demonstrated. New proteins that could be involved in cross-reactivity with pollen from trees, flowers, and herbs are being described each day. The identification of the proteins involved in this disease and its particular characteristics has allowed the development of better tools for the diagnosis and treatment of the disease. The name OAS was first used by Amlot et al. [4] in 1987 to describe the most common set of symptoms that occurred in individuals reporting food allergy and who had a positive skin prick test for the implicated food. The advance in knowledge of OAS has led to the term "syndrome" being discussed by some researchers, because in the majority of patients the specific underlying mechanism of symptoms can be identified and the specific protein that produces the symptoms allows the risk of systemic reactions, the likelihood of cross-reactivity with other foods or pollen, and the patient's prognosis to be predicted. For these reasons, different terms such as "food contact hypersensitivity," "LTP allergy," or "pollen–food syndrome (PFS)" or "pollen-food allergy syndrome" [5] have been proposed, but OAS is still the term most used.

It is now recognized that oral symptoms may occur as a prelude to generalized reactions caused by a variety of foods and are not confined to those occurring with fruits and vegetables. Also, OAS may be IgE- or non-IgE mediated; of

J. Sánchez (✉)
Group of Clinical and Experimental Allergy (GACE), IPS Universitaria, University of Antioquia, Medellín, Colombia

Foundation for the Development of Medical and Biological Sciences (FUNDEMEB), Cartagena, Colombia

R. Cardona
Group of Clinical and Experimental Allergy (GACE), IPS Universitaria, University of Antioquia, Medellín, Colombia

© Springer International Publishing AG, part of Springer Nature 2018
A. M. Giménez-Arnau, H. I. Maibach (eds.), *Contact Urticaria Syndrome*, Updates in Clinical Dermatology, https://doi.org/10.1007/978-3-319-89764-6_5

57

the IgE-mediated forms, pollen-related and non-related reactions occur that include latex, fruit, mites, snails, and bird egg cross-reactivity [6].

In this chapter, we review different aspects of OAS, focusing on the technological advances that have allowed a more precise etiological management in the daily clinic.

Epidemiology

The prevalence of OAS is influenced by many factors. Some of the main factors are the geographic characteristics of each region and the social customs that influence the diet. Another factor that makes it difficult to assess the prevalence of OAS is that many patients experience mild symptoms and simply avoid the offending food without medical evaluation. Medical knowledge about the disease also influences the calculation of its frequency; because it is not uncommon to classify acute episodes of OAS as "urticaria" or simply "food allergy," there is a high probability that there is a subreport of unknown proportions.

As we said before, there was previously controversy about the definition of OAS. Another term used for this syndrome is pollen–food allergy (PFS); the patient is sensitized with a pollen antigen through the airways and exhibits an allergic reaction to a food antigen with a structural similarity to pollen (class 2 food allergy). In addition to PFS, latex–fruit syndrome (LFS) is also well known as a disease exhibiting OAS. Clinically, also, some patients with a positive skin prick test complain of oral discomfort immediately after the ingestion of egg on the oral challenge test but show no spread of allergic symptoms to the entire body even if they continue to eat it. Some authors considered that PFS and LFS are not the same as OAS because systemic and severe reactions may be observed by some pollen-related food allergens (Api g 1, Gly m 4). Those authors suggest that OAS should be strictly confined to the oral cavity and that any extra-oral or systemic symptoms should result in a diagnosis of food anaphylaxis, PFS, or LFS [7, 8] and, to avoid confusion related to the term OAS, they suggest that food allergy caused by a cross-reaction between pollen antigens and fruit or vegetable antigens should be called by the term "pollen–food allergy syndrome" (PFS), because it is more specific [9, 10]. In this chapter, for practical reasons we call the reaction group (PFS, OAS, LFS) by the same name, OAS.

However, it is important to say that the different ways of defining OAS may have clinical implications, leading to patient care scenarios in which the misdiagnosis of OAS could result in inadequate treatment of potentially fatal food anaphylaxis. Ma et al. [10] found 13% of allergists made a misdiagnosis of OAS in children with peanut allergy and that 25% did not consider prescribing epinephrine. This survey also found that 20% of allergists applied the term OAS to patients who presented systemic symptoms caused by fruit intake. Any controversy in the definition of OAS will likely be restricted to the variety of its clinical presentations, because the current understanding of OAS underlying pathophysiology supports different clinical outcomes, in part from the many different types of antigens capable of causing oral allergy symptoms and the unique nature of the antigens themselves. For example, thermolabile proteins usually cause local reactions (PR-10, profilin), whereas the thermostable proteins (e.g., lipid transfer proteins, LTPs) that can be absorbed in their unmodified structure can cause systemic reactions such as anaphylaxis [4].

In 1993, Ortolani et al. [11] conducted a review of OAS studies to create a summary of symptoms elicited in allergic subjects by eating fruits and vegetables. Based on this review and as added in the survey by Ma et al. [10], in addition to the typical oropharyngeal symptoms, 8.7% of patients experience systemic symptoms outside the gastrointestinal tract, 3% experience systemic symptoms without oral symptoms, and 1.7% experience anaphylactic shock. However, as already mentioned, these percentages vary according to our definition of OAS and the geographic characteristics of each population.

Taking into consideration these points, some retrospective studies suggest that the prevalence of OAS in adults is approximately 8% [10], and in a population with atopic dermatitis, about 45% to 80% [4]. Although controversial, these symptoms may progress to systemic symptoms outside the gastrointestinal tract in 8.7% of patients and to anaphylactic shock in 1.7% [10]. Taking into consideration the cross-reactivity between fruits and vegetables and pollen, it is not surprising that in studies including patients with pollen allergy the prevalence is high (47–70%) [12, 13]. However, cross-reactivity patterns vary with geographic region. In central and northern Europe, birch, grasses, and mugwort pollen are the most common sensitizers in those patients with OAS. In the Mediterranean region, for approximately 20% of sensitized individuals with OAS, the most common sensitizers are grasses, ragweed, and *Parietaria* [13]. Variations between regions also determine the differences in which foods are responsible for symptoms of OAS, in Central and Northern Europe being tree nuts and fruits, particularly those of the Rosaceae family, important food allergens [14], in Southern Europe, fruits, and in Japan, the tomato [5]. There is little written about OAS in populations from other countries different from Europe and United States. In the tropic area of Latin America, sensitization to pollen is less than 12% in atopic patients, but in the subtropical areas sensitization is about 30% [15]. This difference could explain why OAS in the tropics in Latin America is reported in less than 2% of patients with allergies, but in the subtropical areas it is about 12%. This frequency of sensitization is lower than previously reported in Europe, but the distribution of high and low prevalence of OAS is similar.

Mechanisms

Cross-reactivity occurs when a specific antibody is formed in response to one epitope that reacts with another similar or identical epitope on another antigen. OAS is usually caused by proteins with a broad cross-reactivity between pollen and some foods. These cross-reactive proteins have high identity and are usually panallergens that are widely distributed throughout the plant and animal kingdoms.

Food allergens that induce OAS are usually broken down by digestive enzymes such as those in gastric juice, and for this reason the symptoms are usually limited to the oral cavity. Because these food allergens differ in properties of known food allergens that are resistant to digestive enzymes and induce sensitization through the intestine, the term "class 2 food allergy" [16] has been used for OAS allergens to distinguish them from food allergy caused by conventional intestinal sensitization (class 1 food allergy). Some of the important characteristics of class 2 food allergy are that allergens may be aeroallergens because of their cross-reactivity with pollen proteins [16].

Figure 5.1 includes the most common proteins associated with OAS pathogenesis. Protein characteristics are involved in the clinical presentation and outcome, depending on whether the cross-reactive protein is a heat-labile PR-10 protein, a partially labile profilin, or a relatively heat-stable lipid transfer protein (LTP). Taking into account that a detailed description of all the proteins that have been associated with OAS is beyond the scope of this chapter, we briefly describe here the proteins that are primarily associated with cross-reactivity with pollen. It is also noted that some allergens might induce OAS in the absence of pollen allergy.

Profilins

Profilins are monomeric, actin-binding proteins that abound in trees, grasses, and weeds [17]. Depending on the population, profilins are recognized by 8% to 20% of patients allergic to pollen. Sensitization to profilins causes reactivity to a wide range of aeroallergens, food allergens, and it has also been suggested that they may induce an IgE autoreactivity [17, 18]. Bet v 2 is a profilin, and patients sensitized to it are frequently associated with OAS symptoms after ingestion of pear, apple, celery, and carrot.

Pathogenesis-Related Proteins

Pathogenesis-related (PR) proteins have been classified into 14 pathogenesis-related protein families, and a small group has been identified as plant allergens. Of these, the PR 10 protein family is the

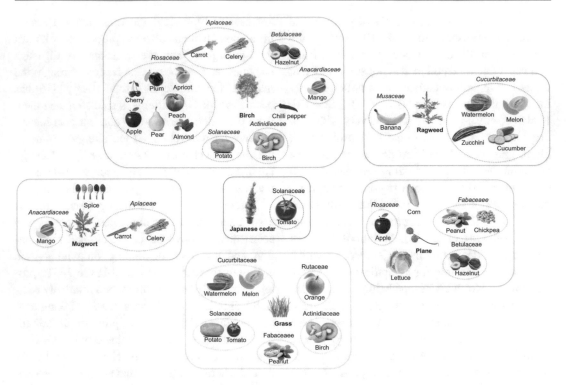

Fig. 5.1 Main fruits and vegetables reported to show cross-reactivity with pollens

most important in OAS: Bet v 1 is a member of this family. In Europe's temperate zones, sensitization to Bet v 1 is the leading cause of pollen allergy. In this population, between 50% and 90% of individuals allergic to birch pollen developed sensitivity to foods such as apples, carrot, hazelnut, and celery in response to cross-reactive allergens against Bet v1 [19]. However, in other populations such as the tropic area of Latin America, sensitization to this protein is quite low [20].

The PR14 family includes lipid transfer proteins (LTPs), and some of these proteins have important cross-reactivity with allergens of the Rosaceae fruits (apples, pears) and the Prunoideae fruits (peaches, apricots, plums, cherries); the LTPs are found in greater concentration in the fruit peel. Allergy to LTPs confers an increased risk of anaphylaxis compared to that seen with PR10 reactivity. Unlike profilins and PR10, LTPs are very stable to heat, so cooking food does not destroy the allergen, making this particular food not well tolerated [21].

Cross-reactive carbohydrate determinants (CCDs) can induce IgE and are present in vegeta-

ble glycoproteins such as celery, tomato, peanut, and potato and are also found in ragweed, timothy grass, and birch pollen. Whether reactivity to CCDs can cause clinical symptoms is still a matter of investigation [20].

Diagnosis

Diagnosis of OAS is based on a positive history of typical symptoms after ingestion of the implicated food. However, the medical history is not always clear enough to make the diagnosis, and identifying the allergen involved can be a clinical challenge.

After contact with the allergen, local oropharyngeal symptoms of angioedema, wheals, erythema, and pruritus are usually present in patients with OAS [22]. In a significant percentage of patients, these symptoms may be accompanied by abdominal pain, respiratory distress, generalized urticaria, and anaphylaxis [23]. A medical history of atopic diseases such as rhinitis, conjunctivitis, dermatitis, and/or asthma is not uncommon and may occur because of the cross-reactivity among pollen and proteins in fruits and vegetables.

The symptoms usually appear in the second or third decade of life but, as we explained before, the real prevalence is still unknown and varies among countries depending on geography, pollen exposure, and dietary patterns [24].

Cooking usually reduces the allergenicity of most food proteins and also reduces the severity of symptoms most times, with some exceptions depending on which protein induces the symptoms [20]. Although symptoms can occur at any time on exposure to the offending vegetables, symptoms are often more pronounced if the exposure occurs during the pollen season [25].

Differential Diagnosis

Differential diagnosis should be made with IgE and non-IgE reactions: swallowing problems such as eosinophilic esophagitis or gastrointestinal disorders may result in complaints about throat symptoms, but usually these symptoms are easy to differentiate from an immediate allergic reaction. Spices and food additives may cause non-IgE-mediated reactions, but usually produce acute symptoms with subsequent tolerance by the patient. Sometimes other allergic reactions can induce clinical symptoms similar to OAS, but usually doubts can be clarified with a good clinical interrogation.

Atopy Evaluation

Sensitization to food or pollen can be confirmed by the skin prick test or evaluation of allergen-specific IgE in serum. A positive test with a clinical history has a high specificity, but negative results do not rule out OAS because proteins of fruits and vegetables from commercial extracts for skin testing are heat labile and can be easily degraded with time. In 1942 Tuft and Blumstein described for the first time the prick-by-prick using fresh extract of fruit juices for the skin prick test (SPT) [26]. When considered collec-

tively, both commercial extracts for SPT and the fresh fruit skin prick test are highly variable according to the food being tested, but the prick-by-prick with fresh extract can be more sensitive than a commercial SPT to detect sensitization to vegetables and fruits [27]. Skin testing with commercial extracts from other foods such as cereals and nuts has high sensitivity and specificity.

The use of purified or recombinant allergens could help in the diagnosis [28], but these diagnostic products are not universally available for the prick test or in vitro test. However, they could be very useful to identify allergens and their role in cross-reactivity. With recombinant or natural separate allergens for the in vitro test, it is possible to predict for some foods the severity of the reaction and whether the patient is tolerant to cooked foods.

Other tests, such as the basophil activation test, have not proved to be very useful [29]. Another potential technique explored for the diagnosis of OAS is the sulfidoleukotriene release assay, which combines the cellular antigen stimulation test with an enzyme-linked immunosorbent assay (CAST-ELISA) [30], but similar to the basophil test, the specificity and sensitivity are unknown for OAS proteins.

Oral Food Challenges

Today, diagnostic testing for OAS continues to vary in sensitivity and specificity, largely as a result of the multiple OAS-causing antigens. The oral challenge is considered to be the "gold standard" test to confirm the presence of allergy to a particular food, but some considerations should be observed when performing an oral food challenge in patients with suspected OAS [31]; the reactivity in the OAS depends on the maturation of vegetables in particular. The lyophilization recently used in the blinding process of the food used in the test can destroy relevant allergens, resulting in a false-negative challenge, so fresh fruits are preferred. Whether the fruit peel is included may also affect results. The use of capsules as part of the blinding process eliminates direct contact with the mucosa, which is considered essential to initiate the reaction in OAS. The degree of processing of an individual food can determine how much allergen is within the food product, and this may affect reactivity. Therefore it is advisable to try to reproduce the provocation with the food that produces the patient's symptoms, but in case of a negative result and if the doubt persists, repeating the test and administering fresh food, uncooked if possible, should be considered [32].

In some cases, it may be necessary to perform challenges cautiously with other possible cross-reactive foods to which the patient has not yet been exposed, although with the identification of the specific allergen that produce the symptoms, this may be less frequently performed.

In a study comparing the OAS history with oral challenge, Rodriguez et al. [33], showed that of 53 patients with a history of OAS to melon, only 25 had a positive result to an open food challenge (OFC), and of those, only 17 had a positive DBPCFC (double-blind placebo control food challenge) test. Given these results, many diagnostic tests have been compared with DBPCFC as the standard to reflect true disease. However, as mentioned earlier, several authors consider that the DBPCFC is not useful to confirm an OAS because some blinding processes may not guarantee oral contact with enough provoking antigen as OAS antigenicity is labile. Supporting this idea, Anhoej et al. [34] found that a good clinical history of OAS to apple had negative and positive predictive values of 100% and 92%, respectively, when compared with OFC. As a result, some studies compare the sensitivity and specificity of diagnostic testing using clinical history as the gold standard. Both considerations are reviewed here [27, 35].

Management

Similar to other allergic reactions, OAS treatment focuses on three points: avoidance, pharmacotherapy, especially during emergency management with injectable epinephrine, and immunomodulation [31].

The main treatment is easy to recommend but difficult to meet: avoidance. Although most patients with symptoms of OAS will choose to avoid the implicated foods, identifying the main allergen implicated is necessary to avoid other foods with possible cross-reactivity, but as most of the time this is not possible empirical restrictions are made [10].

Clinical cross-reactivity, particularly among members of the Rosaceae fruits family, has been shown to be significant between 46% and 63%, leading these authors to recommend that tolerance by other family members should be specifically investigated unless the patient has recently eaten them without any symptoms. Open food challenges with potentially cross-reactive foods should be considered for patients who have had a systemic reaction.

Although this is currently a debated topic in the literature, some patients with OAS may experience systemic symptoms outside the gastrointestinal tract such as anaphylaxis [10]. For this possibility, some authors suggest that patients with OAS should always have self-injectable epinephrine. However, considering that these symptoms occur in less than 1% of OAS patients, other authors consider that generalizing this recommendation to all patients is unnecessary and only patients who have experienced generalized symptoms should be treated in the same way as any other food-allergic patient with instructions on providing an auto-injectable adrenaline device.

Many patients with OAS tolerate the food in the cooked state. Cooking causes denaturation of the relevant proteins and loss of conformational structure [25], resulting in loss of IgE-binding ability. However, it is difficult to ensure that all cooked foods will be well tolerated by the patient, as this depends in part on how the food is prepared and some allergens maintain their allergenic ability.

The role of immunotherapy has been reexamined as a potential therapy. In the cross-reactivity between some of the fruits, vegetables, and pollen allergens, some studies have observed that pollen immunotherapy for respiratory symptoms of patients can also lead to an improvement in gastrointestinal symptoms after the intake of food with those who share panallergens [38].

Based on a case report of fresh fruit tolerance after a year of pollen immunotherapy described by Kelso et al. [8], other studies have examined the effects of subcutaneous and sublingual immunotherapy on OAS with controversial results. This therapy still cannot be routinely recommended for the treatment of OAS.

Another approach is induction of tolerance to food or oral desensitization. This therapy has been proved to allow the patient to tolerate food and also to prevent severe reactions to accidental exposures. However, published studies report conflicting results [36, 37], with efficacy between 30% and 84%, but in most cases the effect disappeared if the patients discontinued the treatment [37–39].

Conclusion

Since the first case report, OAS has been a challenging diagnosis because of its many clinical, diagnostic, and therapeutic considerations. Molecular-based diagnostics has allowed a better understanding of the diverse presentations seen in clinical practice. With the advent of purified and recombinant allergens and microarray technology, a rapid and accurate diagnosis is possible, resulting in the characterization of an individual's sensitivities. For patients with OAS, knowledge of specific sensitization patterns has consequences for both risk assessment and dietary management.

References

1. Hauser M, Roulias A, Ferreira F, Egger M. Panallergens and their impact on the allergic patient. Allergy Asthma Clin Immunol. 2010;6(1):1.
2. Webber CM, England RW. Oral allergy syndrome: a clinical, diagnostic, and therapeutic challenge. Ann Allergy Asthma Immunol. 2010;104(2):101–8; quiz 9-10, 17.
3. Sánchez J, Amaya E, Acevedo A, Celis A, Caraballo D, Cardona R. Prevalence of inducible urticaria in patients with chronic spontaneous urticaria: associated risk factors. J Allergy Clin Immunol Pract. 2017;5:464–70.
4. Amlot PL, Kemeny DM, Zachary C, Parkes P, Lessof MH. Oral allergy syndrome (OAS): symptoms of IgE-mediated hypersensitivity to foods. Clin Allergy. 1987;17(1):33–42.
5. Kondo Y, Urisu A. Oral allergy syndrome. Allergol Int. 2009;58(4):485–91.
6. Konstantinou GN, Grattan CE. Food contact hypersensitivity syndrome: the mucosal contact urticaria paradigm. Clin Exp Dermatol. 2008;33(4):383–9.
7. Detjen P. Oral allergy syndrome or anaphylaxis? Ann Allergy Asthma Immunol. 1996;77(3):254.
8. Kelso JM. Oral allergy syndrome? J Allergy Clin Immunol. 1995;96(2):275.
9. Valenta R, Kraft D. Type 1 allergic reactions to plant-derived food: a consequence of primary sensitization to pollen allergens. J Allergy Clin Immunol. 1996;97(4):893–5.
10. Ma S, Sicherer SH, Nowak-Wegrzyn A. A survey on the management of pollen-food allergy syndrome in allergy practices. J Allergy Clin Immunol. 2003;112(4):784–8.
11. Ortolani C, Pastorello EA, Farioli L, Ispano M, Pravettoni V, Berti C, et al. IgE-mediated allergy from vegetable allergens. Ann Allergy. 1993;71(5):470–6.
12. Dreborg S, Foucard T. Allergy to apple, carrot and potato in children with birch pollen allergy. Allergy. 1983;38(3):167–72.
13. Cuesta-Herranz J, Lázaro M, Figueredo E, Igea JM, Umpiérrez A, De-Las-Heras M. Allergy to plant-derived fresh foods in a birch- and ragweed-free area. Clin Exp Allergy. 2000;30(10):1411–6.
14. Asero R, Antonicelli L, Arena A, Bommarito L, Caruso B, Crivellaro M, et al. EpidemAAITO: features of food allergy in Italian adults attending allergy clinics: a multi-centre study. Clin Exp Allergy. 2009;39(4):547–55.
15. Sánchez J, Sánchez A. Epidemiology of food allergy in Latin America. Allergol Immunopathol (Madr). 2015;43(2):185–95.
16. Breiteneder H, Molecular EC. biochemical classification of plant-derived food allergens. J Allergy Clin Immunol. 2000;106(1 Pt 1):27–36.
17. Valenta R, Duchene M, Ebner C, Valent P, Sillaber C, Deviller P, et al. Profilins constitute a novel family of functional plant pan-allergens. J Exp Med. 1992;175(2):377–85.
18. Valenta R, Duchêne M, Pettenburger K, Sillaber C, Valent P, Bettelheim P, et al. Identification of profilin as a novel pollen allergen; IgE autoreactivity in sensitized individuals. Science. 1991;253(5019):557–60.
19. Klinglmayr E, Hauser M, Zimmermann F, Dissertori O, Lackner P, Wopfner N, et al. Identification of B-cell epitopes of Bet v 1 involved in cross-reactivity with food allergens. Allergy. 2009;64(4):647–51.
20. Hofmann A, Burks AW. Pollen food syndrome: update on the allergens. Curr Allergy Asthma Rep. 2008;8(5):413–7.
21. Ebner C, Hoffmann-Sommergruber K, Breiteneder H. Plant food allergens homologous to pathogenesis-related proteins. Allergy. 2001;56(Suppl 67):43.

22. Ortolani C, Ispano M, Pastorello E, Bigi A, Ansaloni R. The oral allergy syndrome. Ann Allergy. 1988;61(6 t 2):47–52.

23. Kleine-Tebbe J, Vogel L, Crowell DN, Haustein UF, Vieths S. Severe oral allergy syndrome and anaphylactic reactions caused by a Bet v 1- related PR-10 protein in soybean, SAM22. J Allergy Clin Immunol. 2002;110(5):797–804.

24. Fernández-Rivas M, Benito C, González-Mancebo E, de Durana DA. Allergies to fruits and vegetables. Pediatr Allergy Immunol. 2008;19(8):675–81.

25. Bohle B, Zwölfer B, Heratizadeh A, Jahn-Schmid B, Antonia YD, Alter M, et al. Cooking birch pollen-related food: divergent consequences for IgE- and T cell-mediated reactivity in vitro and in vivo. J Allergy Clin Immunol. 2006;118(1):242–9.

26. Tuft L, Blumstein G. Studies in food allergysensitization to fresh fruits: clinical and experimental observations. Journal of Allergy. 1942;13:574–8.

27. Ortolani C, Ispano M, Pastorello EA, Ansaloni R, Magri GC. Comparison of results of skin prick tests (with fresh foods and commercial food extracts) and RAST in 100 patients with oral allergy syndrome. J Allergy Clin Immunol. 1989;83(3):683–90.

28. Asero R, Monsalve R, Barber D. Profilin sensitization detected in the office by skin prick test: a study of prevalence and clinical relevance of profilin as a plant food allergen. Clin Exp Allergy. 2008;38(6):1033–7.

29. Gamboa PM, Sanz ML, Lombardero M, Barber D, Sánchez-Monje R, Goikoetxea MJ, et al. Component-resolved in vitro diagnosis in peach-allergic patients. J Investig Allergol Clin Immunol. 2009;19(1):13–20.

30. Ballmer-Weber BK, Weber JM, Vieths S, Wüthrich B. Predictive value of the sulfidoleukotriene release assay in oral allergy syndrome to celery, hazelnut, and carrot. J Investig Allergol Clin Immunol. 2008;18(2):93–9.

31. American College of Allergy At, & Immunology. Food allergy: a practice parameter. Ann Allergy Asthma Immunol. 2006;96(3 Suppl 2):S1–68.

32. Ballmer-Weber BK, Holzhauser T, Scibilia J, Mittag D, Zisa G, Ortolani C, et al. Clinical characteristics of soybean allergy in Europe: a double-blind, placebo-controlled food challenge study. J Allergy Clin Immunol. 2007;119(6):1489–96.

33. Rodriguez J, Crespo JF, Burks W, Rivas-Plata C, Fernandez-Anaya S, Vives R, et al. Randomized, double-blind, crossover challenge study in 53 subjects reporting adverse reactions to melon (Cucumis melo). J Allergy Clin Immunol. 2000;106(5):968–72.

34. Anhoej C, Backer V, Nolte H. Diagnostic evaluation of grass- and birch-allergic patients with oral allergy syndrome. Allergy. 2001;56(6):548–52.

35. Cadot P, Kochuyt AM, van Ree R, Ceuppens JL. Oral allergy syndrome to chicory associated with birch pollen allergy. Int Arch Allergy Immunol. 2003;131(1):19–24.

36. Asero R. Effects of birch pollen-specific immunotherapy on apple allergy in birch pollen-hypersensitive patients. Clin Exp Allergy. 1998;28(11):1368–73.

37. Asero R. How long does the effect of birch pollen injection SIT on apple allergy last? Allergy. 2003;58(5):435–8.

38. Bucher X, Pichler WJ, Dahinden CA, Helbling A. Effect of tree pollen specific, subcutaneous immunotherapy on the oral allergy syndrome to apple and hazelnut. Allergy. 2004;59(12):1272–6.

39. Kinaciyan T, Jahn-Schmid B, Radakovics A, Zwölfer B, Schreiber C, Francis JN, et al. Successful sublingual immunotherapy with birch pollen has limited effects on concomitant food allergy to apple and the immune response to the Bet v 1 homolog Mal d 1. J Allergy Clin Immunol. 2007;119(4):937–43.

Wheals and Eczema: Pathogenic Mechanism in Immediate Contact Reactions

Eduardo Rozas-Muñoz and Esther Serra-Baldrich

Introduction

Immediate contact reactions (ICRs) are a heterogeneous group of inflammatory conditions characterized by the elicitation of symptoms within minutes to hours after skin contact with specific triggers. Included are two main clinical presentations: contact urticaria (CoU) in patients presenting with wheals/angioedema, and protein contact dermatitis (PCD) in patients presenting predominantly with dermatitis/eczema. However, CoU and PCD are not exclusive, and in some cases, both processes can manifest at the same time [1, 2]. After contact with an agent, patients may present with wheals during the first minutes and dermatitis/eczema within hours or days after. In immediate contact reactions, whether of urticaria/angioedema (CoU) or eczema/dermatitis (PCD) type, generalized lesions or systemic symptoms build the complete contact urticaria syndrome (CUS) [1, 2]. This chapter summarizes the most important aspects regarding the mechanisms of these two conditions.

Nonimmunological, immunological, and uncertain mechanisms have been proposed as possible pathogenic mechanisms in CoU; an immunological mechanism involving a combination of type I and type IV allergic skin reactions, induced mainly by proteins, has been proposed in PCD. Understanding the possible mechanisms will help our approach to the different clinical manifestations and diagnostic procedures performed to confirm the diagnosis.

Contact Urticaria

CoU is characterized by the presence of wheals, angioedema, or both, developing within 30 to 60 min after skin contact with an exogenous agent. Wheals, also known as hives, are pruritic and transient erythematous swelling papules that characteristically disappear in less than 24 h without leaving any trace of their presence. Angioedema, by contrast, refers to the less well-defined lesions that usually affect face, lips, extremities, and genitals. Both lesions result from increased vascular permeability and leakage of fluid, proteins, and inflammatory cells into the skin.

The mechanism by which the different triggers can induce this phenomenon are not well understood, and several hypotheses have been proposed. These mechanisms are generally classified into two main groups: nonimmunological (nonimmunological contact urticaria, NICoU) and immunological (immunological contact urticaria, ICoU). It is possible also that more than one mechanism may be involved in certain cases.

E. Rozas-Muñoz (✉) · E. Serra-Baldrich
Department of Dermatology, Hospital de la Santa
Creu i Sant Pau, Barcelona, Spain

© Springer International Publishing AG, part of Springer Nature 2018
A. M. Giménez-Arnau, H. I. Maibach (eds.), *Contact Urticaria Syndrome*, Updates in Clinical
Dermatology, https://doi.org/10.1007/978-3-319-89764-6_6

Nonimmunological Contact Urticaria

Nonimmunological mechanisms, also known as pseudo-allergic, are believed to be the most common mechanisms of CoU, and include all forms of CoU that are not mediated by effectors of adaptive immunity [2, 3]. Patients with NICoU do not need previous sensitization, and the reaction can be considered a form of skin irritation. Symptoms are usually confined to the skin area that is exposed to the trigger, and include local itch, tingling, a burning sensation, erythema, and wheals or angioedema. This variability in the symptoms is influenced by the concentration, vehicle, molecular structure, and mode of exposure of the agent, and also by the site of skin contact where it has been applied, the face, back, and arms being more reactive than palms and soles [4–10].

A long list of agents capable of inducing this type of reaction include preservatives in cosmetics, fragrances, and topical medications, foodstuffs, toiletries, metals, chemicals, animals, and plants [11, 12]. These different agents, as mentioned earlier, induce an increased vascular permeability in the skin by the release of vasoactive substances without involving immunological processes. Although the exact mechanism by which these agents induce this reaction are not well understood, the most common mediators that have been proposed are histamine, prostaglandins (PGD), sensitive nerves, and ultraviolet light (UV) (Fig. 6.1).

Histamine is known to be the most important mediator of acute and chronic urticaria, but its role in NICoU seems to be secondary. Histamine release from mast cells and basophils is capable of inducing the inflammatory response and the pruritus sensation seen in humans, and in animal models, and several agents known to induce NICoU such as benzoic and cinnamic acid, cinnamic aldehyde, dimethylsulfoxide, and diethyl fumarate can cause histamine release. However, skin reactions induced by these agents could not be blocked by anti-H1, but with antiinflammatory drugs (indomethacin, diclofenac, or acetylsalicylic acid),

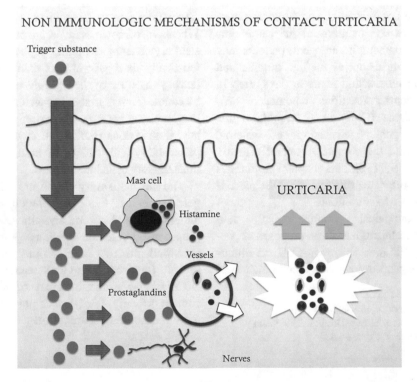

NON IMMUNOLOGIC MECHANISMS OF CONTACT URTICARIA

Trigger substance

Mast cell

Histamine

URTICARIA

Vessels

Prostaglandins

Nerves

Fig. 6.1 Nonimmunological mechanisms of contact urticaria

which also can attenuate the skin reaction when used as pretreatment [7, 13–17].

For these reasons the role of PGD seems to be more important. Prostaglandins promote vasodilatation and increase microvascular permeability independent of the release of histamine. Erythema and wheals can be elicited after intradermal injection of PGD in animal and human skin. Increase in plasma levels of PGD2 without an increase in the levels of histamine has been observed after topical application of several inducers of NICoU, such as sorbic acid, benzoic acid, and nicotinic acid. The increase is dose dependent and directly correlated with the intensity of the cutaneous vasodilatation. Animal models have suggested that the vasodilatation induced by PGD may be mediated by nitric oxide, as the reaction is inhibited by nitric oxide synthase inhibitors [18, 19]. In addition, the presence of glutathione-requiring PGD, an essential enzyme in the metabolism of PGD2, in the cytoplasm of dermal macrophages and Langerhans cells has suggested that these cells may also have an important role [20–29].

Sensory nerves have also been studied in NICoU. Activation of sensory nerves induces the release of several inflammatory mediators such as substance P, neurokinin A, or calcitonin gene-related peptide, which are known to induce vasodilatation and protein and cell extravasation. However, neural desensitization with capsaicin does not inhibit NICoU, indicating that neurogenic inflammation is probably not involved [30–32].

Finally, ultraviolet light (UV) may also have a role. Ultraviolet light has antiinflammatory effects on the cutaneous immune system, and improvement of NICoU has been seen after exposure to UVA and UVB [11, 33–37]. The mechanism by which UV improves CoU is unknown, but the clearance of lesions in areas not exposed to radiation suggests a systemic effect [38]. In evaluating patients for suspected NICoU, the skin site where the test (open test and chamber test) is performed should be considered, because a site irradiated by UV can produce a false-negative result that can last for 2 to 3 weeks [33, 37, 38].

Immunological Contact Urticaria

Contact urticaria induced by immunological mechanisms (ICoU) is less common than NICoU but seems to be better characterized [39]. It is thought to represent a type I hypersensitivity reaction of the Gell and Coombs classification. One or repeated exposures to a specific agent (allergen), most commonly a protein, induces a specific immunological response. The allergen is recognized by specific TH_2 lymphocytes, which stimulates plasma cell production of IgE class antibodies.

These specific IgE class antibodies pass through the blood to the different tissues and bind strongly to the FcεRI on the surface of mast cells, basophils, and other antigen-presenting cells [40–45]; this explains the generalized and systemic symptoms that some patients may present (CoU syndrome).

In a subsequent reexposure, the allergen binds to the IgEs inducing cross-linking of the FcεRI receptors [46]. The consequent cross-linking activates several intracellular signaling pathways that trigger the release of both preformed and newly synthesized mediators. The most important mediator is histamine; however, others such as leukotrienes, prostaglandins, proteases, heparin, platelet-activating factor, substance P, and a wide range of cytokines are also involved [25–29]. The release of these substances leads to increased vascular permeability, smooth muscle contraction, stimulation of mucous production, and chemotaxis of various inflammatory cells such as eosinophils, basophils, and lymphocytes that amplify and maintain the inflammatory process [29, 47, 48].

Prior sensitization is always required in ICoU. Stratum corneum damage and the percutaneous penetration ability of the agent seem to be the most important factors for cutaneous sensitization [49–51]. However, not all agents that penetrate the skin are capable of inducing an IgE response. A minimum size, and specific chemical structure, are also necessary, which is the reason that proteins or polypeptides of large molecule size are the most common substances to induce ICoU. In low molecular weight molecules (haptens), the covalent

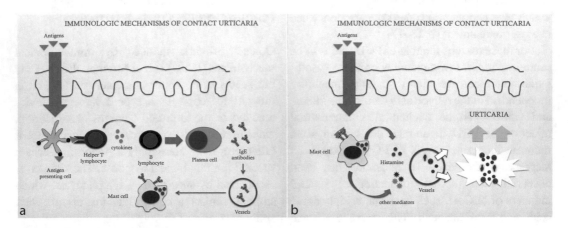

Fig. 6.2 (**a**, **b**) Immunologic mechanisms of contact urticaria

linkage to a carrier protein, usually albumin, is required to induce the process. The ability to induce the immunological response also depends on the genetic susceptibility of each individual. It is understandable, then, that atopic patients present ICoU more frequently, as they are known to have an immunological disturbance that causes IgE-mediated sensitization [52] (Fig. 6.2).

In contrast to NICoU, which usually presents with local symptoms, ICoU may present with generalized lesions and systemic symptoms such as rhinitis, conjunctivitis, asthma, gastrointestinal symptoms, and even anaphylaxis [3, 46]. Symptoms can occur not only by direct contact of the allergen with the skin, but also via the respiratory or gastrointestinal tract. The severity of the symptoms depends on the degree of allergen exposure and patient sensitization. This broad spectrum of clinical manifestations led Maibach and Johnson in 1975 to propose the term "contact urticaria syndrome" [1].

As in NICoU, there are long lists of agents capable of inducing this reaction, the most frequent being food and animal proteins and natural rubber latex.

Uncertain Mechanisms or Mixed Mechanism

In some cases the agents may induce CoU with features of NICoU and ICoU. The best example of this situation is ammonium persulfate, an oxidizing hair bleach, to which some individuals have had CoU reactions after the first exposure, suggesting an NICoU, but also presented with systemic symptoms favoring ICoU [3].

Protein Contact Dermatitis

Protein contact dermatitis is an immediate skin reaction characterized by the presence of urticarial (wheals and angioedema) and eczematous lesions (dermatitis) that occur after skin contact to an exogenous agent. The urticarial lesions usually appear within minutes after skin contact, although the dermatitis usually occurs after hours or days. In contrast to CoU wherein the inflammation is only located in the dermis or subcutaneous tissue, PCD also involves the epidermis with the characteristic clinical and histopathological features of eczematous contact dermatitis. This resemblance with irritant and allergic contact dermatitis, and the presence of nonspecific symptoms such as itching, tingling, burning sensation, and erythema, which may also occur isolated, has made the diagnosis of PCD a real challenge. In fact, its first description was done in 1976 by Hjorth and Roed-Petersen in a series of patients with occupational contact dermatitis on the hands, and only in 1983 did Veien and colleagues further characterize the disease, describing its most important features, including a chronic recurrent dermatitis caused by contact with a proteinaceous material, an acute urticarial or vesicular eruption occurring minutes after contact with the causative protein, and positive immediate testing results with usually negative patch-test results [53, 54].

Although the precise mechanisms that induce this phenomenon are still unclear, a combination of a type I and a type IV allergic skin reaction induced by large molecules such as proteins has been proposed.

Type I allergic skin reactions may explain the flares of urticarial eruptions seen shortly after contact with the causative agent, and the type IV allergic skin reaction, the dermatitis (eczema), seen afterward [55–57]. It is possible that the same allergen may induce both types of clinical manifestations, by a combined type I and type IV hypersensitivity reaction; however, in some cases the dermatitis may be of the irritant type at the beginning, predisposing the patients to develop a type I and/or type IV hypersensitivity reaction later [58–60]. This finding may explain the positive prick test and negative patch test seen in some patients and also the higher incidence seen in atopic patients, who also develop eczema by similar mechanisms.

The causative agent of PCD is thought to be a larger protein molecule rather than a hapten (low molecular weight substance), as it is in other hypersensitivity reactions such as allergic contact dermatitis; however, large proteins are unable to pass through the skin, suggesting that previous damage to the skin barrier must occur to elicit the reaction [2].

The skin serves as a protective barrier, preventing the access of foreign substances to the body, and in normal situations only extremely small compounds (<500 Da) are able to penetrate the stratum corneum. Protein antigen sensitization of large molecules, via the epicutaneous route, must then first overcome the epidermal barrier. The barrier function of the skin has the following three elements: the stratum corneum (air–liquid barrier), the tight junction (liquid–liquid barrier), and the Langerhans cell (LC) network (immunological barrier). All these three components may have a function in the development of PCD [61–63].

The stratum corneum consists mainly of lipids rich in cholesterol, fatty acids, and ceramides. Removal of these lipids is considered a major reason for skin barrier disruption. The hands of those in certain occupations such as chefs, butchers, bakers, housewives, and fishermen are therefore the most commonly affected sites in PCD, as they are usually chronically exposed to irritants, soaps, and washing, which damage the skin barrier and allow larger protein molecules to pass through the epidermis. In the case of atopic patients, reduced ceramide levels and increased ceramidase expressed by staphylococcal bacteria may also predispose to the condition [63–70].

Experimental models have also enhanced the importance of an altered stratum corneum barrier in the development of PCD, especially in atopic patients. The development of dermatitis has been demonstrated in filaggrin-deficient mice. Filaggrin loss-of-function mutations have further been shown to be associated with enhanced expression of IL-1, which is a known inflammatory cytokine frequently found in contact dermatitis [71]. The contribution of a stratum corneum deficiency to protein antigen sensitization is further supported by the clinical observation of an association of genes controlling desquamation, such as serine protease inhibitor and stratum corneum chymotryptic enzyme [67].

The epidermal tight junctions seem to also be involved. A polymorphism in the claudin-1 gene, which is one of the major components of epidermal tight junctions, was recently reported to be associated with the development of dermatitis in atopic patients [68].

The cutaneous barrier perturbation not only can stimulate proinflammatory cytokine production in the epidermis but also induces LC activation. Langerhans cell dendrites penetrate the tight junction barrier and facilitate the capture of antigens [69].

Langerhans cells then initiate a specific immune response with IgE production by plasma cells and a T-cell type IV hypersensitivity reaction mediated by specific T-cell lymphocytes. In a subsequent exposure, IgE is bound to

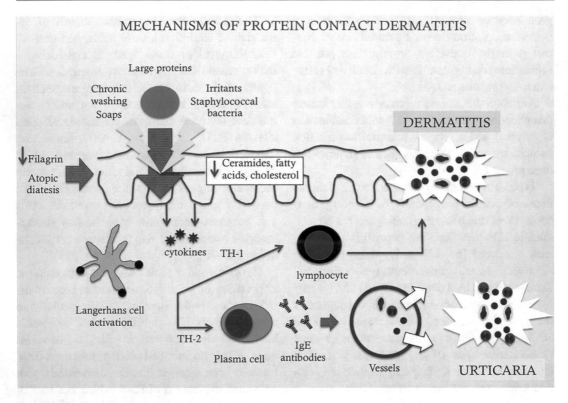

Fig. 6.3 Mechanisms of protein contact dermatitis

Langerhans cells, initiating the type I hypersensitivity reaction manifested as urticaria and also the type IV hypersensitivity reaction manifested as dermatitis. This mechanism leads to local vasodilatation and release of chemokines and inflammatory cells into the epidermis and dermis, with the development of edema, spongiosis, microvesicle formation, erythema, and induration. Other cells that also bear IgE receptors, although not necessarily of high affinity, such as lymphocytes, platelets, and monocytes, may also be involved.

It appears that all the Th1/Th2/Th17 responses are increased and no polarization of Th1/Th2/Th17 responses occurs, a phenomenon also seen in atopic eczema. The predominant Th2 response induced in PCD sensitization with protein antigens is promoted by IL-13, IL-10, IL-21, and IL-9 [70].

The effects of various Toll-like receptor (TLR) ligands on the Th responses have also been investigated. TLR2 is important for the Th1 response, but not the Th2 response, because of interferon-gamma (IFN-γ) production (Th1 response) [72–75] (Fig. 6.3).

Conclusions

Immediate contact reactions/contact urticaria syndrome include a heterogeneous group of inflammatory conditions ranging from urticaria (CoU) to eczema/dermatitis (PCD) that occur after skin contact to specific triggers. Although CoU is characterized by the presence of transient erythematous papules (hives/wheals) that lack epidermal involvement, the PCD hallmark is the epidermal damage that allows large proteins to go through the skin. Contact urticaria seems to be produced by two main mechanisms, nonimmunological and immunological, whereas PCD is produced by a combination of a type I and type IV allergic skin reaction, induced by large molecules.

Further research is required to understand the exact mechanism underlying these complex cutaneous reactions.

Key Messages

Immediate contact reaction is a clinical syndrome that includes contact urticaria and protein contact dermatitis. Contact urticaria is characterized by wheals/angioedema and can be induced through either an immunological or a nonimmunological pathway.

Protein contact dermatitis is characterized by dermatitis/eczema and is induced by a combination of a type I (IgE) and type IV (cellular) skin reaction. Contact urticaria syndrome refers to the presence of generalized or systemic symptoms and may occur in immunological contact urticaria or in protein contact dermatitis.

References

1. Maibach HI, Johnson HL. Contact urticaria syndrome. Contact urticaria to diethyltoluamide (immediate-type hypersensitivity). Arch Dermatol. 1975;111(6):726–30.
2. Gimenez-Arnau A, Maurer M, De La Cuadra J, Maibach H. Immediate contact skin reactions, an update of contact urticaria, contact urticaria syndrome and protein contact dermatitis "A Never Ending Story". Eur J Dermatol. 2010;20(5):552–62.
3. Harvell J, Bason M, Maibach H. Contact urticaria and its mechanisms. Food Chem Toxicol. 1994, February;32(2):103–12.
4. Ylipieti S, Lahti A. Effect of the vehicle on non-immunologic immediate contact reactions. Contact Dermatitis. 1989;21(2):105–6.
5. Lahti A, Poutiainen AM, Hannuksela M. Alcohol vehicles in tests for non-immunological immediate contact reactions. Contact Dermatitis. 1993;29(1):22–5.
6. Hannuksela A, Lahti A, Hannuksela M. Nonimmunologic immediate contact reactions to three isomers of pyridine carboxaldehyde. In: Frosch PJ, Dooms-Goossens A, Lachapelle J-M, Rycroft RJG, Scheper RJ, editors. Current topics in contact dermatitis. Berlin/Heidelberg/New York: Springer; 1989. p. 448–52.
7. Lahti A. Non-immunologic contact urticaria. Acta Derm Venereol Suppl (Stockh). 1980;91(Suppl):1–49.
8. Basketter DA, Wilhelm KP. Studies on non-immune immediate contact reactions in an unselected population. Contact Dermatitis. 1996;35(4):237–40.
9. Larmi E, Lahti A, Hannuksela M. Immediate contact reactions to benzoic acid and the sodium salt of pyrrolidone carboxylic acid. comparison of various skin sites. Contact Dermatitis. 1989;20(1):38–40.
10. Lahti A, Pylvänen V, Hannuksela M. Immediate irritant reactions to benzoic acid are enhanced in washed skin areas. Contact Dermatitis. 1995;33(3):177–82.
11. Gollhausen R, Kligman AM. Human assay for identifying substances which induce non-allergic contact urticaria: the NICU-test. Contact Dermatitis. 1985;13(2):98–106.
12. von Krogh G, Maibach HI. The contact urticaria syndrome–an updated review. J Am Acad Dermatol. 1981;5(3):328–42.
13. Lahti A. Terfenadine does not inhibit non-immunologic contact urticaria. Contact Dermatitis. 1987;16(4):220–3.
14. Lahti A, Oikarinen A, Viinikka L, Ylikorkala O, Hannuksela M. Prostaglandins in contact urticaria induced by benzoic acid. Acta Derm Venereol. 1983;63(5):425–7.
15. Lahti A, Väänänen A, Kokkonen EL, Hannuksela M. Acetylsalicylic acid inhibits non-immunologic contact urticaria. Contact Dermatitis. 1987;16(3):133–5.
16. Johansson J, Lahti A. Topical non-steroidal anti-inflammatory drugs inhibit non-immunologic immediate contact reactions. Contact Dermatitis. 1988;19(3):161–5.
17. Kujala T, Lahti A. Duration of inhibition of non-immunologic immediate contact reactions by acetylsalicylic acid. Contact Dermatitis. 1989;21(1):60–1.
18. Wallengren J. Substance P antagonist inhibits immediate and delayed type cutaneous hypersensitivity reactions. Br J Dermatol. 1991;124(4):324–8.
19. Cheng K, Wu TJ, Wu KK, Sturino C, Metters K, Gottesdiener K, et al. Antagonism of the prostaglandin D2 receptor 1 suppresses nicotinic acid-induced vasodilation in mice and humans. Proc Natl Acad Sci U S A. 2006;103(17):6682–7.
20. Ruzicka T, Auböck J. Arachidonic acid metabolism in guinea pig Langerhans cells: studies on cyclooxygenase and lipoxygenase pathways. J Immunol. 1987;138(2):539–43.
21. Morrow JD, Awad JA, Oates JA, Roberts LJ 2nd. Identification of skin as a major site of prostaglandin D2 release following oral administration of niacin in humans. J Invest Dermatol. 1992;98(5):812–5.
22. Morrow JD, Minton TA, Awad JA, Roberts LJ. Release of markedly increased quantities of prostaglandin D2 from the skin in vivo in humans following the application of sorbic acid. Arch Dermatol. 1994;130(11):1408–12.
23. Downard CD, Roberts LJ 2nd, Morrow JD. Topical benzoic acid induces the increased biosynthesis of prostaglandin D2 in human skin in vivo. Clin Pharmacol Ther. 1995;57(4):441–5.
24. Urade Y, Ujihara M, Horiguchi Y, Ikai K, Hayaishi O. The major source of endogenous prostaglandin D2 production is likely antigen-presenting cells. localization of glutathione-requiring prostaglandin D synthetase in histiocytes, dendritic, and Kupffer cells in various rat tissues. J Immunol. 1989;143(9):2982–9.
25. Larkò O, Lindstedt G, Lundberg PA, Mobacken H. Biochemical and clinical studies in a case of contact urticaria to potato. Contact Dermatitis. 1983;9(2):108–14.

26. Lewis RA, Austen KF. Mediation of local homeostasis and inflammation by leukotrienes and
other mast cell-dependent compounds. Nature.
1981;293(5828):103–8.

27. Schwartz LB, Austen KF. Structure and function of
the chemical mediators of mast cells. Prog Allergy.
1984;34:271–321.

28. Wallengren J, Ekman R, Möller H. Substance P
and vasoactive intestinal peptide in bullous and
inflammatory skin disease. Acta Derm Venereol.
1986;66(1):23–8.

29. Sabroe RA, Greaves MW. The pathogenesis
of chronic idiopathic urticaria. Arch Dermatol.
1997;133(8):1003–8.

30. Bernstein JE, Swift RM, Soltani K, Lorincz
AL. Inhibition of axon reflex vasodilatation by
topically applied capsaicin. J Invest Dermatol.
1981;76(5):394–5.

31. Larmi E, Lahti A, Hannuksela M. Effects of capsaicin
and topical anesthesia on nonimmunologic immediate
contact reactions to benzoic acid and methyl nicotinate. In: Frosch PJ, Dooms-Goossens A, Lachapelle
J-M, Rycroft RJG, Scheper RJ, editors. Current topics
in contact dermatitis. Berlin/Heidelberg/New York:
Springer; 1989. p. 441–7.

32. Lundblad L, Lundberg JM, Anggård A, Zetterström
O. Capsaicin-sensitive nerves and the cutaneous
allergy reaction in man. possible involvement of
sensory neuropeptides in the flare reaction. Allergy.
1987;42(1):20–5.

33. Larmi E, Lahti A, Hannuksela M. Ultraviolet
light inhibits nonimmunologic immediate contact reactions to benzoic acid. Arch Dermatol Res.
1988;280(7):420–3.

34. Czarnetzki BM, Rosenbach T, Kolde G, Frosch
PJ. Phototherapy of urticaria pigmentosa: clinical
response and changes of cutaneous reactivity, histamine and chemotactic leukotrienes. Arch Dermatol
Res. 1985;277(2):105–13.

35. Kolde G, Frosch PJ, Czarnetzki BM. Response of
cutaneous mast cells to PUVA in patients with urticaria pigmentosa: histomorphometric, ultrastructural,
and biochemical investigations. J Invest Dermatol.
1984;83(3):175–8.

36. Larmi E. Systemic effect of ultraviolet irradiation
on non-immunologic immediate contact reactions
to benzoic acid and methyl nicotinate. Acta Derm
Venereol. 1989;69(4):296–301.

37. Larmi E. PUVA treatment inhibits nonimmunologic immediate contact reactions to benzoic acid and methyl nicotinate. Int J Dermatol.
1989;28(9):609–11.

38. Larmi E, Lahti A, Hannuksela M. Effect of ultraviolet
B on nonimmunologic contact reactions induced by
dimethyl sulphoxide, phenol and sodium lauryl sul-
phate. Photo-Dermatology. 1989;6(6):258–62.

39. Lahti A. Immediate contact reactions. In: Rycroft
RJG, Menné T, Frosch PJ, editors. Textbook
of contact dermatitis. Berlin: Springer; 1995.
p. 68–72.

40. Kraft S, Wessendorf JH, Hanau D, Bieber
T. Regulation of the high affinity receptor for IgE
on human epidermal Langerhans cells. J Immunol.
1998;161(2):1000–6.

41. Capron M, Capron A, Dessaint JP, Torpier G,
Johansson SG, Prin L. Fc receptors for IgE on human
and rat eosinophils. J Immunol. 1981;126(6):2087–92.

42. Spiegelberg HL. Structure and function of Fc receptors for IgE on lymphocytes, monocytes, and macrophages. Adv Immunol. 1984;35:61–88. Review

43. Boltansky H, Kaliner MA. Cells demonstrating Fc receptors for IgE. Surv Immunol Res.
1984;3(2–3):99–102.

44. Yodoi J, Ishizaka K. Lymphocytes bearing Fc receptors for IgE. I. presence of human and rat T lymphocytes with Fc epsilon receptors. J Immunol.
1979;122(6):2577–83.

45. Joseph M, Auriault C, Capron A, Vorng H, Viens P. A
new function for platelets: IgE-dependent killing of
schistosomes. Nature. 1983;303(5920):810–2.

46. Garssen J, Vandebriel RJ, Kimber I, van Loveren
H. Hypersensitivity reactions: definitions, basic
mechanisms and localizations. In: Vos JG, Younes M,
Smith E, editors. Allergic hypersensitivities induced
by chemicals, recommendations for prevention. Boca
Raton: CRC Press; 1996. p. 19–58.

47. Finkelman FD, Katona IM, Urban JF Jr, Holmes J,
Ohara J, Tung AS, Sample JV, et al. IL-4 is required
to generate and sustain in vivo IgE responses.
J Immunol. 1988;141(7):2335–41.

48. Ricci M, Matucci A, Rossi OT. Cells, cytokines, IgE
and allergic airways inflammation. J Investig Allergol
Clin Immunol. 1994;4(5):214–20.

49. Hsieh KY, Tsai CC, Wu CH, Lin RH. Epicutaneous
exposure to protein antigen and food allergy. Clin Exp
Allergy. 2003;33(8):1067–75.

50. Li XM, Kleiner G, Huang CK, Lee SY, Schofield B,
Soter NA, et al. Murine model of atopic dermatitis
associated with food hypersensitivity. J Allergy Clin
Immunol. 2001;107(4):693–702.

51. Strid J, Hourihane J, Kimber I, Callard R, Strobel
S. Disruption of the stratum corneum allows potent
epicutaneous immunization with protein antigens
resulting in a dominant systemic Th2 response. Eur
J Immunol. 2004;34(8):2100–9.

52. Williams HC. Clinical practice. Atopic dermatitis. N
Engl J Med. 2005;352(22):2314–24.

53. Hjorth N, Roed-Petersen J. Occupational protein contact dermatitis in food handlers. Contact Dermatitis.
1976;2:28–42.

54. Veien NK, Hattel T, Justresen O, Northolm A. Causes
of eczema in the food industry. Dermatosen in
Beruf und Umwelt. Occup Environ Dermatoses.
1983;31:84–6.

55. Levin C, Warshaw E. Protein contact dermatitis:
allergens, pathogenesis and management. Dermatitis.
2008;19(5):241–51.

56. Mulder PGH, Munte K, Devillers ACA, et al.
Diagnostic tests in children with atopic dermatitis and
food allergy. Allergy. 1998;53:1087–91.

57. Kanerva L, Pajari-Backas M. IgE-mediated RAST-negative occupa-tional protein contact dermatitis from taxonomically unrelated fish species. Contact Dermatitis. 1999;41:295–6.
58. Janssens V, Morren M, Dooms Goossens A, DeGreef H. Protein contact dermatitis, myth or reality. Br J Dermatol. 1995;132:1–6.
59. Barbaud A, Poreaux C, Penven E, Waton J. Occupational protein contact dermatitis. Eur J Dermatol. 2015;25(6):527–34.
60. Haas N, Hamann K, Grabbe J, et al. Expression of the high affinity IgE-receptor on human Langerhans' cells. Elucidating the role of epidermal IgE in atopic eczema. Acta Derm Venereol. 1992;72:271–2.
61. Vester L, Thyssen JP, Menné T, Johansen JD. Occupational food-related hand dermatoses seen over a 10 year period. Contact Dermatitis. 2012;66:264–7.
62. Koch S, Kohl K, Klein E, et al. Skin homing of Langerhans cell precursors: adhesion, chemotaxis, and migration. J Allergy Clin Immunol. 2006;117:163–8.
63. Homey B, Steinhoff M, Ruzicka T, Leung DY. Cytokines and chemokines orchestrate atopic skin inflammation. J Allergy Clin Immunol. 2006;118:178–89.
64. Choi W, Lee J, Kim J, Kim Y, Tae G. Efficient skin permeation of soluble proteins via flexible and functional nano-carrier. J Control Release. 2012;157:272–8.
65. Berardesca E, Barbareschi M, Veraldi S, Pimpinelli N. Evaluation of efficacy of a skin lipid mixture in patients with irritant contact dermatitis, allergic contact dermatitis or atopic dermatitis : a multicenter study. Contact Dermatitis. 2001;45:280–5.
66. Yokouchi M, Kubo A, Kawasaki H, Yoshida K, Ishii K, Furuse M, Amagai M. Epidermal tight junction barrier function is altered by skin inflammation, but not by filaggrin-deficient stratum corneum. J Dermatol Sci. 2015;77(1):28–36.

67. Wang LF, Lin JY, Hsieh KH, Lin RH. Epicutaneous exposure of protein antigen induces a predominant TH2-like response with high IgE production in mice. J Immunol. 1996;156:4079–82.
68. Furuse M, Hata M, Furuse K, Yoshida Y, Haratake A, Sugitani Y, Noda T, Kubo A, Tsukita S. Claudin-based tight junctions are crucial for the mammalian epidermal barrier: a lesson from claudin-1-deficient mice. J Cell Biol. 2002;156:1099–111.
69. I-Lin L, Li-Fang W. Epicutaneous sensitization with protein antigen. Dermatol Sin. 2012;30:154–9.
70. He R, Oyoshi MK, Wang JY, Hodge MR, Jin H, Geha RS. The prostaglandin D2 receptor CRTH2 is important for allergic skin inflammation after epicutaneous antigen challenge. J Allergy Clin Immunol. 2010;126:784.
71. Hänel KH, Pfaff CM, Cornelissen C, Amann PM, Marquardt Y, Czaja K, et al. Control of the physical and antimicrobial skin barrier by an IL-31-IL-1 Signaling network. J Immunol. 2016;196(8):3233–44.
72. Spergel JM, Mizoguchi E, Brewer JP, Martin TR, Bhan AK, Geha RS. Epicutaneous sensitization with protein antigen induces localized allergic dermatitis and hyperresponsiveness to methacholine after single exposure to aerosolized antigen in mice. J Clin Invest. 1998;101:1614.
73. Spergel JM, Mizoguchi E, Oettgen H, Bhan AK, Geha RS. Roles of TH1 and TH2 cytokines in a murine model of allergic dermatitis. J Clin Invest. 1999;103:1103.
74. Bruijnzeel-Koomen C. Food induced skin diseases. Environ Toxicol Pharmacol. 1997;4(1–2):39–41.
75. Inomata N, Nagashima M, Hakuta A, Aihara M. Food allergy preceded by contact urticaria due to the same food: involvement of epicutaneous sensitization in food allergy. Allergol Int. 2015;64(1):73–8.

Immediate Skin Contact Reactions Induced by Proteins

Kayria Muttardi and Emek Kocatürk

Introduction

Proteins are large, naturally occurring molecules with a polymeric structure. Their direct contact with the skin can cause two main types of immediate skin reactions: contact urticaria (CoU) and protein contact dermatitis (PCD). Both encompass contact urticaria syndrome (CUS) [1].

CoU refers to a wheal and flare reaction that occurs within 30 min of direct contact of a substance with the skin. It tends to resolve completely within hours and can be triggered by both proteins and chemicals [2]. PCD is distinct and was initially reported in 1976 by Hjorth and Roed-Peterson [3], who described an eczematous rash on the arms and forearms of Danish food handlers [3]. In this chapter we discuss the presentation and pathogenesis of, and review both the common and more rare protein triggers for, these skin contact reactions.

Epidemiology

Most of our knowledge is based on case reports and case series, and therefore it is difficult to accurately estimate the global incidence of CoU and PCD. It is suggested that CoU is underreported and is likely to be common [4, 5].

Occupational registers provide a good source of data, but it is important to be aware of geographic differences. For instance, data from the Finish Register of Occupational Disease showed that CoU is the second most common presentation of occupational contact disease (29.5%), following contact allergic dermatitis (70.5%) [6]. Cow dander was found to be the most frequently causative protein, attributed to the higher exposure of Finnish farmers to cow dander, as cows are kept inside for most of the year. In comparison, a retrospective study conducted at a clinic specializing in occupational dermatology in Melbourne, Australia, showed a much lower prevalence (8.3%) of occupational CoU, with the main occupations involved being healthcare workers, food handlers, and hairdressers [7]. They also found that atopy was associated with CoU to latex protein and foodstuffs. This is also echoed in other reports in which an association between atopy and PCD was reported as common and noted in 50% of affected patients [7].

Therefore a lower threshold of suspicion for protein-related CUS is required for occupations such as food handlers and those working in

K. Muttardi (✉)
West Hertfordshire NHS Trust, Department of Dermatology, Hertfordshire, UK
e-mail: k.muttardi@doctors.net.uk

E. Kocatürk
Okmeydanı Training and Research Hospital, Department of Dermatology, İstanbul, Turkey

© Springer International Publishing AG, part of Springer Nature 2018
A. M. Giménez-Arnau, H. I. Maibach (eds.), *Contact Urticaria Syndrome*, Updates in Clinical Dermatology, https://doi.org/10.1007/978-3-319-89764-6_7

agriculture, farming, and floriculture, as well as hunters, veterinarians, and biologists [8]. In addition, it is important to consider those with an atopic tendency working in these sectors as being at additional risk of protein-related CUS.

Clinical Presentation and Differential Diagnosis

As mentioned previously, CoU presents with a wheal and flare reaction that occurs within 30 min of direct contact of a substance with the skin and resolves completely within hours. This reaction can be triggered by proteins and nonprotein substances. The patient often provides a good history and, although this is generally limited to the contact area, other sites such as the face or a more generalized urticaria can occur. Chapter 3 discusses this in more detail.

PCD tends to present differently, with signs of a chronic or recurrent eczema that is usually limited to the hands but may extend to the arms, neck, and face [9]. In some patients the eczema only affects the fingertips or pulps ("pulpitis"); localizations can be observed as with garlic and onion, affecting only the first, third, and fourth fingers of the nondominant hand [10]. A chronic paronychia has also been described with erythema, swelling, and skin changes of the proximal nail fold in food handlers [11] and in those exposed to latex [12]. Of course, the presentation of eczema alone includes a wide range of differential diagnoses including atopic eczema, irritant contact dermatitis, and allergic contact dermatitis. Both PCD and allergic contact dermatitis can occur simultaneously; for example, PCD from proteins in onion and garlic and allergic contact dermatitis from the diallyl disulfide present in them [13]. Therefore, a certain index of suspicion is needed by the clinician, especially for those with the occupations outlined here and symptoms that are refractory to topical treatment. Atopy may coexist in 50% of patients presenting with PCD [14].

Some clues from the history include patients who may notice vesiculation and urticaria after being in contact with the causative protein.

Table 7.1 Stages of the "contact urticaria syndrome"

Stage	Clinical manifestation
Stage 1	Localized urticaria: nonspecific symptoms (itching, tingling, burning)
Stage 2	Generalized urticaria with or without angioedema
Stage 3	Extracutaneous involvement (rhinoconjunctivitis, bronchospasm, orolaryngeal or gastrointestinal symptoms)
Stage 4	Anaphylactic shock

Source: Von Krogh and Maibach [18]

Similarly, noticing an improvement of the eczema during holidays or periods off work can be a good clue to an occupationally related exposure.

Other symptoms can also occur depending on the characteristics of the causative protein [15]. Rhinoconjunctivitis and asthma can accompany skin signs in bakers who are constantly exposed to flour [16]. In some patients, gut symptoms and "oral allergy syndrome" can be triggered by a nonimmunological or an immunological IgE-mediated reaction to the causative protein if it is in contact with the mouth or from a cross reaction to a similar protein found in food [11, 17]. Anaphylaxis has also been reported. The systemic symptoms associated with CUS are outlined in Table 7.1, as described by Von Krogh and Maibach [18].

Responsible Protein Triggers

A wide range of causative proteins (molecular weight, 100,300 to several hundred thousands) from different sources have been reported in CoU and PCD. For the purposes of this chapter, they are grouped into four major groups for discussion:

Group 1: fruits, vegetables, spices, plants, and woods
Group 2: animal proteins
Group 3: grains
Group 4: enzymes

Considering the breadth of causative proteins, one can begin to understand the variety of different occupations that can be affected. One occupation that constantly appeared to be among the most affected in epidemiological studies is healthcare workers. The majority of those allergies were caused by latex CoU, when rubber latex powdered glove use was commonplace in the 1970s. We therefore discuss latex separately.

Latex

Epidemiology and Risk Factors

Natural rubber latex (NRL) is a milky, white liquid containing the polymer *cis*-1,4-polyisoprene, derived from the laticifer cells of the rubber tree, *Hevea brasiliensis*. The scope of the problem with NRL is highlighted by prevalence studies, based on skin prick testing, which indicate that 2% to 17% of exposed healthcare workers are sensitized to latex whereas the sensitization rate in the general population is less than 1% [19]. Frequent exposures to latex products are statistically significantly correlated with a higher prevalence of latex allergy in healthcare workers [20]. Other significantly affected groups included hairdressers [21] and veterinarians [22] because of their frequent use of latex gloves. Additionally, a high prevalence of latex allergy is found in patients with spina bifida and other congenital abnormalities who require regular urological catheterization [23, 24].

Among those that are most severely affected are patients with spina bifida, who demonstrate a high prevalence of latex-specific antibodies, making this group at risk of intraoperative anaphylaxis to latex [25]. The most severe reactions were documented in the US in the 1980s when 15 patients died during barium enema examinations from mucosal contact with a latex balloon that was used [26].

Other risk factors apart from the groups outlined here include atopic patients and those with prolonged exposure to NRL with a damaged epidermis, for example, wet hands, irritant eczema [27, 28].

As a consequence, interventions were introduced to manage this problem, including the use of substitutions such as non-powdered and non-latex gloves. This step has resulted in a decline in the incidence of allergy to natural rubber latex since the late 1990s, but the allergy it is still somewhat prevalent and important to consider in certain cohorts [29, 30].

Natural Rubber Latex Proteins and Allergy

NRL fluid from the *Hevea brasiliensis* tree contains 2% proteins [31]. During the manufacture of latex products, the latex undergoes several chemical processes to produce an inert and versatile polyisoprene. The manufacturing process also includes a leaching phase to remove excess chemicals and proteins. Despite this, residues of both chemicals and protein remain on products, causing a source of allergy [31]. It is also suggested that some proteins are changed during the manufacturing process such that they become more allergenic [32]. Furthermore, these NRL protein antigens have been shown to bind to cornstarch in powders that are used to make powdered gloves, therefore posing a higher risk for skin and airway sensitization [33].

Of the approximately 240 polypeptides in NRL derived from *Hevea brasiliensis*, nearly 60 are antigenic, and of those 13 proteins have been well characterized, labeled Hev b1–Hev b13 [34]. These NRL proteins mostly function as defense-related proteins and are known to result in IgE-mediated allergic reactions [34].

These NRL proteins are found in many everyday products including these:

- Rubber gloves
- Balloons
- Condoms and diaphragms
- Rubber bands
- Bandages
- Dental dams

Possible allergy to these products and others containing NRL can present in three ways. The first is with a true allergy to latex protein, which usually refers to positive latex-specific IgE antibodies leading to a type I hypersensitivity reaction in previously sensitized subjects. Patients usually present immediately or shortly after the contact of NRL with the skin, mucosa, or lungs, either with localized hives and itching at the site of contact with NRL protein or a more widespread urticarial rash. NRL proteins can also become aeroallergens by attaching to starch in powders and if inhaled can lead to symptoms such as asthma, rhinoconjunctivitis, and angioedema [25, 26]. In severe cases, anaphylaxis has been documented.

It is also important to note that the severity of IgE-mediated reactions can worsen with repeated exposures and therefore even patients with mild symptoms should avoid NRL exposure in the future. Although gloves are the most common form of exposure, it is important to consider other sources of true latex allergy in patients who give a history of itching and swelling of the mouth following contact with a balloon, itching and swelling of the tongue or oral mucosa after going to the dentist, or itching and swelling after vaginal or rectal examination or after use of a condom [35].

The second way in which allergy to NRL can also present is the form of allergic contact dermatitis, a delayed-type IV hypersensitivity reaction that usually presents 4 to 36 h after exposure to latex. The symptoms are those of eczema and dermatitis, particularly of the hands when in contact with gloves, but dermatitis can be present anywhere on the body at the site of contact (Fig. 7.1a, b). The allergens in this type of reaction are mostly chemicals used in the rubber

manufacturing process rather than the NRL proteins [36]. Thiurams, carbamates, and mercaptobenzothiazole are the most common rubber additive chemicals that cause contact dermatitis. However, some cases of protein contact dermatitis, which can present identically to allergic contact dermatitis to chemicals, have been documented secondary to NRL proteins [37, 38]. Table 7.2 helps to define these clinical entities.

Lastly, some patients may present with irritant contact dermatitis, a form of irritant eczema that usually occurs 12–24 h after contact with rubber gloves but is not a true allergy to NRL protein. The eczema usually affects the hands in a specific pattern with worse eczema between the finger webs. It is usually the result of the following:

- Frequent hand washing
- Incomplete drying
- Contact with chemicals or hand sanitizers
- Sweating and frictional irritation from gloves

Latex Protein Cross-Reactivity

Approximately 50% of latex allergic subjects show laboratory or clinical symptoms of allergy (cross-reactivity) to one or more fruits [35]. This phenomenon is also known as latex–fruit or latex–plant/pollen syndrome, and it occurs as a result of common plant defense-related protein reactions between the latex plant and some fruits [39]. Bananas, avocados, kiwi, and chestnut appear to elicit the most clinical cross-reactivity, but many others such as apple,

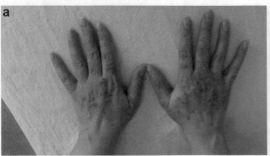
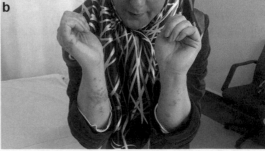

Fig. 7.1 (**a, b**) Type 4 allergy to latex in a housewife. The responsible allergens in this patient were thiuram mix and carba mix. Note the typical involvement of the forearms, which are in contact with the gloves

Table 7.2 Summary of clinical reactions to Natural Rubber Latex (NRL)

Reactions	Mechanism	Clinical presentation	Timing of reaction	Other features	Testing
Latex allergy including immunological contact urticaria (CoU)	Type I (IgE) hypersensitivity	Hives Asthma Rhinoconjunctivitis Angioedema Anaphylaxis	Immediate or shortly after (usually within 30 min)	Can have cross reactions with kiwi, banana, avocado	RAST latex sp. IgE- serum Skin prick testing Rarely provocation testing
Allergic contact dermatitis	Type IV hypersensitivity	Eczema, usually localized but can be widespread	Delayed, usually 4–36 h	–	Patch testing reveals allergy to chemical – most commonly thiuram, carba mixMBT
Protein contact dermatitis (PCD)	Type I and type IV hypersensitivity reactions	Eczema, usually localized but can be widespread Rare cases reported with latex- more common with other proteins	Delayed but can have immediate contact exacerbation, usually presents with recurrent eczema	Occasionally urticarial exacerbation of eczema when in contact with NRL	RAST latex sp. IgE- serum Skin prick testing Patch testing
Irritant contact dermatitis	Nonimmune irritation secondary to friction, sweat, or frequent hand washing	Localized eczema, usually to the hands and particularly worse in between finger webs	Delayed, usually 12–24 h	Usually improves with soap substitute drying hands well and regular moisturizing	Patch testing negative

potato, tomato, and others including some plants have been documented [40]. Clinical manifestations range from urticaria and angioedema to oral allergy syndrome and also in some cases anaphylaxis [41].

Latex Allergy Testing

Thorough NRL testing is important, and a good history seeking risk factors such as atopy, occupation, previous hand dermatitis, and details of symptoms, including their pattern and timing as outlined in Table 7.2, should be sought. Both immediate type I hypersensitivity to latex proteins and allergic contact dermatitis to rubber chemicals can present together in the same patient, and therefore it is important to do both RAST-specific IgE testing to latex protein and patch testing to initially assess a patient. Patients

who have latex-reactive IgE antibody without a clinical history may have cross-reactive antibodies of no clinical significance [42].

If the specific IgE tests are negative and the patient is suspected of having an immediate-type reaction or PCD to latex proteins, then skin prick testing with a dilute latex antigen should be performed. Serological testing for the presence of anti-latex IgE antibody has a sensitivity of 75–90% and specificity of 33–98%, depending on the type of assay and substrate antigen; therefore, a negative test does not exclude latex allergy as this test measures serological antibodies that decrease after allergen avoidance [43]. However, skin prick testing is more sensitive and is therefore the gold standard test for diagnosis, but its drawback is that it does hold a slight risk of anaphylaxis if the patient has a severe allergy to NRL protein. Therefore, very dilute concentrations of latex antigen are used [42].

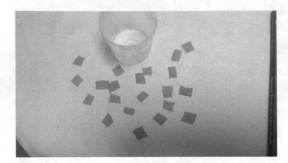

Fig. 7.2 Preparation of latex gloves for skin prick testing. Testing is performed by placing a drop of diluted antigen solution on the skin and gently pricking the skin with a lancet. The results are assessed 15 min after the skin prick and if negative then a more concentrated dilution can be used

Skin prick testing can be conducted with commercial skin prick test extracts (from Stallergenes in France and Lofarma in Italy) and or by using nonstandardized, office-made extracts produced from mixing glove squares with saline and diluting this [44] (Fig. 7.2). Testing is performed by placing a drop of diluted antigen solution on the skin and gently pricking the skin with a lancet. The results are assessed 15 min after the skin prick, and if negative then a more concentrated dilution can be used. If all tests are negative, then irritant contact dermatitis or CoU to other substances should be considered. Rarely, some departments would conduct provocation tests using latex gloves, but as this test is unregulated and has a high risk of anaphylaxis it is not preferred.

Latex Allergy Prevention

Latex is ubiquitous, found in many healthcare and household products, and therefore complete avoidance can be very difficult [45]. Primary prevention to prevent sensitization include a universal shift to using non-powdered latex-free gloves [46]. In addition, replacement of latex-laden medical and home devices with synthetic ones such as those containing chloroprene, nitrile, polyisoprene, and polyurethane [1] has already resulted in a significant decline in latex allergy incidence since the early 1990s, as discussed previously. Secondary prevention and identification of those already having an latex allergy is equally

important. Proper pre-procedural questioning and assessment if necessary to screen for latex allergy are required. Patients should be counseled appropriately for avoidance of NRL products, including condoms, balloons, and latex gloves.

When exposure is unavoidable, patients should be aware of choosing products that have a reduced latex content [47]. They should be counseled for the possibility of latex–fruit syndrome, and for those with a high risk of severe reactions, to advise wearing a medical alert identification and being provided with training on EpiPen use.

At the moment there is no cure for latex allergy, but several studies have demonstrated positive results with sublingual immunotherapy. A review conducted in 2012 by Nettis et al. demonstrated that all but one of eight studies with sublingual immunotherapy demonstrated positive results, but the number of patients remain low, and currently there are no guidelines recommending latex immunotherapy [48]. However, this is still a promising area. In addition as latex allergy is an IgE-mediated condition, the advent of omalizumab (anti-IgE antibody) and its successful off-license use in the treatment of latex allergy has been widely reported, providing a glimpse of hope for the near future for those suffering from severe NRL allergy [49, 50].

Other Protein Triggers

Overall, it is food proteins including those from seafood, meat, fruits, and vegetables that are the most common causes of CoU and PCD in daily life. We discuss other protein triggers for CoU and PCD in four groups as outlined here.

Group 1: Fruits, Vegetables, Plants, and Spices

PCD and CoU to proteinaceous material in fruits and vegetables are particularly seen among people with food-related occupations such as cooks and caterers [51]. Additionally, there have been some presentations among housewives [15]. Typical PCD presentations include eczema particularly affecting the fingertips and finger pulps of the nondominant hand, usually used to hold the foods while cutting or chopping with the dominant hand. However, bilateral hand eczema, perioral eczema, and even more extensive arm and face involvement with dermatitis have been seen (Fig. 7.3a).

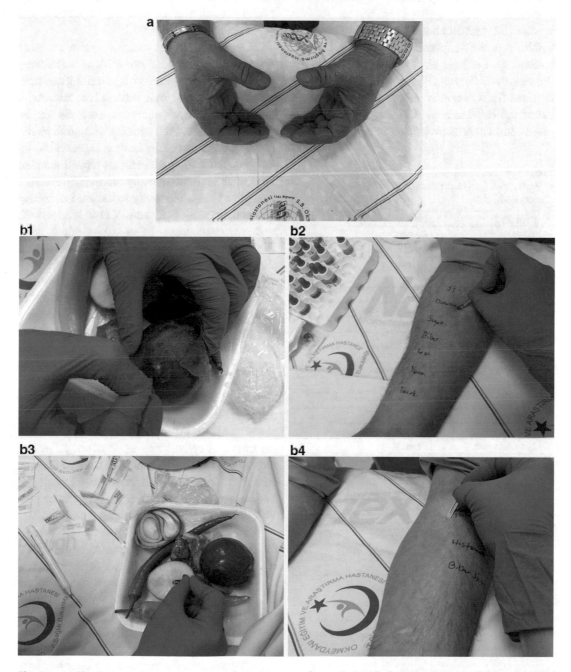

Fig. 7.3 (a) Hand eczema in a cook. In this case positive patch test results were found with thiuram mix and carba mix, but avoiding latex gloves did not resolve the dermatitis. Possible coexistence of protein contact dermatitis was suspected. (b) *1–4:* Skin prick testing with foods the cook mostly handled was performed, yielding negative results. However, it is important to be aware that it is not uncommon for the causative protein to not be detected, as most food-related occupations handle a wide variety of fruit, vegetables, and spices at any given time

Reports of CoU syndrome presenting with wheals and respiratory symptoms including rhinitis, asthma, and conjunctivitis have also been associated with many fruits, vegetables, and spices, including paprika in a biscuit factory worker [52] and artichokes in a worker at a vegetable processing plant [53]. Most of these patients tend to have positive skin prick tests for the reported allergen (Fig. 7.3b, 1–4). Table 7.3 outlines fruits, vegetables, and spices that have been implicated in both PCD and CoU [15]. The more common ones include onion, garlic, ginger,

Table 7.3 Proteins from plants, fruits, vegetables, and spices reported to cause contact urticaria and/or protein contact dermatitis

Protein source	Protein source
Almond	Lemon
Apple	Lettuce
Apricot	Mango
Asparagus	Melon
Banana	Mushroom
Bean	Natural rubber latex
Bishop's weed	Olive
Caraway	Onion
Carrot	Orange
Castor bean	Papaw skin
Cauliflower	Paprika
Celery	Parsley
Chicory	Parsnip
Chives	Peach
Chrysanthemum	Peanuts
Coriander	Pear
Cress	Pecan nuts
Cucumber	Pineapple
Cumin	Potato
Curry	Rocket
Dill	Ruccola
Eggplant	Sapele wood
Endive	Spathe flowers
Fig	Spinach
Garlic	Tomato
Gerbera	Walnut
Green pepper	Watercress
Hazelnut	Watermelon
Hedge mustard	Weeping fig
Horseradish	Yucca
Kiwi	

Source: Adapted from Amaro et al. [15] (see Ref. [15] for full publication details)

shiitake mushrooms, and tomatoes [54, 55]. However, it is important to be aware that it is not uncommon for the causative protein to not be detected because most food-related occupations handle a wide variety of fruit, vegetables, and spices at any given time [56].

Cross-reactivity to proteins can also cause other clinical manifestations such as oral allergy syndrome, which presents with swelling and itching of the lips and oral mucosal surfaces with pollen-related food allergens such as apple, cherry, and hazelnut in patients with birch pollen allergy [57]. This results from cross reactions by allergens from the pathogenesis-related ten protein, which is found in many plants [58]. Another example of cross-reactivity in the clinical setting is in patients with CoU and PCD to lettuce, who tend to cross-react to a Compositae mix. Therefore patch testing for a mix of Compositae plants is now often used as an adjuvant to diagnosing lettuce-induced PCD, because lettuce protein allergens degrade quickly, making testing of lettuce alone unreliable [59].

Plants and flowers have also been reported as causing CoU and PCD symptoms among gardeners, florists, and researchers [60]. Common causes of allergy include weeping fig (*Ficus benjamina*), yucca plant (*Yucca aloifolia*), dragon trees, ceriman, and Paul flower [61]. Decorative plants have also been seen to cause CoU, including tulips, chrysanthemums, and dried flowers, such as *Limonium titanium* [62]. In addition, a case of PCD to sapele wood has been reported in a carpenter, adding this occupation to those possibly at risk of plant protein-related allergy [63].

When investigating patients for CoU from food proteins, it is also important to be aware that nonimmune-mediated CoU can occur with certain foods by producing a nonimmunological release of vasoactive substances such as histamine and prostaglandins directly from mast cells, leading to hives and itching [18]. These nonimmune CoU reactions are not usually directed against plant proteins but tend to occur more with food flavorings, fragrances, and preservative agents (benzoic acid, sorbic acid, balsam of Peru, cinnamic acid) [64].

Group 2: Animal Proteins

Proteins from animals are a major cause of CoU and PCD, especially among farmers, butchers, slaughterhouse workers, veterinarians, and those working with animals in research and in zoos [65]. The exact prevalence is unknown and varies regionally depending on the local custom and foods. Data from the Finnish register of occupational disease suggest that approximately 50% of occupational CoU and PCD is related to animal proteins [66]. The allergens from most mammals, milk, and some insects are lipocalins, which are proteins that serve many functions [65, 67]. These proteins have a degree of homology among species, making them very weakly allergenic, and if triggering an immune response they do so via the Th-2 and specific IgE immune response [65, 68].

Veterinarians are at risk of CoU and respiratory symptoms from exposure to proteins in animal dander, saliva, semen, and amniotic fluid during procedures [22, 69]. Laboratory animals including rat, mice, guinea pigs, and hamsters have also been reported to cause CoU and PCD in researchers. Interestingly, researchers are more affected than pet keepers of the same animals [70, 71]. It is suggested that this may be because researchers are exposed to more saliva and blood from animals in a similar way to veterinarians [65]. Zookeepers and breeders are also at additional risk of CoU and PCD from insects, who carry potent protein allergens in their midgut and wings [72]. Rarer cases include a case of CoU in a zookeeper to giraffe dander [73] and five cases of PCD to pet ferrets [9].

Proteins from fish and other seafood species are the most common cause of occupational hand dermatitis among cooks [55, 74]. In many cases the implicated seafood is tolerated when taken orally as food but triggers CoU and respiratory symptoms when in contact with the skin [75]. Cases of fishing bait maggots (*Nereis diversicolor*, *Calliphora vomitoria*, *Chironomus thummi thummi*, and *Lumbrineris impatiens*) as a cause of CoU and PCD in fishermen have also been described [15].

Edible meats including poultry, lamb, cow, pork, and also dairy products have all been reported to cause CoU and PCD, with pork being the most commonly reported meat [65, 76]. Table 7.4 summarizes animal proteins reported in association with CoU and PCD.

Group 3: Proteins from Grains

Of the grain proteins documented to cause PCD (Table 7.5), wheat and rye proteins are the most common allergens, presenting largely in bakers [77]. IgE-mediated asthma (bakers asthma) and rhinitis to wheat protein have also been widely documented. Although the exact mechanism remains unknown, several key wheat allergens, wheat 27-kDa allergen, peroxidase, and purple acid phosphatase have been identified as causative [78]. Another phenomenon that is still rare but increasing are cases of CoU syndrome, wheat allergy, and wheat-dependent exercise-induced urticaria and anaphylaxis in association with hydrolyzed wheat protein (Crotein Q, trimonium hydrolyzed collagen), which are found in various cosmetics (creams, shampoos, soaps) [79–81].

Group 4: Enzymes

Enzymes are widely used in many industry processes and household products. Therefore, most cases of CoU and PCD reactions related to enzymes are occupational among soap makers, bakers, and people working with chemicals in factories [83]. However, there have been a few cases related to enzyme exposure from household products. Overall, IgE-mediated asthma and respiratory symptoms are more common presentations than skin complaints in association with both occupational and nonoccupational enzyme exposure [83].

α-Amylase-related reactions are the most widely reported among the enzymes. Bacterial and fungal α-amylases are used in the baking industry to enhance carbohydrate fermentation by yeast [84]. As a consequence, cases of PCD to alpha-amylase have been reported in bakers,

Table 7.4 Proteins from animals reported to cause contact urticaria and/or protein contact dermatitis

Protein source	Protein source
Amniotic fluid	Seafood
	Codfish
	Mackerel
	Horse mackerel
	Plaice
	Herring
	Perch
	Rainbow trout
	Salmon
	Baby squid
	White fish
	Whitebait
	Whiting
	Angler fish
	Tuna fish
	Fluke
	Dory
	Fish mix
	Haddock
	Red mullet
	Sea bream
	Sole
	Sea eel
	Cuttlefish
	Abalone
	Clam
	Mussel
	Oyster
	Shrimp
	Lobster
	Scampi
	Prawn
	Shellfish
	Crab
	Squid
Amphibian serum	Seminal fluid
Blood	Skin
Pig	Chicken
Cow	Turkey
Lamb	
Horse	
Brains – Frog	Wool
Cockroach	Worms/Larvae
	Nereis diversicolor
	Calliphora vomitoria
	Midge larvae
	Lumbrineris impatiens

(continued)

Table 7.4 (continued)

Protein source	Protein source
Dairy products	
Cow's milk	
Dog's milk	
Cheese	
Cheese products	
Dander	
Cow	
Giraffe	
Egg yolk	
Hydrolyzed collagen	
Liver	
Calf/Ox	
Chicken	
Lamb	
Locust	
Meat	
Cow	
Pork	
Chicken	
Horse	
Lamb	
Frog	
Parasites	
Anisakis simplex	
Placenta, calf	
Pig	
Blood	
Gut	
Mesenteric fat	
Saliva	

Source: Adapted from Amaro et al. [15] (see Ref. [15] for full reference details)

Table 7.5 Proteins from grains reported to cause contact urticaria and/or protein contact dermatitis

Protein source	Protein source
Rye	Oat
Wheat	Cornstarch
Barley	Rice [82]

Source: Adapted from Amaro et al. [15]

Table 7.6   Enzymes reported to cause contact urticaria and /or protein contact dermatitis

Enzyme	Uses
α-Amylase	Processes for baking and brewing Starch processing Laundry detergent Biofuel production Textile industry
Glucosamylase	Baking and brewing
Lactase	Dairy industry
Lysozyme	Pharmaceutical industry (sore throat remedies, infant formulas, contact lens solutions)
Cellulase	Laundry detergent Coffee bean drying Pulp and paper industry Biofuel production
Xylanase	Baking Wood pulp bleaching Plant fiber degumming Poultry food additive
Collagenase	Topical wound debridement treatments
Protease	Baking and brewing Laundry detergents Meat processing
Papain	Baking and brewing Laundry detergents Dairy industry Meat tenderizing Contact lenses cleaning Silk refining Leather industry
Lipase	Cheese making Laundry detergents Paper industry
Catalase	Food industry Dairy and cheese industry

Source: Adapted from Table 19.1 by Stanciu et al. [83]

some also presenting with IgE-mediated asthma (bakers asthma).

Aside from amylase, other enzymes have been reported to cause CoU, PCD, and asthma; the most important ones are summarized alongside their uses in Table 7.6 [83]. Rarer interesting cases include seven cases of women developing CoU and anaphylaxis from a vaginal suppository containing lysozyme [85], a case of recurrent periorbital edema related to a papain-containing contact lens solution [86], and four factory workers with CoU and respiratory problems secondary to xylanase and cellulase [87, 88].

New Sources of Protein Exposure

The rapid evolvement of the beauty industry in recent years has led to an increase in cases of nonoccupational CoU and PCD from proteins [89]. Detailed questioning of patients about cosmetic practices is crucial as the source of the allergen maybe found in the cosmetic product or procedure. A recent fatal case of anaphylaxis relating to high concentrations of NRL in bonding glues for hair extensions was reported in a 28-year-old who was known to be allergic to nuts and had a positive skin prick test to latex [90].

Creams are also increasingly becoming a source of CoU and PCD. A recent report published 18 cases of wheat allergy and wheat-dependent exercise-induced anaphylaxis to hydrolyzed wheat proteins in soap, noting also associated contact urticaria in these patients [91]. These cases provide good evidence to support the theory of epicutaneous sensitization of proteins [92]. Further studies have also demonstrated that in patients with contact urticaria and allergy to certain hydrolyzed wheat proteins, cross reactions with other hydrolyzed wheat proteins can occur, which can be life threatening in those with severe CUS and anaphylaxis [93].

Two more recent examples of cosmetic sources of protein contact reaction are a case of CoU caused by alpha-lactalbumin from mare's milk in a cosmetic cream [94] and the first case of CSU stage 3 secondary to honey that caused sensitization during a skin care treatment [95].

A group in France recently also published an interesting case of eyelid contact dermatitis caused by hydroxypropyl tetrahydropyrantriol (trade name, Pro-Xylane) [96], which is a sugar–protein hybrid made from xylose sugars found in beech trees. It was originally developed by Lancôme in 2006 and has since been used widely in anti-aging creams and serums for reason of its known effect of stimulating glycosaminoglycans; however, no other cases have been described so far [96].

Some of the allergenic proteins from plant, fruit, vegetable, animal, and fish sources are yet to be identified. In addition, it is still not fully understood as to why the same protein allergen can produce two different immediate contact reactions.

Diagnosis

A thorough and detailed history is the key first step in making a diagnosis of CoU and PCD. In addition, it helps focus earlier testing to the key allergens. For CoU, it is important to first understand if this reaction to proteins is occurring via an immunological IgE mechanism or a nonimmunological mechanism. In vitro, specific RAST testing can detect cases of IgE-mediated allergy, but it is only available for a few proteins including latex. Beyond that skin prick testing (in vivo) is the gold standard for diagnosis. If this is negative, then a skin provocation test can be undertaken. However, skin provocation testing is less standardized and less predictable and therefore associated with a risk of serious reactions. Provocation testing should only be performed by trained individuals with resuscitation equipment available [8].

Patch testing can also be done to exclude allergic contact dermatitis from other chemicals, which can mimic or coexist with PCD. Further details on diagnosis of CoU and PCD are discussed in Chapters 10 and 11.

Management

The first step of management of CoU and CPD is to identify the correct allergen and counsel patients on complete avoidance of the triggering allergen [14]. Advice should also include risks of cross reactions such as latex–fruit syndrome.

Avoidance tends to result in improvement of symptoms; however, occasionally complete avoidance may be difficult and can often require the patient to change their occupation or role within their job. Second-generation antihistamines can help alleviate urticaria symptoms. For PCD, which usually affects the hands, topical corticosteroids and moisturizers can help treat the dermatitis until avoidance is maintained.

References

1. Gimenez-Arnau A, Maibach HI. Contact urticaria syndrome. Florida: Taylor & Francis Group, LLC; 2015.
2. Warner RM, Taylor S, Yung-Hian L. Agents causing contact urticaria. Clin Dermatol. 1997;15:623–35.
3. Hjorth N, Roed-Petersen J. Occupational protein contact dermatitis in food handlers. Contact Dermatitis. 1976;2:28–42.
4. Elpern DJ. The syndrome of immediate reactivities (contact urticaria syndrome). A historical study from a dermatology practice. I. Age, sex, race and putative substances. Hawaii Med J. 1985;44:426–39.

5. Nilsson E. Contact sensitivity and urticaria in "wet" work. Contact Dermatitis. 1985;13:321–8.
6. Kanerva L, Jolanki R, Toikkanen J, Estlander T. Statistics on occupational contact urticaria. In: Smita A, Lahti A, Maibach HI, editors. Contact urticaria syndrome. Boca Raton: CRC Press; 1997. p. 57–69.
7. Williams JD, Lee AY, Matheson MC, Frowen KE, Noonan AM, Nixon RL. Occupational contact urticaria: Australian data. Br J Dermatol. 2008;159:125–31.
8. Johansen JD, Lepoittevin JP, Thyssen JP. Quick guide to contact dermatitis. Berlin Heidelberg: Springer; 2016.
9. Amsler E, Bayrou O, Pecquet C, Francès C. Five cases of contact dermatitis to a trendy pet. Dermatology. 2012;224(4):292–4.
10. Janssens V, Morren M, Dooms-Goossens A, Degreef H. Protein contact dermatitis: myth or reality? Br J Dermatol. 1995;132:1–6.
11. Tosti A, Guerra L, Morelli R, Bardazzi F, Fanti PA. Role of foods in the pathogenesis of chronic paronychia. J Am Acad Dermatol. 1992;27:706–10.
12. Kanerva L. Occupational protein contact dermatitis and paronychia from natural rubber latex. J Eur Acad Dermatol Venereol. 2000;14:504–6.
13. Laing ME, Barry J, Buckley AM, Murphy GM. Immediate and delayed hypersensitivity reactions to food and latex in a chef. Contact Dermatitis. 2006;55:193–4.
14. Doutre M-S. Occupational contact urticaria and protein contact dermatitis. Eur J Dermatol. 2005;15:419–24.
15. Amaro C, Goossens A. Immunological occupational contact urticaria and contact dermatitis from proteins: a review. Contact Dermatitis. 2008;58:67–75.
16. Morren M, Janssens V, Dooms-Goossens A, et al. A – Amylase, a flour additive: an important cause of protein contact dermatitis in bakers. J Am Acad Dermatol. 1993;29:723–8.
17. Hernández-Bel P, de la Cuadra J, García R, Alegre V. Protein contact dermatitis: review of 27 cases. Actas Dermosifiliogr. 2011;102(5):336–43.
18. Von Krogh C, Maibach HI. The contact urticaria syndrome. An update review. J Am Acad Dermatol. 1981;5:328–42.
19. Liss GM, Sussman GL. Latex sensitization: occupational versus general population prevalence rates. Am J Ind Med. 1999;35:196–200.
20. Liss GM, Sussman GL, Deal K, et al. Latex allergy: epidemiological study of 1351 hospital workers. Occup Environ Med. 1997;54:335–42.
21. Valsecchi R, Leghissa P, Zerbinati N. Contact urticaria from latex in hairdressers. Eur J Inflamm. 2003;1:143–4.
22. Valsecchi R, Leghissa P, Cortinovis R. Occupational contact dermatitis and contact urticaria in veterinarians. Contact Dermatitis. 2003;49:167–8.

23. Eiwegger T, Dehlinke E, Schwindt J, et al. Early exposure to latex products mediates latex sensitization in spina bifida but not in other diseases with comparable latex exposure rates. Clin Exp Allergy. 2006;36:1242–6.
24. Ylitalo L. Natural rubber latex allergy in children, PhD Thesis, Acta Universitatis Tamperensis 719, University of Tampere, Tampere, Finland, 2000.
25. Taylor JS, Erkek E. Latex allergy: diagnosis and management. Dermatol Ther. 2004;17:289–301.
26. Fezcko PJ, Simms SM, Bakirci N. Fatal hypersensitivity during a barium enema. Am J Roentgenol. 1989;153:276–7.
27. Niggemann B, Kulig M, Bergmann R, et al. Development of latex allergy in children up to 5 years of age – a retrospective analysis of risk factors. Pediatr Allergy Immunol. 1999;9:36–9.
28. Ylitalo L, Turjanmaa K, Palosuo T, et al. Natural rubber latex allergy in children who had not undergone surgery and children who had undergone multiple operations. J Allergy Clin Immunol. 1997;100:606–12.
29. Bensefa-Colas L, Telle-Lamberton M, Faye S, Bourrain JL, Crépy MN, Lasfargues G, Choudat D, RNV3P members, Momas I. Occupational contact urticaria: lessons from the French National Network for Occupational Disease Vigilance and Prevention (RNV3P). Br J Dermatol. 2015;173(6):1453–61.
30. Ibler KS, Jemec GB, Garvey LH, Agner T. Prevalence of delayed-type and immediate-type hypersensitivity in healthcare workers with hand eczema. Contact Dermatitis. 2016;75(4):223–9.
31. Mellström GA, Boman AS. Gloves: types, materials, and manufacturing. In: Mellström GA, Wahlberg JE, Maibach HL, editors. Protective gloves for occupational use. Boca Raton: CRC Press; 1994.
32. European Commission. Health and Consumer Protection Directorate General (internet).Opinion on Natural Rubber Latex Allergy 27th June 2000. Available from: http://ec.europa.eu/health/ph_risk/committees/scmp/documents/out31_en.pdf. Accessed on 8 Aug 2017.
33. Yeang HY. Natural rubber allergens: new developments. Curr Opin Clin Immunol. 2004;4:99–10.
34. American Latex Allergy Association (internet). Latex allergens registered by WHO-IUIS. Available from http://latexallergyresources.org/sites/default/files/article-attachments/sec9_latexAllergens.pdf. Accessed 11 Aug 2017.
35. Asthma and Allergy Foundation of America (internet). Latex allergy. http://www.aafa.org/page/latex-allergy.aspx. Accessed 11 Aug 2017.
36. Shah D, Chowdhury MMU. Rubber allergy. Clin Dermatol. 2011;29:278–86.
37. Barbaud A, Poreaux C, Penven E, Waton J. Occupational protein contact dermatitis. Eur J Dermatol. 2015;25(6):527–34.
38. Kanerva L, Alanko K, Jolanki R, Kanervo K, Susitaival P, Estlander T. The dental face mask – the

most common cause of work-related face dermatitis in dental nurses. Contact Dermatitis. 2001;44:261–2.

39. Dias-Perales A, Sanchez-Monge R, Blanco C, et al. What is the role of the hevein-like domain of fruit class I chitinases in their allergenic capacity? Clin Exp Allergy. 2002;32:448–54.

40. Blanco C. Latex-fruit syndrome. Curr Allergy Asthma Rep. 2003;3:47–53.

41. Soares J, Dias A, Peixoto S, Pereira A, Quaresma M. Particularities in a child with cashew nut allergy. Glob Pediatr Health. 2014;1:2333794X14552898 (Epub).

42. Poley GE, Slater JE, HS N. Latex allergy from the current reviews of allergy and immunology. J Allergy Clin Immunol. 2000;105(N6, 1):1054–62.

43. Hamilton RG, Biagini RE, Krieg EF. Diagnostic performance of food and drug administration–cleared serologic assays for natural rubber latex-specific IgE antibody: the multi-center latex skin testing study task force. J Allergy Clin Immunol. 1999;103:925–30.

44. Hamilton RG, Adkinson NF Jr. Natural rubber latex skin testing reagents: safety and diagnostic accuracy of non-ammoniated, ammoniated and latex glove extracts. J Allergy Clin Immunol. 1996;98:872–83.

45. Jezierski M. Creating a latex-safe environment: Riddle Memorial Hospital's response to protect patients and employees. J Emerg Nurs. 1997;23:191–8.

46. Crippa M, Belleri L, Mistrello G, et al. Prevention of latex allergy among healthcare workers and in general population: latex protein content in devices commonly used in hospitals and general practice. Int Arch Occup Environ Health. 2006;79:550–7.

47. Heilman DK, Jones RT, Swanson MC, Yunginger JW. A prospective, controlled study showing that rubber gloves are the major contributor to latex aeroallergen levels in the operating room. J Allergy Clin Immunol. 1996;98:325–30.

48. Nettis E, Delle Donne P, Di Leo E, et al. Latex immunotherapy: state of the art. Ann Allergy Asthma Immunol. 2012;109:160.

49. Moscato G, Pala G, Sastre J. Specific immunotherapy and biological treatments for occupational allergy. Curr Opin Allergy Clin Immunol. 2014;14(6):576–81.

50. Leynadier F, Doudou O, Gaouar H, et al. Effect of omalizumab in health care workers with occupational latex allergy. J Allergy Clin Immunol. 2004;113:360–1.

51. Wakelin SH. Contact urticaria. Clin Exp Dermatol. 2001;26:132–6.

52. Foti C, Carino M, Cassano N, et al. Occupational contact urticaria from paprika. Contact Dermatitis. 1997;37:135.

53. Quirce S, Tabar AI, Olaguibel JM, Cuevas M. Occupational contact urticaria syndrome caused by globe artichoke (Cynara scolymus). J Allergy Clin Immunol. 1996;97:710–1.

54. Aalto-Korte K, Susitaival P, Kaminska R, Makinen-Kiljunen S. Occupational protein contact dermatitis from shiitake mushroom and demonstration of shiitake-specific immunoglobulin E. Contact Dermatitis. 2005;53:211–3.

55. Lukacs J, Schliemann S, Elsner P. Occupational contact urticaria caused by food- a systematic clinical review. Contact Dermatitis. 2016;75:195–204.

56. Brancaccio RR, Alvarez MS. Contact allergy to food. Dermatol Ther. 2004;17:302–13.

57. Webber CM, England RW. Oral allergy syndrome: a clinical, diagnostic, and therapeutic challenge. Ann Allergy Asthma Immunol. 2010;104:101–8.

58. Breiteneder H, Ebner C. Molecular and biochemical classification of plant-derived food allergens. J Allergy Clin Immunol. 2000;106:27–36.

59. Paulsen E, Andersen KE. Lettuce contact allergy. Contact Dermatitis. 2015;74:67–75.

60. Paulsen E, Skov PS, Andersen KE. Immediate skin and mucosal symptoms from pot plants and vegetables in gardeners and greenhouse workers. Contact Dermatitis. 1998;39:166–70.

61. Kanerva L, Estlander T, Petman L, Mäkinen-Kiljunen S. Occupational allergic contact urticaria to yucca (Yucca aloifolia), weeping fig (Ficus benjamina), and spathe flower (Spathiphyllum wallisii). Allergy. 2001;56:1008–11.

62. Quirce S, García-Figueroa B, Olaguíbel JM, Muro MD, Tabar AI. Occupational asthma and contact urticaria from dried flowers of Limonium tataricum. Allergy. 1993;48(4):285–90.

63. Alvarez-Cuesta C, Gala Ortiz G, Rodrı'guez Dı'az E, et al. Occupational asthma and IgE-mediated contact dermatitis from sapele wood. Contact Dermatitis. 2004;51:88–98.

64. Lahti A. Non-immunologic contact urticaria. Acta Derm Venereol Suppl (Stockh). 1980;Suppl 91:1–49.

65. Susitaival P. Animals and animal products as a cause of contact urticaria and protein contact dermatitis. In: Gimenez-Arnau A, Maibach HI, editors. Contact urticaria syndrome. Florida: Taylor & Francis Group, LLC; 2015. p. 141–50.

66. Finnish Institute of Occupational Diseases. Register of occupational diseases. Information of the register available at https://osha.europa.eu/en/topics/osm/reports/finnish_system_009.stm. Accessed 24 Aug 2017.

67. Virtanen T, Zeiler T, Mäntyjärvi R. Important animal allergens are lipocalin proteins: why are they allergenic? Int Arch Allergy Immunol. 1999;120:247–58.

68. Virtanen T, Kinnunen T, Rytkönen-Nissinen M. Mammalian lipocalin allergens – insight into their enigmatic allergenity. Clin Exp Allergy. 2011;42:494–504.

69. Susitaival P, Kirk J, Schenker M. Self-reported hand dermatitis in California Veterinarians. Am J Contact Dermat. 2001;12:103–8.

70. Aoyama K, Ueda A, Manda F, et al. Allergy to laboratory animals: an epidemiological study. Br J Ind Med. 1992;49(1):41–7.

71. Bhabha FK, Nixon R. Occupational exposure to laboratory animals causing a severe exacerbation of atopic eczema. Autralas J Dermatol. 2012;53(2):155–6.

72. Lopata A, Fenemore B, Jeebhay M, Gäde G, Potter P. Occupational allergy in laboratory workers caused by the African migratory grasshopper Locusta migratoria. Allergy. 2005;60:200–5.

73. Herzinger T, Scharrer E, Placzek M, Przybilla B. Contact urticaria to giraffe hair. Int Arch Allergy Immunol. 2005;138:324–7.

74. Vester L, Thyssen JP, Menné T, Johansen JD. Occupational food-related hand dermatoses seen over a 10-year period. Contact Dermatitis. 2012;66:264–70.

75. Onesimo R, Giorgio V, Pili S, et al. Isolated contact urticaria caused by immunoglobulin E-mediated fish allergy. Isr Med Assoc J. 2012;14(1):11–3.

76. Jovanovic M, Oliwiecki S, Beck MH. Occupational contact urticaria from beef associated with hand eczema. Contact Dermatitis. 1992;27(3):188–9.

77. Houba R, Heederik D, Doekes G. Wheat sensitization and work-related symptoms in the baking industry are preventable. An epidemiologic study. Am J Respir Crit Care Med. 1998;158(5 Pt 1):1499–503.

78. Matsuo H, Uemura M, Yorozuya M, Adachi A, Morita E. Identification of IgE-reactive proteins in patients with wheat protein contact dermatitis. Contact Dermatitis. 2010;63(1):23–30.

79. Coenraads PJ. Sensitization potential of hydrolysed wheat proteins. Contact Dermatitis. 2016;74(6):321–2.

80. Pootongkam S, Nedorost S. Oat and wheat as contact allergens in personal care products. Dermatitis. 2013;24(6):291–5.

81. Fukutomi Y, Taniguchi M, Nakamura H, Akiyama K. Epidemiological link between wheat allergy and exposure to hydrolyzed wheat protein in facial soap. Allergy. 2014;69(10):1405–11.

82. Di Lernia V, Albertini G, Bisighini G. Immunologic contact urticaria syndrome from raw rice. Contact Dermatitis. 1992;27:196.

83. Stanciu M, Sassville D. Contact urticaria, dermatitis and respiratory allergy caused by enzymes. In: Gimenez-Arnau A, Maibach HI, editors. Contact urticaria syndrome. Florida: Taylor & Francis Group, LLC; 2015. p. 169–88.

84. Moreno-Ancillo A, Domínguez-Noche C, Gil-Adrados AC, Cosmes PM. Bread eating induced oral angioedema due to alpha-amylase allergy. J Investig Allergol Clin Immunol. 2004;14:346–7.

85. Pichler WJ, Campi P. Allergy to lysozyme/egg white-containing vaginal suppositories. Ann Allergy. 1992;69(6):521–5.

86. Chaplin MF, Bucke C. Enzyme technology. Cambridge: Cambridge University Press; 1990. p. 280.

87. Kanerva L, Tarvainen K. Allergic contact dermatitis and contact urticaria from cellulolytic enzymes. Am J Contact Dermatitis. 1990;1:244–5.

88. Tarvainen K, Kanerva L, Tupasela O, Grenquist-Nordén B, Jolanki R, et al. Allergy from cellulase and xylanase enzymes. Clin Exp Allergy. 1991;21:609–15.

89. Verhulst L, Goossens A. Cosmetic components causing contact urticaria: a review and update. Contact Dermatitis. 2016;75(6):333–44.

90. Pumphrey RS, Duddridge M, Norton J. Fatal latex allergy. J Allergy Clin Immunol. 2001;107:558.

91. Kobayashi T, Ito T, Kawakami H, Fuzishiro K, Hirano H, Okubo Y, Tsuboi R. Eighteen cases of wheat allergy and wheat-dependent exercise-induced urticaria/anaphylaxis sensitized by hydrolyzed wheat protein in soap. Int J Dermatol. 2015;54(8):e302–5.

92. Inomata N, Nagashima M, Hakuta A, Aihara M. Food allergy preceded by contact urticaria due to the same food: involvement of epicutaneous sensitization in food allergy. Allergol Int. 2015;64(1):73–8.

93. Nakamura M, Yagami A, Hara K, Sano-Nagai A, Kobayashi T, Matsunaga K. Evaluation of the cross-reactivity of antigens in Glupearl 19S and other hydrolysed wheat proteins in cosmetics. Contact Dermatitis. 2016;74:346–52.

94. Verhulst L, Kerre S, Goossens A. The unsuspected power of mare's milk. Contact Dermatitis. 2016;74:376–7.

95. Katayama M, Inomata N, Inagawa N, et al. A case of contact urticaria syndrome stage 3 after honey ingestion, induced by epicutaneous sensitization during skin care with honey. Contact Dermatitis. 2016;74:189–91.

96. Assier A, Wolkenstein P, Chosidow O. First case of contact dermatitis caused by hydroxypropyl tetrahydropyrantriol used in an anti-ageing cream. Contact Dermatitis. 2017;1:60–1.

Immediate Skin Contact Reactions Induced by Chemicals

Elena Giménez-Arnau

Introduction

Chemicals That Trigger Nonimmunological and Immunological Contact Urticaria

Immediate skin contact reactions are characterized by the instantaneous development of itchy flares, wheals, and/or dermatitis on the skin following external contact with a substance. These reactions usually manifest as contact urticaria (CoU), contact urticaria syndrome (CUS), or protein contact dermatitis (PCD) [1]. CoU generally appears within approximately 30 min and clears completely within hours, without residual signs of irritation. An ever-expanding list of causes has been reported, of which most are proteins (molecular weight 10,000 to several hundred thousand daltons), but also chemical compounds of low molecular weight (LMW) (<1,000 Da).

LMW chemical agents can be responsible for immediate contact skin symptoms in the different categories of CoU. According to the underlying mechanisms involved, CoU is classified as nonimmunological or immunological. A third category exists for reactions with mixed features or undetermined pathomechanisms [2]. This third category is much less common and is not covered herein.

Nonimmunological CoU (NICoU) is the most common form of the disease. NICoU occurs without prior exposure to an eliciting substance and without previous sensitization. Chemicals inducing NICoU are frequently encountered in our environment as biocides or preservatives, fragrances, and flavorings in cosmetic products, toiletries, drugs, topical medicaments, and foodstuffs [3, 4], although other miscellaneous chemicals and metals can also be responsible for these reactions. Most individuals react to these substances with local erythema and/or edema within 45 min after application, albeit with widely varying intensities of skin reaction [5]. The pathogenesis is not clearly understood but seems to involve the release of vasogenic mediators without involvement of immunological processes (Fig. 8.1a). Because of the lack of response to antihistamines and positive responses to acetylsalicylic acid and nonsteroidal anti-inflammatory drugs, it has been proposed that the physiopathology involves prostaglandin release from the epidermis rather than histamine release from mast cells [6, 7].

Conversely, immunological CoU (ICoU) is an immediate type I hypersensitivity reaction, mediated by allergen-specific immunoglobulin (Ig) E in previously sensitized individuals [2]. Thus, ICoU requires sensitization and appears after repeated contacts with the trigger substance. It is

E. Giménez-Arnau (✉)
Dermatochemistry Laboratory, Institut de Chimie de Strasbourg (CNRS UMR 7177), Université de Strasbourg, Strasbourg, France
e-mail: egimenez@unistra.fr

© Springer International Publishing AG, part of Springer Nature 2018
A. M. Giménez-Arnau, H. I. Maibach (eds.), *Contact Urticaria Syndrome*, Updates in Clinical Dermatology, https://doi.org/10.1007/978-3-319-89764-6_8

Fig. 8.1 General
mechanisms of
nonimmunological
contact urticaria
(NICoU) (**a**) and
immunological contact
urticaria (ICoU) (**b**)

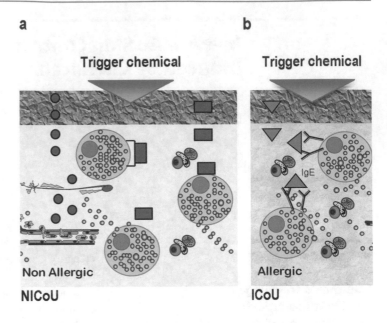

more frequent in people with previous atopic symptoms. Histamine release is the major mechanism of action observed. This mechanism includes allergen penetration through the epidermis and binding to IgE at the surface of mast cells and basophiles, causing degranulation and release of histamine and other vasoactive substances such as prostaglandins, leukotrienes, and kinins [8] (Fig. 8.1b). In rare cases, IgG or IgM has been also incriminated. The consequences are potentially more serious than for NICoU, as reactions may not remain localized to the area of contact, and generalized urticaria, or even involvement of organs such as the respiratory and gastrointestinal tract, may follow and lead to anaphylactic shock.

A large number of causes have been documented as producing ICoU. The most common agents inducing ICoU are food proteins (animal or vegetal), animal proteins, and natural rubber latex, and these have been largely reviewed [9, 10]. However, LMW chemicals including drugs, biocides, and preservatives, and metals or industrial compounds can also produce ICoU. These chemicals are very often present in drugs, cosmetics [11], and industrial preparations. Extensive lists of proteins and chemicals are

reported as causing ICoU, but only some of these being reported as occupational [2, 10, 12]. Most publications about CoU concern case reports or small series, and epidemiological studies are scarce. However, some data indicate that ICoU is not rare, although frequently underestimated. The ultimate evidence corroborating that a compound is responsible for ICoU is the measurement of specific IgE in the serum of the patient by the radioallergosorbent test (RAST) whenever possible. The patient's serum is incubated with the agent bound to a solid phase, and the amount of specific IgE recognizing and binding to the agent is quantified with radiolabeled anti-IgE [13]. Determination of specific IgE by RAST will confirm type I hypersensitivity, but its ordinary detection is restricted to some compounds, particularly when they are nonproteinaceous.

Table 8.1 summarizes the most often reported LMW chemical agents producing immediate nonimmunological and immunological skin reactions [1, 12]. The most important LMW chemicals responsible for NICoU and ICoU are described in this chapter and classified into the major families of products, fragrances and cosmetic ingredients, biocides and preservatives and drugs, together with other categories.

Table 8.1 Chemical compounds reported as triggering nonimmunological contact urticaria (NICoU) and immunological contact urticaria (ICoU) skin reactions [1, 12]

Compound name	Product category	NICoU	ICoU	Unclassified[a]
Acetic acid	Other			×
Acetyl acetone	Other		×	
Acetylsalicylic acid	Drugs			×
Acid anhydrides	Other		×	
Acrylic acid[b]	Other		×	
Acrylic monomers	Other		×	
Aescin[b]	Drugs		×	
Albendazole	Drugs		×	
Alcohols (amyl, ethyl, propyl, isopropyl, benzyl)	Biocides-preservatives			×
Aliphatic polyamide	Other		×	
Allantoin[b]	Fragrances-cosmetics		×	
Aluminum (metal)	Other			×
Aminophenazone	Drugs			×
p-Aminodiphenylamine (dye)	Other		×	
Aminothiazole[b]	Other		×	
Ammonia	Biocides-preservatives		×	
Amoxicillin	Drugs			×
Ampicillin	Drugs		×	
α-Amyl cinnamaldehyde	Fragrances-cosmetics	×		
Anisyl alcohol	Fragrances-cosmetics	×		
Aziridine	Other		×	
Azithromycin	Drugs		×	
Bacitracin	Drugs		×	
Balsam of Peru	Fragrances-cosmetics	×		
Basic blue 99 (hair dye)	Other		×	
Benzaldehyde	Fragrances-cosmetics	×		
Benzocaine	Drugs			×
Benzoic acid	Biocides-preservatives	×		
Benzonitrile	Other		×	
Benzophenone	Fragrances-cosmetics	×		
Benzoyl peroxide	Drugs		×	
Bisphenol A	Other		×	
Bronopol	Biocides-preservatives	×		
Butylated hydroxytoluene[b]	Biocides-preservatives		×	
Butylhydroxytoluol	Other			×
Camphor	Biocides-preservatives	×		
Capsaicin	Drugs	×		
Carbamates	Other			×
Cassia oil	Fragrances-cosmetics	×		
Cephalosporins	Drugs		×	
Cetyl alcohol (emulsifier)	Fragrances-cosmetics			×
Chloramine	Biocides-preservatives		×	
Chloramphenicol	Drugs		×	
Chlorhexidine	Biocides-preservatives		×	
Chlorocresol	Biocides-preservatives	×	×	
Chloroform	Other	×		
Chlorothalonil	Other		×	

(continued)

Table 8.1 (continued)

Compound name	Product category	NICoU	ICoU	Unclassified[a]
Chlorpromazine	Drugs			×
Chromium (metal)	Other		×	
Cinnamaldehyde	Fragrances-cosmetics	×		
Cinnamic acid	Fragrances-cosmetics	×		
Cinnamic alcohol	Fragrances-cosmetics	×		
Cinnamon oil	Fragrances-cosmetics			×
Cisplatin (platinum salts)	Drugs		×	
Cobalt (metal)	Other		×	
Colophony (plant derivative)	Other		×	
Copper (metal)	Other			×
Coumarin	Fragrances-cosmetics	×		
Dibutylphthalate	Other		×	
Di-(2-ethylhexyl) phthalate	Other		×	
Diethyl fumarate	Other			×
Diethyltoluamine	Other		×	
Dimethylammonium chloride	Other			×
Dimethyl sulfoxide	Other	×		
Dinitrochlorobenzene	Drugs			×
Diphenylcyclopropenone	Drugs		×	
Diphenylmethane-4,4′-diisocyanate	Other		×	
Donepezil	Drugs		×	
Epoxy resins	Other		×	
Eugenol	Fragrances-cosmetics	×		
Formaldehyde	Biocides-preservatives	×	×	
Formaldehyde resin	Other		×	
Fumaric acid	Other			×
Gentamicin	Drugs		×	
Geraniol	Fragrances-cosmetics	×		
Gold (metal)	Other			×
Hydroxycitronellal	Fragrances-cosmetics	×		
Imidazolidinyl urea	Biocides-preservatives	×		
Iodochlorhydroxyquin	Drugs		×	
Iridium (metal)	Other		×	
Isoeugenol	Fragrances-cosmetics	×		
Kathon CG	Biocides-preservatives	×		
Ketoprofen	Drugs			×
Levomepromazine	Drugs		×	
Lidocaine	Drugs			×
Lindane	Drugs		×	
Mechlorethamine	Drugs		×	
Menthol	Fragrances-cosmetics	×		
Mercurochrome	Biocides-preservatives		×	
Mercury (metal)[b]	Other		×	
Methimazole	Drugs		×	
Methylethyl ketone	Other		×	
Mezlocillin	Drugs		×	
Monoamylamine	Drugs		×	
Neomycin	Drugs		×	

(continued)

Table 8.1 (continued)

Compound name	Product category	NICoU	ICoU	Unclassified[a]
Nickel (metal)	Other		×	
Nicotinic acid esters	Drugs	×		
Nylon	Other		×	
Palladium (metal)	Other			×
Panthenol (hair product)	Other			×
Parabens[b]	Biocides-preservatives		×	
Penicillins	Drugs		×	
Pentamidine isothionate	Drugs		×	
Phenothiazides	Drugs		×	
2-Phenoxyethanol	Biocides-preservatives			×
p-Phenylenediamine (hair dye)	Other		×	
Phenyl mercuric acetate	Biocides-preservatives		×	
Phenyl mercuric propionate	Biocides-preservatives		×	
Pilocarpine	Drugs			×
Polyethylene glycol	Biocides-preservatives			×
Polypropylene	Other			×
Polysorbates (emulsifier)[b]	Fragrances-cosmetics		×	
Promethazine	Drugs			×
Propylene glycol	Fragrances-cosmetics	×		
Propyphenazone	Drugs			×
Pyrazolones	Drugs		×	
Pyrrolidone carboxylate	Fragrances-cosmetics	×		
Resorcinol	Fragrances-cosmetics	×		
Rhodium (metal)	Other	×		
Ruthenium (metal)	Other	×		
Rifampicin	Drugs		×	
Sodium benzoate	Biocides-preservatives	×		
Sodium hypochlorite	Biocides-preservatives		×	
Sorbic acid	Biocides-preservatives	×		
Sorbitan monolaurate (emulsifier)[b]	Fragrances-cosmetics		×	
Sorbitan monostearate (emulsifier)[b]	Fragrances-cosmetics		×	
Sorbitan sesquioleate (emulsifier)[b]	Fragrances-cosmetics		×	
Stearyl alcohol (emulsifier)	Fragrances-cosmetics			×
Steroids	Drugs			×
Streptomycin	Drugs		×	
Sulbactam	Drugs		×	
Tin (metal)	Other	×		
Trichloroethanol	Other			×
Turpentine (plant derivative)	Other	×		
Vanillin	Fragrances-cosmetics	×		
Vinyl pyridine	Other			×
Virginiamycin	Drugs		×	
Wool alcohol	Fragrances-cosmetics		×	
Xylene	Other			×
Zinc (metal)	Other	×		

[a]Immediate contact reaction, unclassified nonimmunological/immunological
[b]Described as (non-clear evidence)

Fragrances and Cosmetics Ingredients

NICoU reactions to fragrances and to cosmetics ingredients are well known [14]. They have been often reported to some of the constituents of the Fragrance Mix I (FMI) and to balsam of Peru [15].

The FMI, developed in the late 1970s, and the Fragrance Mix II (FMII) developed in 2005, are the most valuable screening tools for the detection of delayed hypersensitivity to fragrances [16, 17]. Indeed, the components of FMI (α-amyl cinnamaldehyde, cinnamaldehyde, cinnamic alcohol, eugenol, isoeugenol, geraniol, hydroxy-citronellal, and the natural extract oak moss) and FMII (hydroxyisohexyl 3-cyclohexene carboxaldehyde, citral, α-hexyl-cinnamaldehyde, citronellol, farnesol, and coumarin) are the most common skin sensitizers identified as responsible for delayed-type allergic contact dermatitis to fragrances. Consequently, clinical relevance to these chemicals must be carefully examined because individuals may develop simple NICoU or CoU associated with delayed hypersensitivity. Chemical structures of FMI and FMII ingredients are shown in Fig. 8.2.

Safford et al. conducted a study on 20 patients positive to the FMI in 48 h and classified the FMI ingredients according to the decreasing ability to induce CoU as follows: cinnamaldehyde, cinnamic alcohol, isoeugenol, hydroxycitronellal, and geraniol [18]. Cinnamaldehyde and cinnamic alcohol were the strongest urticaria inducers for nonallergic patients.

CoU from cinnamaldehyde has been reported by several authors [3], leading even to anaphylaxis [19]. Among the many components of balsam of Peru, cinnamaldehyde is described as well as the strongest agent inducing NICoU, followed by cinnamic acid, benzoic acid, and benzaldehyde [20].

Balsam of Peru is derived from the sap of the tree *Myroxylon pereirae* (MP). It is composed of 250 constituents, of which 189 are of known chemical structure [21]. MP has been used in topical medicaments for its antibacterial properties, and in many countries it has been abandoned for that use because of its sensitizing potential. However, it may still occur in natural and herbal products, being used as a flavor or perfume ingredient. Extracts and distillates of MP are still used in perfumes [22]. It is thus possible that these can cause allergic reactions in MP-sensitized individuals.

Cinnamaldehyde is the main component of cassia oil (~90%) and cinnamon bark oil (~75%). It is also the main component of artificial cinnamon oil. Smaller quantities are found in many other essential oils. In nature, the *trans*-isomer is predominant. It is a yellowish liquid with a characteristic spicy odor, strongly reminiscent of cinnamon. Being an α,β-unsaturated aldehyde, it undergoes many reactions, such as hydrogenation to cinnamic alcohol. Its oxidation occurs readily on exposure to air yielding cinnamic acid. Cinnamic acid has been also used in perfumery, and as a flavoring ingredient in pharmaceutical preparations and in food products. Forsbeck and Skog found CoU from cinnamic acid 5% in petrolatum in three of five patients with immediate skin reactions to balsam of Peru [20].

Geraniol is an olefinic terpene mainly present in palmarosa, geranium, and rose oils. It is a colorless liquid, with a flowery rose-like odor. A case of a patient with CoU from geraniol has been reported to be caused by immunological mechanisms. The patient developed widespread urticaria and flare reactions on the face and neck at the 72-h reading of the patch test [23]. Oxidation processes produce the aldehydes geranial and neral, and in addition, hydroperoxides. Autoxidation greatly influences the sensitizing effect of geraniol, becoming a potent allergen [24].

Eugenol and *isoeugenol* are phenylpropene compounds. *Eugenol* is the main component of several essential oils; clove leaf oil and cinnamon leaf oil may contain more than 90%. Eugenol occurs in small amounts in many other essential oils. It is a colorless to slightly yellow liquid with a spicy, clove odor. It is widely used in dental practice to relieve pain arising from various sources, such as pulpitis and dentinal hypersensitivity. It is also used in toothache drops, mouthwash, and antiseptics. Eugenol in dental

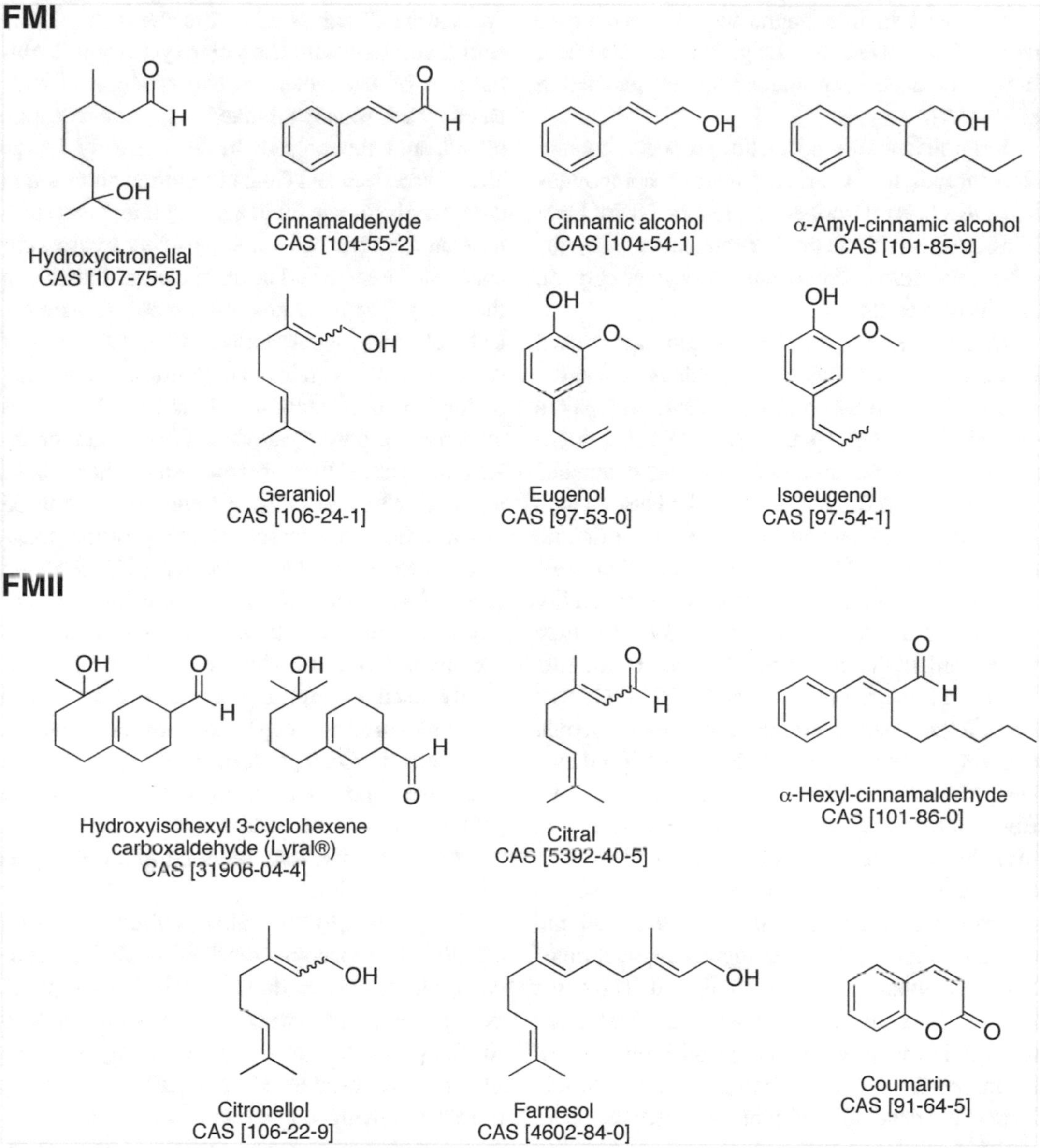

FMI

Hydroxycitronellal
CAS [107-75-5]

Cinnamaldehyde
CAS [104-55-2]

Cinnamic alcohol
CAS [104-54-1]

α-Amyl-cinnamic alcohol
CAS [101-85-9]

Geraniol
CAS [106-24-1]

Eugenol
CAS [97-53-0]

Isoeugenol
CAS [97-54-1]

FMII

Hydroxyisohexyl 3-cyclohexene
carboxaldehyde (Lyral®)
CAS [31906-04-4]

Citral
CAS [5392-40-5]

α-Hexyl-cinnamaldehyde
CAS [101-86-0]

Citronellol
CAS [106-22-9]

Farnesol
CAS [4602-84-0]

Coumarin
CAS [91-64-5]

Fig. 8.2 Chemical structures of the components of fragrance mix (FMI) and FMII

preparations has been reported to cause CoU, gingivitis, stomatitis venenata, and allergic hand eczema in dental personnel [25, 26]. It is considered to be a less common sensitizer than isoeugenol, cinnamaldehyde, or cinnamic alcohol. *Isoeugenol* occurs in many essential oils, mostly with eugenol, but not as the main component. Commercial isoeugenol is a mixture of *cis-* and *trans*-isomers, in which the thermodynamically more stable *trans*-isomer dominates. It is a yel-

lowish, viscous liquid with a fine clove odor. Isoeugenol is a strong allergen [27]; it caused contact allergy in 1.7% of 2261 consecutive tested eczema patients in an European multi-center study [28]. It is found in many cosmetic products and may be present in relative highly concentrations.

Coumarin is an aromatic lactone naturally occurring in Tonka beans and other plants, determining, for example, the odor of woodruff. It is widely used in fine fragrances for spicy green notes. Considered for long time a sensitizer, impurities have been blamed for the sensitizing effect [29].

Fragrances and cosmetic products contain also ingredients other than odorant compounds that have been described to produce NICoU and ICoU. Among these are benzophenone, polysorbates, sorbitan sesquioleate, propylene glycol, and wool alcohols.

Benzophenones are photo-screen agents used in sunscreens and cosmetics, such as anti-aging creams, hair sprays and shampoos, and paints and plastics. Benzophenones have been documented to cause numerous adverse cutaneous reactions, including contact and photo-contact dermatitis, contact and photo-contact urticaria, and anaphylaxis. In recent years these chemicals became particularly well known for their ability to provoke allergy and photo-allergy [30]; they were named the American Contact Dermatitis Society's Allergen of the Year for 2014. CUS at stage IV has been reported in the case of people applying sunscreen and self-tanning products, benzophenone-3 being the major cause [31]. Benzophenone-3, also named oxybenzone, is often incorporated into sunscreen formulations to offer enhanced UVA protection because its absorption spectrum extends to less than 350 nm. Cases of anaphylaxis from topical application of benzophenone-3 have been published. The cases resulted in a generalized wheal and flare reactions and syncope after widespread application of a sunscreen or sunless tanning product with this filter. CoU developed after more limited exposure [31, 32].

Polysorbates are a class of emulsifiers used in some pharmaceuticals and food preparations, but they are also often used in cosmetics to solubilize essential oils into water-based products. Oily liquids, they derive from esterification of ethoxylated sorbitan with fatty acids. The nomenclature used for polysorbates is characteristic. For example, polysorbate 80, also called polyoxyethylene 20 sorbitan monooleate. The number 20 following the "polyoxyethylene" part refers to the total number of oxyethylene $-(CH_2CH_2O)-$ groups found in the molecule. The number following the "polysorbate" part is related to the type of fatty acid associated with the polyoxyethylene sorbitan part of the molecule. Monolaurate is indicated by 20, monopalmitate by 40, monostearate by 60, and monooleate by 80. Already in the 1970s, Maibach and Conant reported an urticaria case to polysorbate 60 in a male patient with redness on the forehead when applying hydrocortisone 1% cream [33]. The chemical responsible in the cream was determined to be polysorbate 60, an emulsifying agent mixture of stearate esters of sorbitol and sorbitol anhydrides, consisting mainly on the monoester. It is also known as Tween 60 or polyoxyethylene 20 sorbitan monostearate. Since then, several cases have been reported. More recently, a biologically induced urticaria from polysorbate 80 in a psoriasis treatment in Spain has been reported [34]. *Sorbitan sesquioleate*, a sorbitol-based emulsifier, is actually added to the FMI ingredients to constitute the mixture. Sorbitol-based emulsifiers are commonly used in topical corticosteroids, topical antibiotics, and antifungals, moisturizing creams, and lotions. Contact dermatitis from sorbitol derivatives appears to be increasingly prevalent [35]. This trend goes hand-in-hand with the ICoU to sorbitan sesquioleate reported in a corticosteroid ointment [36].

Propylene glycol, also called propane-1,2-diol, is a viscous colorless alcohol (chemically classed as a diol), nearly odorless but possessing a weak sweet taste. It is mainly used for the production of unsaturated polyester resins. It is also used as a humectant food additive (E1520), a hygroscopic compound used to keep products moist, as a moisturizer in cosmetics, food, toothpaste, mouthwash, and tobacco products, as the main ingredient in deodorant sticks, as an antifreeze liquid, and as a solvent in many pharmaceuticals and topical formulations. Propylene glycol is one of the major ingredients of the cartridges used in electronic cigarettes where it is aerosolized in the atomizer. It has been associated with irritant and allergic contact dermatitis as well as CoU in humans. These sensitization effects can be manifested at propylene glycol concentrations as low as 2% [37]. Still, the Cosmetic Ingredient Review Panel found that propylene glycol is safe if used in cosmetic products at concentrations not exceeding 50% [38]. The work of Maibach and Conant cited here describing an urticaria case to polysorbate 60 concerned a hydrocortisone cream containing propylene glycol [33]. CoU could not be concluded in experiments with open propylene glycol application. Only one report describes NICoU after topical application [39, 40].

Wool alcohols are the principal component of lanolin, a natural product obtained from the fleece of sheep. Sebum is extracted from the wool, cleaned, and refined to produce anhydrous lanolin, which consists of wool alcohols, fatty alcohols, and fatty acids. Currently, wool alcohols are considered the main sensitizers in lanolin. Wool alcohols, wool fat, anhydrous lanolin, lanolin alcohol, wool wax, and wool grease are just some of the terms used interchangeably with lanolin. Lanolin is a good emulsifier, meaning that it binds well with water and is particularly useful in the manufacture of pharmaceutical and cosmetic formulations. Wool alcohols are found in many pharmaceutical preparations, cosmetics, and toiletries, and also have some industrial uses. The general incidence of lanolin allergy in consecutively tested eczema patients is about 2% to 3% [41].

Biocides and Preservatives

Preservatives are added to water-containing products (e.g., cosmetics) to inhibit the growth of nonpathogenic and pathogenic microorganisms that may cause degradation of the product or be harmful to the consumer. After fragrances, they are the most important cause of allergic contact dermatitis, being this very well documented [42]. CoU is less common. The literature consists essentially of case reports, and studies on actual incidence and prevalence are lacking.

Chemicals with preservative properties that are worth describing in the CoU context are discussed here. It is not always clear, depending on the underlying mechanisms involved, if the reactions are involving the immune system. Chemical structures are shown in Fig. 8.3.

Sorbic acid, or 2,4-hexadienoic acid, is a colorless solid slightly soluble in water. It is an antimicrobial agent often used as a preservative in food and drinks (E200). In general, the salts (sodium, potassium, and calcium sorbates, E201–E203) are preferred over the acid form because they are more soluble in water, but the active form is the acid. CoU from sorbic acid is thought to be rare, but a few reports can be found in the literature. Some authors have described that creams and shampoos containing sorbic acid caused erythema, slight itching, and sometimes edema [43–45]. As is sorbic acid, *benzoic acid* is a natural preservative, having antibacterial and antifungal properties. It is well recognized to cause NICoU with concentration-dependent reactions [46]. Present also in balsam of Peru, it induced CoU at 5% in patients with immediate contact reactions to balsam of Peru [20]. It is commonly used also as a preservative in acidic food products. Thus, cases have been reported in food additives, and benzoic and sorbic acids elicit NICoU at concentrations in use in salad dressings or other food products [45, 47].

Formaldehyde (HCHO) and its releasers constitute an important class of preservatives in consumer goods. HCHO is the simplest of the aldehydes category of compounds. It is a frequent and potent sensitizer and a strong ubiquitous allergen, including from non-cosmetics sources of contact. Its bactericidal and fungicidal properties confer it a place of choice for preservation of cosmetics, but its use has been reduced because of the bad press it has as an irritant, sensitizer, and carcinogen [48]. Exposure to HCHO in the EU is thus subjected to restrictions. Free HCHO may be used as a preservative in all cosmetic products (maximum authorized concentration 0.2%, but only 0.1% in products for oral hygiene) except aerosol cosmetics. EU regulation 1223/2009 permits the use in nail hardeners up to a maximum concentration of 5%. Annex VI of the Cosmetics Directive 76/768 EC further stipulates that all finished products containing HCHO or substances that release it must be labeled with the warning "contains formaldehyde" wherein the concentration of free HCHO in the finished product exceeds 0.05% [49]. On January 1, 2016,

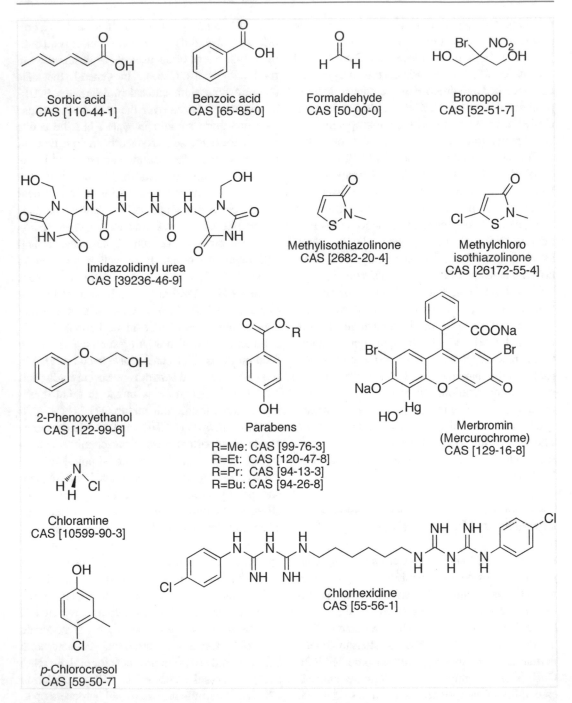

Fig. 8.3 Chemical structures of the most important preservatives and biocides

the EU officially adopted its reclassification under the CLP (Classification, Labelling and Packaging) Regulations EC 1272/2008, as a Class 1B carcinogen and Class 2 mutagen. For its continued use in cosmetics, the criteria specified for CMR 1A and 1B must be met, including the Scientific Committee on Consumer Safety (SCCS) to declare it safe for use in cosmetic products. The SCCS has published recently an opinion that states that nail hardeners with a maximum concentration of 2.2% free HCHO can be used. Even if it is a strong sensitizer, reported immediate reactions to HCHO are mainly classified as NICoU because they seem not to be mediated by IgE [49]. However, there is still no consensus in the reports that have appeared as to whether the mechanism is immunological or nonimmunological [50]. Most of the literature on generalized urticaria, respiratory compromise, and anaphylaxis concerns exposure to HCHO-containing disinfectants used for root canals and other dental procedures [51, 52]. There have been few reports on allergy to HCHO associated with IgE, and single cases of HCHO-specific IgE-mediated urticaria exist in the literature [51–53]. Thus, probably HCHO should be classified as a substance that shows mixed features of NICoU and ICoU, as the mechanism remains unclear.

As an alternative to the use of HCHO, chemical compounds that slowly release it in the presence of water and under usage conditions, the so-called *formaldehyde-releasers*, are commonly employed as preservatives in cosmetics (water-based preparations) instead of free HCHO. Examples are *bronopol* and *imidazolidinyl urea*. Unfortunately, many formaldehyde releasers used in cosmetics are also skin sensitizers, as caused by released HCHO but also by reactive intermediates other than HCHO that could be involved in the formation of the hapten–protein antigenic complex, a key step of the sensitization process, and thus explaining their sensitizing potential per se [54].

Methylisothiazolinone (MI) and *methylchloroisothiazolinone* (MCI) are the active ingredients of the biocide Kathon CG (MI/MCI 1:3 combination), used since the 1980s and one of the most common sources of allergic contact dermatitis caused by preservatives [55, 56]. Following the introduction in the EU of a 15 ppm use limit in cosmetics, contact allergy to MI/MCI significantly decreased to a prevalence rate of about 2% after the 1990s. The sensitizing potential of the mixture was mostly attributed to the chlorinated derivative MCI, shown to be the stronger sensitizer, whereas the nonchlorinated MI was reported to be a much weaker allergen. Thus, in the early 2000s, MI alone started to be

used as preservative in industrial products and in 2005 in cosmetics, but at higher concentrations than in the MI/MCI mixture because of its lower biocide potential. As a consequence, over recent years there has been an alarming increase in the prevalence of allergic contact dermatitis to MI [57, 58]. Occupational cases of contact dermatitis to MI first were reported from paints [59], followed by nonoccupational cases essentially seen from wet wipes for hygiene and cosmetics [60]. Severe cases of airborne and systemic dermatitis have appeared recently from exposure to MI present particularly in water-based wall paints [61]. At the same time, MI/MCI contact allergy has increased significantly during the past few years [62]. It has been proposed that the rise in MI/MCI contact allergy was likely linked to the higher consumer exposure to MI, and most probably resulted from a previous sensitization of individuals to MI. Because the occurrence of consumer products containing only MI is only in the recent few years, questions were raised about the MI and MCI cross-reaction pattern. Studies of chemical reactivity in situ in a reconstructed human epidermis model showed that reaction mechanisms for MI and MCI were different, making it difficult to explain cross-reactivity [63]. CoU cases caused by isothiazolinones are rare and are generally classified as NICoU [64].

CoU to other biocides such as *benzyl alcohol*, *2-phenoxyethanol*, and *polyethylene glycols*, used as preservatives in a wide number of cosmetics and topical preparations, has also been reported [65–68]. CoU from alcohols was reviewed in the 1990s, with cases classified as nonimmunological and some as immunological based on open skin tests [69].

Other important biocides have been correlated to ICoU such as parabens, and many antiseptics such as mercurochrome, chloramine, chlorhexidine, and chlorocresol.

Parabens (methyl, ethyl, propyl, butyl) are a series of parahydroxybenzoates or esters of parahydroxybenzoic acid (also known as 4-hydroxybenzoic acid). Parabens are effective preservatives in many types of formulas, especially in cosmetic products. They are also used as food additives. In individuals with normal skin, parabens are, for the most part, nonirritating and nonsensitizing. Routine testing in the European standard series yields low prevalence rates of sensitization [70, 71]. At the usual concentration of 0.1–0.3% in cosmetics, parabens rarely cause adverse reactions. They have been reported to cause localized CoU when applied to the skin, and an IgE immune-mediated mechanism is suspected.

Mercurochrome is the trade name of merbromin, an organomercuric disodium salt and a fluorescein, used as a topical antiseptic. Because mercury is highly toxic, it is no longer sold in the US from 1998 and in France from 2006. Mercurial compounds are known as causing allergic contact dermatitis, and immediate hypersensitivity is rarely induced. A few cases have been reported in which immediate hypersensitivity to mercuric fluorescein compounds has been proved by skin test and histamine liberation [72, 73].

Chloramines are derivatives of ammonia by substitution of one, two, or three hydrogen atoms with chlorine atoms. Monochloramine (commonly called *chloramine*) is an inorganic compound with the formula NH_2Cl. Chloramine is commonly used as a sterilizer, disinfectant, and chemical reagent. It has been described as an occupational hazard for pharmaceutical workers, nurses, and cleaners. Goossens et al. reported the first case of immediate positive epicutaneous tests to chloramine powder solutions used by a nurse [74]. All skin tests performed on the patient were suspicious of an immediate-type reaction. The immunological nature of the clinical manifestations was investigated by RAST on serum of the patient. High levels of IgE antibodies to chloramine were found, those previously bound to human serum albumin (HSA). The clinical manifestation on the patient was confirmed by radioimmunoassay and classified as a stage 3 CUS. Chloramine is often confused with chloramine-T as both are employed as sterilizer, antiseptic, and disinfectant agents. However, they are two different chemicals. Chloramine-T is a *N*-chlorinated deprotonated sulfonamide, white powder, in contrast to chloramine, a simple monochlorinated amine that is a colorless liquid usually handled as a diluted aqueous solution.

Allergic asthma caused by chloramine-T is well known and the reactions are IgE mediated. Kramps et al. were able to demonstrate the presence of specific IgE antibodies in the serum of asthmatic-chloramine T-allergic patients [75]. However, skin symptoms of IgE-dependent CoU have also been reported in the case of a hospital bath attendant in Finland. The performed RAST to chloramine-T showed specific IgE antibodies, with values being defined as positive [76].

Chlorhexidine is a synthetic chlorophenyl-bis-biguanide compound, containing two chloroguanide chains linked by a hexamethylene chain. It is a strong base and a di-cation at physiological pH. Usually insoluble in water, it needs to be formulated with gluconic or acetic acid to form water-soluble digluconate or diacetate esters. Chlorhexidine, especially as digluconate ester, is widely used in many dental topical applications (toothpaste, dental gel, mouthwash solutions) as it binds oral mucosa, inhibiting dental plaque formation. It is also used as disinfectant and antiseptic of minor cuts and wounds. It can cause both type I immediate allergy and type IV delayed allergy. Despite its common usage, the sensitization rate seems low, but this is certainly underestimated. It may induce immediate-type sensitivity reactions either by topical application or by insertion of coated catheters in surgical fields. The mechanism suspected is an IgE-mediated pathomechanism in sensitized individuals [77]. Many healthcare workers are exposed to hand washes containing chlorhexidine. In the United Kingdom, four cases of occupational IgE-mediated allergy to chlorhexidine were identified, the diagnosis being made on an appropriate clinical history with positive serum-specific IgE to chlorhexidine and/or positive skin prick testing [78]. The main aspects of chlorhexidine toxicity have been reviewed elsewhere [79].

Chlorocresol (*p*-chlorocresol) is a chlorinated phenol used as an antiseptic and preservative. It forms colorless crystals at room temperature and is slightly soluble in water. For medical use it is dissolved in alcohol combined with other phenols. Several case reports involve chlorocresol as a cause of CoU, but whether this occurs through an immunological mechanism is not clear [80, 81].

Drugs

Drugs, small reactive chemicals, can induce both NICoU and ICoU within minutes to 1 h after exposure. These drugs include mainly antibiotics, because of direct contact of nurses and healthcare personnel during their preparation, or employees during their production in the pharmaceutical industry. Penicillins and cephalosporins are the most incriminated (Fig. 8.4). All these seem to have an immunological physiopathology and are discussed following. For most of the other drugs reported, observed immediate contact reactions cannot be definitely classified as nonimmunological or immunological. Often, skin tests do not allow distinguishing between an IgE-dependent reaction and a nonspecific histamine release, and research of specific IgE by using the radioallergosorbent test (RAST) is only available for some drugs. One example is given by lidocaine.

Lidocaine is a common amino amide-type local anesthetic applied topically. It is also an antiarrhythmic drug applied intravenously. An immediate positive patch test and prick test demonstrated its involvement in the simultaneous presence of CoU and allergic contact dermatitis in the same patient [82, 83].

Ketoprofen   ((*RS*)-2-(3-benzoylphenyl)-propionic acid), an important cause of photo-contact dermatitis, has also been described as responsible for CoU [84]. It is one of the propionic acid class of nonsteroidal antiinflammatory drugs (NSAID) with analgesic effects.

Other immediate reactions have been observed in personnel of psychiatry services during the manipulation of *phenothiazines*, antipsychotic drugs related to the thiazine class of heterocyclic compounds, such as chlorpromazine and *promethazine*. The latter is a first-generation antihistamine of the phenothiazine family. It is a chiral compound and is found as a mixture of

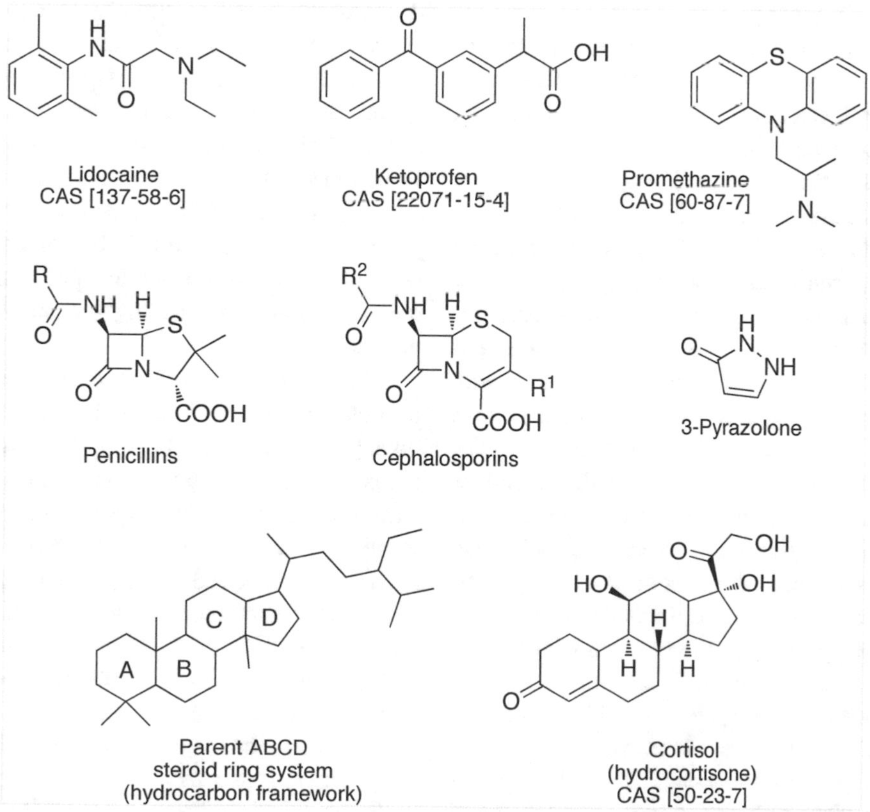

Fig. 8.4 Chemical structures of drugs involved in immediate skin contact reactions

enantiomers. Among the many professional areas where case reports of CoU have been recorded, workers in the pharmaceutical and chemical industries are of considerable concern, as they are in contact with highly reactive substances (some listed in Table 8.1) used for synthesis, for example, that have been also described as inducers of immediate skin reactions. The pathogenesis of NICoU to all these chemicals is not clearly defined. Different urticariogens may act by different mechanisms. For example, dimethyl sulfoxide can both damage blood vessels and cause mast cell degranulation. However, antihistamines do not inhibit reactions to dimethyl sulfoxide and other NICoU triggering agents, although ethylsalicylic acid and nonsteroidal antiinflammatory drugs do, both orally and topically, suggesting a role for prostaglandins [7].

However, the main drugs responsible for occupational CoU are antibiotics and, particularly, penicillin, ampicillin, amoxicillin, and cephalosporins. Antibiotics are very often associated with ICoU [85].

The term *penicillin* is often used to refer to benzylpenicillin (penicillin G, found in 1928), procaine benzylpenicillin, benzathine benzylpenicillin, and phenoxymethylpenicillin. The core of the molecule has the formula $R-C_9H_{11}N_2O_4S$, where R is a variable side chain that differentiates the penicillins from one another. The key structural feature is the four-membered β-lactam ring, essential for antibacterial activity. Thus, all penicillin antibiotics contain a common nucleus (6-aminopenicillanic acid) composed of a β-lactam ring fused with a thiazolidine ring, this complex connected to a side chain. An intact β-lactam ring is necessary for bactericidal activity, and the side chain determines the spectrum of antibacterial activity, the susceptibility to destruction when exposed to acids and β-lactamases, and pharmacokinetics properties. Allergic reactions are estimated to occur in approximately 2% of patients treated with penicillin. Severe reactions to penicillin such as anaphylaxis can occur and are potentially life threatening. Penicillin is a hapten and becomes immunogenic only when it binds to a protein. The β-lactam ring covalently binds to lysine residues of proteins and forms the penicilloyl group, known as the "major

determinant" because it is the major penicillin metabolic product. Penicillin metabolites also form disulfide bonds with sulfhydryl groups of cysteine, producing the "minor determinants," so called because they are formed in smaller quantities. Thus, immediate allergic reactions to penicillin are mediated through IgE antibodies against either the major or minor determinants or both. Based on this, penicillin skin testing techniques have been developed demonstrating the presence or absence of specific IgE antibodies against major and minor determinants. The use of benzylpenicilloyl-poly-L-lysine can test IgE antibodies against major determinants. Histamine is used as a positive control, and saline is used as a negative control. Skin detection of serum IgE specific for major penicillin determinants has a high positive predictive value but fails to identify patients with penicillin allergy. It has been suggested that, ideally, skin testing to major and minor penicillin determinants would improve diagnosis. Methods of preparation of reagents for minor determinants have been published, and penicillin G has been used as a partial source of minor determinants. Alternatives to benzylpenicilloyl-poly-L-lysine and minor determinant mixtures are commercially available for skin testing [86]. Penicillin skin testing is believed to be safe if done properly; although severe reactions such as anaphylaxis have been reported, these were produced because of violation of the test protocols such as doing intracutaneous testing without first doing prick testing.

After penicillins, *cephalosporins* are the most important β-lactams inducing IgE-mediated reactions [87]. Allergy has been reported with use of a specific cephalosporin, as a cross-reaction between different cephalosporins or as a cross-reaction to other β-lactam antibiotics. Unlike determinants derived from penicillins, cephalosporin allergenic determinants have not been well identified, and thus standardized diagnostic skin testing is not available. Nevertheless, skin testing with diluted solutions of cephalosporins can be valuable in confirming IgE-mediated hypersensitivity reactions [88, 89].

Pyrazolone is a five-membered ring lactam. It is a derivative of pyrazole that has a keto (=O) group. There are three isomers: 3-, 4-, and 5-pyrazolone. Pyrazolones are NSAIDs and the most frequent drugs inducing selective reactions thought to be mediated by specific IgE. Sensitivity of diagnostic tests is poor, probably because knowledge of the structures involved is incomplete. Research is today ongoing on pyrazolone metabolites and its relevance to hypersensitivity reactions [90].

Steroids are organic compounds with four rings arranged in a specific molecular configuration. The core structure is composed of 17 carbon atoms, bonded in four fused rings: three cyclohexane rings (A, B, C) and one cyclopentane ring (D). Steroids vary by the functional group attached to this core and by the oxidation state of the rings. Corticosteroids (i.e., cortisol or hydrocortisone) are potent antiinflammatory and immunomodulator agents used in treatment of various inflammatory diseases, including allergic diseases. They can in some cases induce immediate or delayed hypersensitivity reactions. Topical corticosteroids are well-known contact sensitizers. However, diagnosing an allergic reaction is still a challenge for clinicians. Although knowledge of delayed hypersensitivity as a secondary effect of topical use is improving, little is known about immediate reactions to systemic corticosteroids [91]. Cases of urticaria from hydrocortisone have been reported, in atopic patients after hydrocortisone injection or infusion, and in patients treated with hydrocortisone sodium succinate. All cases are thought to be IgE mediated [92, 93].

Other Chemicals

Chemicals not belonging to the families of compounds already described but necessary to mention are shown in Fig. 8.5.

Epoxy resins are LMW pre-polymers, which normally contain at least two epoxide groups. The epoxide group is also known as the glycidyl or oxirane group. Cyclic acid anhydrides are synthetic highly reactive LMW compounds widely used as curing agents for epoxy resins and in the production of polyester resins. Commonly used anhydrides are phthalic, tetrahydrophthalic,

methyl tetrahydrophthalic, hexahydrophthalic, methyl hexahydrophthalic, and maleic and trimellitic anhydrides. Cyclic acid anhydrides often cause allergic respiratory diseases, and in the literature only single case reports of CoU of a few patients were found. However, occupational CoU has been described by a Finnish study as workers may be exposed in powder or liquid form during manufacturing processes [94]. Data are presented for 21 subjects who had been exposed to organic acid anhydrides and examined during the period 1990–2006. The majority of the patients had been exposed to an epoxy resin containing methyl hexahydrophthalic anhydride. Specific IgE results were in line with the prick tests, and the large reaction was seen for the acid anhydride to which the patient had been exposed. Phthalic anhydride IgE was positive in 19 of 20 patients.

Another important constituent of epoxy resins that has been incriminated as producing immediate reactions is *bisphenol A*. It is an organic synthetic compound belonging to the diphenylmethane derivatives group and bisphenols, with two hydroxyphenyl groups. It is a colorless solid soluble in organic solvents, but poorly soluble in water. Specific IgE cases have been reported [95, 96].

Acrylates are the salts, esters, and conjugated bases of acrylic acid and its derivatives. They are common monomers (i.e., methyl methacrylate) in polymer plastics. Acrylates easily form acrylate polymers because of the high reactivity of the constituting double bonds. Monomers such as 2-ethylhexyl acrylate, acrylic acid, cyanoacrylates, and methyl methacrylate have been reported to cause immediate skin reactions [97].

Aromatic amines are a broad group of chemicals used in a variety of applications, such as hair dyes, ink for printers, photographic products, and the paper and textile industries. According to their large spectrum of application, skin exposure of the general population to these compounds is high. Safety aspects and toxicity studies have shown that *para*-amino aromatic compounds and their derivatives are strong skin sensitizers, generally related to dyeing products. One of the best known is *para-phenylenediamine* (PPD). PPD is one of the most common primary intermediates

Fig. 8.5 Chemical structures of other low molecular weight (LMW) compounds involved in immediate skin contact reactions

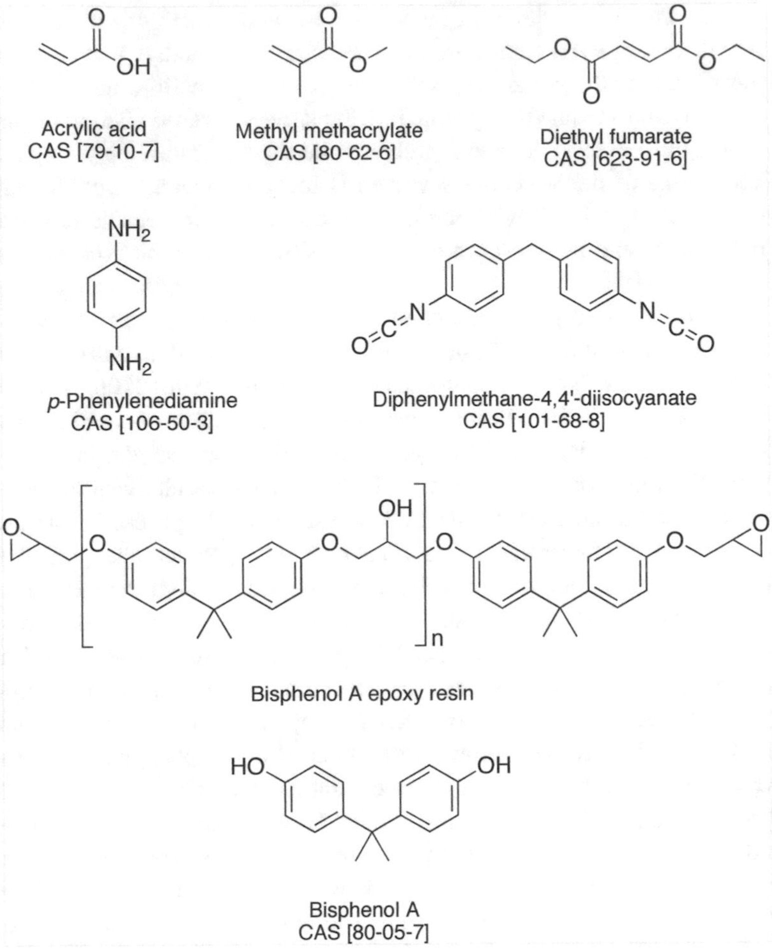

Acrylic acid
CAS [79-10-7]

Methyl methacrylate
CAS [80-62-6]

Diethyl fumarate
CAS [623-91-6]

p-Phenylenediamine
CAS [106-50-3]

Diphenylmethane-4,4'-diisocyanate
CAS [101-68-8]

Bisphenol A epoxy resin

Bisphenol A
CAS [80-05-7]

of oxidative hair dyes and is usually reported as the main sensitizer in hair dye dermatitis. PPD is therefore included in the European Standard Series for diagnostic patch testing of eczema patients and is generally regarded as the screening agent for contact allergy to *para*-amino aromatic compounds but also to azo-aromatic compounds used in textile dyes [98–100]. It can also induce immediate-type reactions, going from local urticaria to fatal systemic reactions and anaphylactic shock [101–103].

Other chemical compounds of LMW reported as inducing ICoU are aliphatic polyamides, methylethyl ketone, widely used as a solvent in plastic manufacturing, and monoamylamine, a vehicle ingredient of topical medicaments. Also reported is benzonitrile, a useful solvent and versatile precursor to many derivatives, carbamate-constituting groups of polyurethanes and diethyl fumarate.

Finally, metals and metallic salts can also cause occupational CoU. Aluminum, chromium, cobalt, iridium salts, nickel, platinum salts, and rhodium have been reported. Among these, platinum salts are important allergens in the catalyst industry, and clinical manifestations may involve both the respiratory system and the skin [104–109].

References

1. Giménez-Arnau A, Maurer M, De la Cuadra J, Maibach HI. Immediate contact skin reactions, an update of contact urticaria, contact urticaria syndrome and protein contact dermatitis-"A never ending story". Eur J Dermatol. 2010;20:552–62.

2. Ale SI, Maibach HI. Occupational contact urticaria. In: Kanerva L, Elsner P, Wahlberg JE, Maibach HI, editors. Handbook of occupational dermatology. Berlin: Springer; 2000. p. 200–16.

3. Lahti A. Non-immunologic contact urticaria. Acta Dermatovener (Stockholm). 1980;60(Suppl. 91):1–49.

4. Kligman AM. The spectrum of contact urticaria: wheals, erythema and pruritus. Dermatologic Clin. 1990;8:57–60.

5. Coverly J, Peters L, Whittle E, Basketter DA. Susceptibility to skin stinging, non-immunologic contact urticaria and skin irritation-is there a relationship? Contact Dermatitis. 1998;38:90–5.

6. Lahti A, Vaananen A, Kokkonen E-L, Hannuksela M. Acetylsalicylic acid inhibits non-immunologic contact urticaria. Contact Dermatitis. 1987;16:133–5.

7. Johansson J, Lahti A. Topical non-steroidal anti-inflammatory drugs inhibit non-immunological immediate contact reactions. Contact Dermatitis. 1988;19:161–5.

8. Wakelin SH. Contact urticaria. Clin Exp Dermatol. 2001;26:132–6.

9. Amaro C, Goossens A. Immunological occupational contact urticaria and contact dermatitis from proteins: a review. Contact Dermatitis. 2008;58:67–75.

10. Goossens A, Amaro C, Géraut C. Urticaire et dermatite de contact aux protéines en pathologie professionnelle. In:Progrès en Dermato-Allergologie. Paris: John Libbey Eurotext; 2007. p. 57–70.

11. Castanedo-Tardan MP, Jacob SE, Baumann LS. Contact urticaria to cosmetic and toiletry ingredients. Cosmetic Dermatol. 2008;21:339–46.

12. Lahti A, Basketter D. Immediate contact reactions. In: Johansen JD, Frosch PJ, Lepoittevin J-P, editors. Contact dermatitis. 5th ed. Berlin: Springer; 2011. p. 137–53.

13. Gleich GJ, Yunginger JW. The radioallergosorbent test: a method to measure IgE antibodies, IgG blocking antibodies, and the potency of allergy extracts. Bull N Y Acad Med. 1981;57:559–67.

14. Vigan M. Urticaire de contact aux cosmétiques. In:Progrès en Dermato-Allergologie. Paris: John Libbey Eurotext; 2007. p. 17–34.

15. Cancian M, Fortina AB, Peserico A. Contact urticaria syndrome from constituents of balsam of Peru and fragrance mix in a patient with chronic urticaria. Contact Dermatitis. 1999;41:3000.

16. Larsen WG. Perfume dermatitis. a study of 20 patients. Arch Dermatol. 1977;113:623–7.

17. Frosch PJ, Pirker C, Rastogi SC, Andersen K, Bruze M, Svedman C, Goossens A, White IR, Uter W, Giménez-Arnau E, Lepoittevin J-P, Menné T, Johansen JD. Patch testing with a new fragrance mix detects additional patients sensitive to perfumes and missed by the current fragrance mix. Contact Dermatitis. 2005;52:207–15.

18. Safford RJ, Basketter DA, Allenby CF, Goodwin BFJ. Immediate contact reactions to chemicals in the fragrance mix and a study of the quenching action of eugenol. Br J Dermatol. 1990;123:595–606.

19. Diba VC, Statham BN. Contact urticaria from cinnamal leading to anaphylaxis. Contact Dermatitis. 2003;48:119.

20. Forsbeck M, Skog E. Immediate reactions to patch tests with balsam of Peru. Contact Dermatitis. 1977;3:201–5.

21. Hausen BM, Simatupang T, Bruhn G, Evers P, Koenig WA. Identification of new allergens constituents and proof of evidence for coniferyl benzoate in balsam of Peru. Am J Contact Dermat. 1995;6:199–208.

22. Api AM. Only Peru Balsam extracts or distillates are used in perfumery. Contact Dermatitis. 2006;54:179.

23. Yamamoto A, Morita A, Tsuji T, et al. Contact urticaria from geraniol. Contact Dermatitis. 2002;46:52.

24. Hagvall L, Bäcktorp C, Svensson S, Nyman G, Börje A, Karlberg AT. Fragrance compound geraniol forms contact allergens on air exposure. identification and quantification of oxidation products and effect on skin sensitization. Chem Res Toxicol. 2007;20:807–14.

25. Kanerva L, Estlander T, Jolanki R. Dental nurse's occupational allergic contact dermatitis from eugenol used as a restorative dental material with polymethylmethacrylate. Contact Dermatitis. 1998;38:339–40.

26. Praven T, Pushpalatha C, Shrenik J, Sowmya SW. An unexpected positive hypersensitive reaction to eugenol. BMJ Case Rep. 2013. https://doi.org/10.1136/bcr-2013-009464.

27. Marzulli FN, Maibach HI. Contact allergy: predictive testing of fragrance ingredients in humans by Draize and maximization tests. J Environ Pathol Toxicol. 1980;3:243–5.

28. Tananka S, Royds C, Buckley D, Basketter DA, Goossens A, Bruze M, Svedman C, Menné T, Johansen JD, White IR, McFadden JP. Contact allergy to isoeugenol and its derivatives: problems with allergen substitution. Contact Dermatitis. 2004;51:288–91.

29. Vocanson M, Valeyrie M, Rozières A, Hennino A, Floc'h F, Gard A, Nicolas JF. Lack of evidence for allergenic properties of coumarin in a fragrance allergy mouse model. Contact Dermatitis. 2007;57:361–4.

30. Heurung AR, Raju SI, Warshaw EM. Benzophenones. Dermatitis. 2014;25:3–10.

31. Emonet S, Pasche-Koo F, Perin-Minisini MJ, Hauser C. Anaphylaxis to oxybenzone, a frequent constituent of sunscreens. J Allergy Clin Immunol. 2001;107:556–7.

32. Yesudian PD, King CM. Severe contact urticarial and anaphylaxis from benzophenone-3 (2-hydroxy-4-methoxy benzophenone). Contact Dermatitis. 2002;46:55–6.

33. Maibach HI, Conant M. Contact urticarial to a corticosteroid cream: polysorbate 60. Contact Dermatitis. 1977;3:350–1.

34. Pérez-Pérez L, García Gavín J, Piñeiro B, Zulaica A. Biologic-induced urticarial due to polysor-

bate 80: usefulness of prick test. Br J Dermatol. 2011;164:1119–20.

35. Asarch A, Scheinmann PL. Sorbitan sesquiolate: an emerging contact allergen. Dermatitis. 2008;19:339–41.

36. Hardy H, Maibach H. Contact urticarial syndrome from sorbitan sesquiolate in a corticosteroid ointment. Contact Dermatitis. 1995;32:114.

37. EWG's Skin Deep® Cosmetics Database. http://www.ewg.org/skindeep.

38. Cosmetic Ingredient Review. http://www.cir-safety.org/ingredient/propylene-glycol.

39. Funk JO, Maibach HI. Propylene glycol dermatitis: re-evaluation of an old problem. Contact Dermatitis. 1994;31:236–41.

40. Andersen KE, Storrs FJ. Skin irritation caused by propylene glycols. Hautarzt. 1982;33:12–4.

41. Warshaw EM, Nelsen DD, Maibach HI, Marks JG, Zug KA, et al. Positive patch test reactions to lanolin: cross-sectional data from the North American Contact Dermatitis Group, 1994 to 2006. Dermatitis. 2009;20:79–88.

42. Lundov MB, Moesby L, Zachariae C, Johansen JD. Contamination versus preservation of cosmetics: a review on legislation, usage, infections, and contact allergy. Contact Dermatitis. 2009;60:70–8.

43. Fryklöf L-E. A note on the irritant properties of sorbic acid in ointments and creams. J Pharm Pharmacol. 1958;10:719–20.

44. Rietschel RL. Contact urticaria from synthetic cassia oil and sorbic acid limited to the face. Contact Dermatitis. 1978;4:347–9.

45. Clemmensen O, Hjort N. Perioral contact urticarial from sorbic acid and benzoic acid in salad dressing. Contact Dermatitis. 1982;8:1–6.

46. Nair B. Final report on the safety assessment of benzyl alcohol, benzoic acid and sodium benzoate. Int J Toxicol. 2001;20:23–50.

47. Hannuksela M, Haahtela T. Hypersensitivity reactions to food additives. Allergy. 1987;42:561–75.

48. Public Health England. Formaldehyde: health effects, incident management and toxicology. 2017. https://www.gov.uk/government/publications/formaldehyde-properties-incident-management-and-toxicology.

49. Eighth Commission Directive 86/199/EC of 26 March 1986 adapting to technical progress Annexes II, IV and VI to council directive 76/768/EC on the approximation of the laws of the member states relating to cosmetic products. Off J Eur Commun 1986; L149:38–45.

50. Von Krogh G, Maibach HI. Contact urticaria. In: Adam RM, editor. Occupational skin disease. New York: Grune & Stratton; 1983. p. 58–69.

51. Torresani C, Periti I, Beski L. Contact urticaria syndrome from formaldehyde with multiple physical urticarias. Contact Dermatitis. 1996;35:174–5.

52. Braun J, Zana H, Purohit A. Anaphylactic reactions to formaldehyde in root canal sealant after endodontic treatment. four cases of anaphylactic shock and three of generalized urticarial. Allergy. 2003;58:1210–4.

53. Ogawa M, Nishinakagawa S, Yokosawa F, Yoshida T, Endo Y. Formaldehyde-specific IgE-mediated urticaria due to formaldehyde in a room environment. Jpn J Occup Med Traumatol. 2009;57:125–9.

54. Kireche M, Giménez-Arnau E, Lepoittevin J-P. Preservatives in cosmetics: reactivity of allergenic formaldehyde releasers toward amino acids through breakdown products other than formaldehyde. Contact Dermatitis. 2010;63:192–202.

55. Schnuch A, Lessmann H, Geier J, Uter W. Contact allergy to preservatives. analysis of IVDK data 1996-2009. Br J Dermatol. 2011;164:1316–25.

56. Thyssen JP, Engkilde K, Lundov MD, Carlsen BC, Menné T, Johansen JD. Temporal trends of preservative allergy in Denmark (1985-2008). Contact Dermatitis. 2010;62:272–3.

57. Gonçalo M, Goossens A. Whilst Rome burns: the epidemic of contact allergy to methylisothiazolinone. Contact Dermatitis. 2013;68:257–8.

58. Lundov MD, Opstrup MS, Johansen JD. Methylisothiazolinone contact allergy – a growing epidemic. Contact Dermatitis. 2013;69:271–5.

59. Thyssen JP, Sederberg-Olsen N, Thomsen JF, Menné T. Contact dermatitis from methylisothiazolinone in a paint factory. Contact Dermatitis. 2006;54:322–4.

60. García-Gavín J, Vansina S, Kerre S, Naert A, Goossens A. Methylisothiazolinone, an emerging allergen in cosmetics? Contact Dermatitis. 2010;63:96–101.

61. Lundov MD, Zachariae C, Menné T, Johansen JD. Airborne exposure to preservative methylisothiazolinone causes severe allergic reactions. BMJ. 2012;345:e8221.

62. Geier J, Lessmann H, Schnuch A, Uter W. Recent increase in allergic reactions to methylchloroisothiazolinone/methylisothiazolinone: is methylisothiazolinone the culprit? Contact Dermatitis. 2012;67:334–41.

63. Debeuckelaere C, Moussallieh FM, Elbayed K, Namer IJ, Berl V, Giménez-Arnau E, Lepoittevin J-P. In situ chemical behaviour of methylisothiazolinone (MI) and methylchloroisothiazolinone (MCI) in reconstructed human epidermis: a new approach to the cross-reactivity issue. Contact Dermatitis. 2016;74:159–67.

64. Gebhardt M, Looks A, Hipler UC. Urticaria caused by type IV sensitization to isothiazolinones. Contact Dermatitis. 1997;36:314.

65. Guin JD, Goodman J. Contact urticaria from benzyl alcohol presenting as intolerance to saline soaks. Contact Dermatitis. 2001;45:182–3.

66. Walker SL, Chalmers RJG, Beck MH. Contact urticaria due to *p*-chloro-*m*-cresol. Br J Dermatol. 2004;151:927–52.

67. Birnie AJ, English JS. 2-Phenoxyethanol-induced contact urticaria. Contact Dermatitis. 2006;54:349.

68. Co-Minh HB, Demoly P, Guillot B, Raison-Peyron N. Anaphylactic shock after oral intake and con-

tact urticaria due to polyethylene glycols. Allergy. 2007;62:92–3.

69. Ophaswongse S, Maibach HI. Alcohol dermatitis: allergic contact dermatitis and contact urticaria syndrome. Contact Dermatitis. 1994;30:1–6.

70. Uter W. The European surveillance system of contact allergies (ESSCA): results of patch testing the standard series. J Eur Acad Dermatol Venereol. 2008;22:174–81.

71. Zug KA, Warshaw EM, Fowler JF, et al. Patch-test results of the North American contact dermatitis group 2005-2006. Dermatitis. 2009;20:149–60.

72. Barranco Sanz P, Martin Muñoz F, Lopez Serrano C, Martin Esteban M, Ojeda Casas JA. Hypersensitivity to mercuric fluorescein compounds. Allergol Immunopathol. 1989;17:219–22.

73. Corrales Torres JL, De Corres F. Anaphylactic hypersensitivity to mercurochrome (merbrominum). Ann Allergy. 1985;54:230–2.

74. Dooms-Goossens A, Gevers D, Mertens A, Vanderheyden D. Allergic contact urticaria due to chloramine. Contact Dermatitis. 1983;9:319–20.

75. Kramps JA, van Toorenenbergen AW, Vooren PH, Dijkman JH. Occupational asthma due to inhalation of chloramine-T. II Demonstration of specific IgE antibodies. Int Arch Allergy Appl Immunol. 1981;64:428–38.

76. Kanerva L, Alanko K, Estlander T, Sihvonen T, Jolanki R. Occupational allergic contact urticaria from chloramine-T solution. Contact Dermatitis. 1997;37:180–1.

77. Sinaiko R, Heinemann C, Maibach HI. Contact urticaria and anaphylaxis to Chlorhexidine. In: Zhai H, Wilhelm KP, Maibach HI, editors. Dermatotoxicology. Boca Raton: CRC Press; 2007. p. 485–95.

78. Nagendran V, Wicking J, Ekbote A, Onyekwe T, Garvey LH. Ig-E mediated chlorhexidine allergy: a new occupational hazard? Occup Med. 2009;59:270–2.

79. Calogiuri GF, Di Leo E, Trautmann A, Nettis E, Ferrannini A, Vacca A. Chlorhexidine hypersensitivity: a critical and updated review. J Allergy Ther. 2013;4:141.

80. Walker S, Chalmers R, Beck M. Contact urticaria due to p-chloro-m-cresol. Br J Dermatol. 2004;151:936–7.

81. Goncalo M, Goncalo S, Moreno A. Immediate and delayed sensitivity to chlorocresol. Contact Dermatitis. 1987;17:46–7.

82. Jovanovic M, Karadaglic D, Brkic S. Contact urticaria and allergic contact dermatitis to lidocaine in a patient sensitive to benzocaine and propolis. Contact Dermatitis. 2006;54:124–6.

83. Waton J, Boulanger A, Trechot PH, Schumtz JL, Barbaud A. Contact urticaria from Emla cream. Contact Dermatitis. 2004;51:284–7.

84. Suzuki T, Kawada A, Yashimoto Y, Isogai R, Aragane Y, Tezuka T. Contact urticaria to ketoprofen. Contact Dermatitis. 2003;48:284–5.

85. Arroliga ME, Pien L. Penicillin allergy: consider trying penicillin again. Cleveland Clinic J Med. 2003;70:313–26.

86. Nola RC, Puy R, Deckert K, O'Hehir RE, Douglass JA. Experience with a new commercial skin testing kit to identify IgE-mediated penicillin allergy. Int Med J. 2008;38:357–67.

87. Kim MH, Lee JM. Diagnosis and management of immediate hypersensitivity reactions to cephalosporins. Allergy Asthma Immunol Res. 2014;6:485–95.

88. Romano A, Mayorga C, Torres MJ, Artesani MC, Suau R, Sanchez F, Perez E, Venuti A, Blanca M. Immediate allergic reactions to cephalosporins: cross-reactivity and selective responses. J Allergy Clin Immunol. 2000;106:1177–83.

89. Kim JE, Kim SH, Jin HJ, Hwang EK, Kim JH, Ye YM, Park HS. IgE sensitization to cephalosporins in health care workers. Allergy Asthma Immunol Res. 2012;4:85–91.

90. Ariza A, García-Martín E, Salas M, Montañez MI, Mayorga C, et al. Pyrazolones metabolites are relevant for identifying selective anaphylaxis to metamizole. Sci Rep. 2016;6:23845.

91. Brandão FM, Goossens A. Topical drugs. In: Johansen JD, Frosch PJ, Lepoittevin J-P, editors. Contact dermatitis. 5th ed. Berlin: Springer; 2011. p. 729–62.

92. Rasanen L, Tarvainen K, Makinen-Kiljunen S. Urticaria to hydrocortisone. Allergy. 2001;56:352–3.

93. Nettis E, Muratore L, Valogiuri G, Ferrannini A, Tursi A. Urticaria to hydrocortisone. Allergy. 2001;56:802–3.

94. Helaskoski F, Kuuliala O, Aalto-Korte K. Occupational contact urticaria caused by cyclic acid anhydrides. Contact Dermatitis. 2009;60:214–21.

95. Kanerva L, Jolanki R, Tupasela O, Halmepuro L, Keskinen H, Estlander T, Sysilampi ML. Immediate and delayed allergy from epoxy resins based on diglycidyl ether of bisphenol a. Scand J Work Environ Health. 1991;17:208–15.

96. Kanerva L, Pelttari M, Jolanki R, Alanko K, Estlander T, Suhonen R. Occupational contact urticarial from diglycidyl ether of bisphenol A epoxy resin. Allergy. 2002;57:1205–7.

97. Kanerva L, Tokannen J, Jolanki R, Estlander T. Statistical data on occupational contact urticaria. Contact Dermatitis. 1996;35:229–33.

98. Koopmans AK, Bruynzeel DP. Is PPD a useful screening agent? Contact Dermatitis. 2003;48:89–92.

99. Seidenari S, Mantovani L, Manzini BM, Pignatti M. Cross-sensitizations between azo dyes and para-amino compound. Contact Dermatitis. 1997;36:91–6.

100. Uter W, Geier J, Lessmann H, Hausen BM. Contact allergy to disperse blue 106 and disperse blue 124 in german and austrian patients, 1995 to 1999. Contact Dermatitis. 2001;44:173–7.

101. Wong GA, King CM. Immediate-type hypersensitivity and allergic contact dermatitis due to para-

phenylenediamine in hair dye. Contact Dermatitis. 2003;48:166.

102. Sosted H, Agner T, Andersen KE, Menné T. 55 cases of allergic reactions to hair dye: a descriptive consumer complaint-based study. Contact Dermatitis. 2002;47:299–303.

103. Goldberg BJ, Hermnn FF, Hirata I. Systemic anaphylaxis due ton an oxidation product of p-phenylenediamine in a hair dye. Ann Allergy. 1987;58:205–8.

104. Helgesen AL, Austad J. Contact urticaria from aluminium and nickel in the same patient. Contact Dermatitis. 1997;37:303–4.

105. Kreciscz B, Kiec-Swierczynska M, Krawczyk P, Chomiczewska D, Palczynski C. Cobalt-induced anaphylaxis, contact urticaria and delayed allergy

I a ceramics decorator. Contact Dermatitis. 2009;60:173–4.

106. Bergman A, Svedberg U, Nilsson E. Contact urticaria with anaphylactic reactions caused by occupational exposure to iridium salt. Contact Dermatitis. 1995;32:14–7.

107. Estlander T, Kanerva L, Tupasela O, Keskinen H, Jolanki R. Immediate and delayed allergy to nickel with contact urticaria, rhinitis, asthma and contact dermatitis. Clin Exp Allergy. 1993;23:306–10.

108. Cristaudo A, Sera F, Severino V, De Rocco M, Di Lella E, Picardo M. Occupational hypersensitivity to metal salts, including platinum, in the secondary industry. Allergy. 2005;60:159–64.

109. Schena D, Barba A, Costa G. Occupational contact urticaria due to cisplatin. Contact Dermatitis. 1996;34:220–1.

Immunoglobulin E: Pathogenic Relevance in Immediate Contact Reactions

Maria Estela Martinez-Escala, Leah Ariella Kaplan, and Ana M. Giménez-Arnau

Introduction

Contact urticaria syndrome (CUS) comprises a heterogeneous group of disorders characterized by the development of immediate contact skin reactions [1]. It manifests clinically with wheals or eczema or both, developed within minutes after contact with eliciting substances. In severe cases, systemic symptoms such as anaphylaxis can develop. CUS includes two different entities: (1) contact urticaria (CoU) and (2) protein contact dermatitis (PCD). Contact urticaria is usually induced by low– and high–molecular weight molecules, and clinically presents wheals that are limited to the areas of exposure and disappear within a few hours without residual lesions. Generalized urticaria might develop. In contrast, PCD, induced by large molecules, commonly affects the hands (fingertips) and occasionally spreads to wrists and arms. Besides the initial presentation with erythema and wheals/angioedema, a late phase of vesicular lesions and lichenification are characteristic [1, 2]. Proteins and chemical agents are the most common substance causing both entities. Among patients with PCD, 50% suffer atopic dermatitis [3]. In general, both clinical forms show negative patch tests, with positive prick/scratch tests in early reading, and occasionally a positive radioallergosorbent test. In PCD, prick-by-prick and prick/scratch tests can show immediate and delayed positive results [2].

The pathogenesis of CoU is divided into nonimmunological and immunological mechanisms. The first is induced by the release of vasogenic mediators, without involvement of the immune system, and therefore a previous sensitization is not required. The immunological mechanism consists of an allergen-specific IgE-mediated reaction, such as type I hypersensitivity, in which a previous sensitization is required [1, 2, 4]. In PCD, the pathogenesis is not understood, but it has been suggested to have a nonimmunological and immunological mechanism. Several theories have been proposed with regard to the immunological mechanisms. One of the most accepted theories suggests a combination of type I and type IV hypersensitivity reactions, which would explain the presence of wheals and eczema as clinical manifestations induced by the same antigen [2]. However, the high frequency of a negative patch test in those patients would not support this theory. Some authors consider that patch test

M. E. Martinez-Escala (✉)
Department of Dermatology, Northwestern University, Feinberg School of Medicine, Chicago, IL, USA
e-mail: mmarti13@nm.org

L. A. Kaplan
Tulane University, New Orleans, LA, USA

A. M. Giménez-Arnau
Hospital del Mar - Institut Mar d'Investigacions Mediques, Universitat Autònoma de Barcelona (UAB), Department of Dermatology, Barcelona, Spain

© Springer International Publishing AG, part of Springer Nature 2018
A. M. Giménez-Arnau, H. I. Maibach (eds.), *Contact Urticaria Syndrome*, Updates in Clinical Dermatology, https://doi.org/10.1007/978-3-319-89764-6_9

results may be false negative because the antigen may require a longer duration of exposure, the protein-based molecules are too large, or higher concentrations are needed to penetrate healthy skin [3, 5, 6]. Other authors have demonstrated that a preceding type I hypersensitivity response may obscure the detection of a type IV hypersensitivity reaction, because the IgE antibody may deplete available antigens to develop a delayed hypersensitivity reaction [6]. Delayed-type hypersensitivity could be simply justified because a positive patch test has been detected in some cases [4, 7–11]. Another theory involves the presence of IgE-presenting Langerhans cells, which are speculated to cause a delayed IgE-mediated reaction resembling atopic dermatitis [3, 12]. Indeed, IgE-bearing Langerhans cells are found in patients with atopic dermatitis, which would also justify the high association of atopic dermatitis with PCD.

In this chapter we aim to review the structure and function of immunoglobulin (Ig) E, the IgE-mediated type I hypersensitive reaction, as the prototype of immediate contact reaction, and the role of IgE favoring this type of immunological response.

Immunoglobulin E

In 1968, Drs. Kimishige and Teruko Ishizaka described IgE, which was the last human antibody to be discovered because it occurs at low levels in the peripheral blood [13, 14]. IgE, as well as IgG, is exclusively mammalian, and both derive from an ancestral antibody closely related to the avian IgY [15]. With the evolution of this ancestral antibody, a functional specialization of each Ig was derived: (1) antibody-mediated opsonization by IgG, and (2) hypersensitivity reactions to parasitic infection by IgE. The decrease of the prevalence of parasitic infections in Western lifestyles causes IgE to have a major part in allergic diseases.

IgE is a 190-kDa glycoprotein with the same basic molecular architecture as other antibodies. The main structure is formed by two identical heavy (H) chains, and two identical light (L) chains, both composed of their constant (C) and variable (V) domains (Fig. 9.1). Compared with IgG, IgE have an extra C domain in their H chain that is equivalent to the flexible hinge region of IgG (Fig. 9.1a, b). This extra domain is important in the stability of the complex between IgE and its high-affinity receptor (FcεRI) on surface cells. The stable complex becomes permanently bound to IgE with a receptor that has a long life, 2 to 3 weeks. As a reference, IgG is able to bind to its receptor for only a few hours [16]. As mentioned earlier, IgE is the least abundant antibody class in serum because most of the IgE is sequestered in tissues. Its half-life is about 2 to 3 days compared to IgG, but increases when IgE is complexed to its high-affinity receptor. In the human lifetime, IgE levels increase from birth and peak between 16 to 19 years of age [17].

IgE can be found in two forms: as a soluble molecule, or in a membrane form. The latter binds to the cytoplasmic membrane via an additional domain that is present in each H chain (extracellular membrane proximal domain) of the IgE. This form of IgE constitutes the antigen receptor of the B cell committed to IgE synthesis, and even though it is attached to the cell membrane, the binding site to the high-affinity receptor expressed on other surface cells is still accessible [18].

Two IgE receptors are described and differentiated by affinity for the Ig: FcεRI, the high-affinity receptor, and FcεRII (or CD23), the low-affinity receptor. FcεRI structurally belongs to the Ig superfamily (Fig. 9.2a). It is abundant in mast cells and basophil membranes as a tetramer $(\alpha\beta\gamma_2)$, and is expressed less in Langerhans cells, monocytes, and platelet and eosinophil membranes as a trimer $(\alpha\gamma_2)$. The humanized anti-IgE antibody (omalizumab) has aided to elucidate the interplay between FcεRI and IgE [19–21]. Serum IgE influences FcεRI cell-surface expression and is related to the total number of FcεRI per cell [22]. As already stated, the IgE can remain bound to FcεRI for 3 weeks, and this union stabilizes the receptor expression on the cell surface [19, 23, 24]. The main effector function of FcεRI in its tetramer form is the immediate hypersensitivity reaction, characterized by mast cell degranulation and lipid mediator synthesis [18, 25].

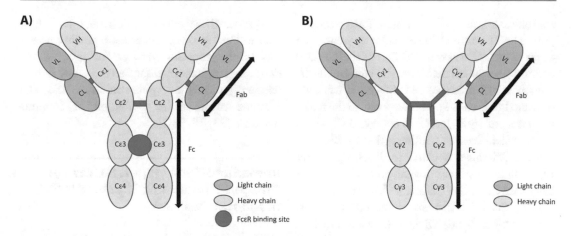

Fig. 9.1 Comparison of immunoglobulin (Ig)E structure with IgG. IgE (**a**) is a 190-kDa glycoprotein and IgG (**b**) is a 150-kDa glycoprotein with two identical heavy chains and two identical light chains. The Cε3–Cε4 are equiva-lent to Cγ2–Cγ3 domains of IgG, and the pair Cε2 is equivalent to the flexible hinge region of IgG. *Fab* antigen-binding fragment, *Fc* crystallizable region fragment

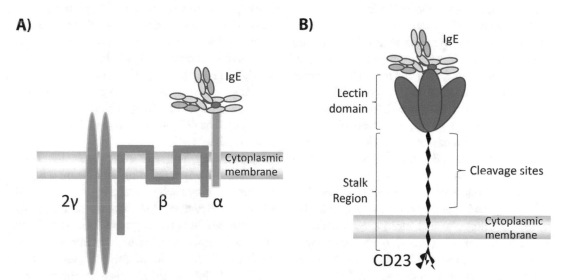

Fig. 9.2 IgE receptor structure. (**a**) High-affinity receptor or FcεRI, which can be expressed as a tetramer with 2γ subunits, 1β and 1α (as it is represented), usually on the surface of effector cells (basophil and mast cell), or as a trimer with 2γ subunits and 1α on antigen-presenting cells (Langerhans cell). (**b**) Low-affinity receptor or CD23 is composed of three head lectin domains and a stalk region that binds to the cell surface. The soluble CD23 is released by cleavage of the stalk region

However, it has also been suggested that FcεRI on antigen-presenting cells favors the transfer of antigen captured by IgE to the lymph nodes, where the antigen will be presented to either naïve Th cells or naïve B cells [25].

FcεRII, also known as CD23, is considered to be the low-affinity receptor. It structurally corre-sponds to the C-type (calcium-dependent) lectin superfamily, and it is characterized as a three-lectin "head" domain that binds to IgE, and a helical coiled-coil "stalk" region which binds to the cytoplasmic membrane through the intracel-lular N-terminal portion (Fig. 9.2b). It is mis-named as a low-affinity receptor because its affinity with a single lectin domain is low; how-ever, when IgE binds to the trimer, its affinity approximates that of the high-affinity receptor [18]. The N-terminal intracellular sequence can differ in their first seven (CD23a) or six (CD23b) amino acids, which determines in which cells the sequence will be expressed. CD23a is basically restricted to B cells and corresponds to the major regulator of IgE levels. Thereby, IgE levels become stabilized by binding IgE to CD23a on B cells, as it induces negative feedback signals for IgE synthesis by the following process: when IgE levels are high, the CD23a molecules are occupied by the IgEs, decreasing the IgE synthesis. On the other hand, when IgE levels are low, CD23 molecules are mostly unoccupied and therefore enhance IgE synthesis [18, 26, 27]. Instead, CD23b is expressed in numerous cells including T cells, dendritic cells, monocytes, neutrophils, and intestinal epithelial cells.

A soluble CD23 fragment can be generated by proteolysis on the stalk region (between the lectin domain and cytoplasmic membrane) of the CD23 molecule, and this may have opposite effects on the regulation (homeostasis) of IgE compared to the CD23 membrane-bound form [28]. By cleaving CD23, IgE production may become upregulated by the lack of feedback inhibition by the IgE–CD23 engagement on B cells. Proteolysis of the stalk region can be induced by endogenous proteases (ADAM 10, a disintegrin and metalloproteinase 10), but also by many allergens that can be enzymatically active (e.g., Der p I, *Dermatophagoides pteronyssinus*), and release CD23 fragments, therefore upregulating the IgE synthesis. CD23 also has a role in antigen presentation in B cells when it interacts with MHC class II. It processes the IgE-captured antigen that, once uploaded to the MHC class II, is presented to the CD4+ T cells. This IgE-mediated antigen presentation can induce 100-fold T- and B-cell responses over sole antigen presentation [29–33]. CD21 is one of the most important cofactors of CD23, and because it is expressed in B cells, follicular dendritic cells, activated T cells, and basophils when pairing with CD23, shows important involvement in the allergic response. It is well known for its role in B-cell survival and the specification of IgE [34].

Besides these two specific receptors, IgE is able to bind to other receptors, including receptors of the constant fragment of IgG, which, depending on their effector function, may induce antigen presentation, polarization to the Th2 immune response, or inhibition of immune response [25, 35–38].

Immediate-Type Hypersensitivity: Antigen-Dependent Effects of IgE in Allergic Response

Hypersensitivity is an overreaction of the immune system that can become life threatening for the patient. It initially requires an exposure to an allergen, an external or even internal antigen, causing, as a consequence, an allergic or autoimmune disease in the individual. Gell and Coombs described four types of hypersensitivity: (1) type I, immediate hypersensitivity classically considered IgE mediated; (2) type II, cytotoxic antibody-mediated (IgG, IgM); (3) type III, immune complex-mediated (IgG, IgM); and (4) type IV, also known as delayed hypersensitivity, which is T-cell mediated [39].

IgE-binding antigens have typically been described with external antigens causing a type I hypersensitivity, such as aeroallergens and food allergens. However, IgE against autoantigens inducing an allergic response has also been described with the term auto-allergy [40]. Because of the topic of this chapter, further details of IgE-mediated hypersensitivity are discussed.

Sensitization Phase (Fig. 9.3)

In type I hypersensitivity, sensitization is a two-step immune response developed after antigen exposure. First, a T-helper (Th) cell differentiates into a Th subset, and second, this subset of Th cells induces a switch class production from IgM to IgE on B cells [41, 42]. This type of immune response is developed by intrinsic properties of the specific allergen and environmental factors, yet host immune factors have an important role

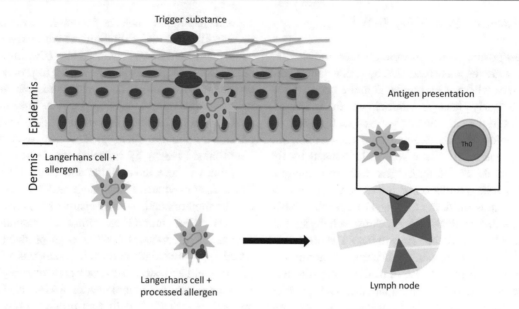

Fig. 9.3 Sensitization phase. The trigger substance is captured by the professional antigen-presenting cells, either by Langerhans cells located in the epidermis or dendritic cells in the dermis. They process the antigen to upload to the MHC class II, and migrate to the peripheral lymph node to present the processed antigen to naïve T-helper cells

and explain why some individuals develop allergies and others do not. Those factors are influenced by genetic predispositions and environmental exposures [41, 42].

Once dendritic cells take up the allergen in the epidermis and dermis, they migrate to peripheral lymph nodes to encounter the naïve Th cells. Different Th-cell subsets have been described with their cytokine profiles including Th1 with interferon (IFN)-γ and interleukin (IL)-12; Th2 with IL-4, IL-5, and IL-13; Th17 with IL-17A and F; Th22 with IL-22; and Th9-producing IL-9. The allergic immune response induced by specific allergens (e.g., aeroallergens or latex) is associated to the Th2 subset along with its IL, as well as IL-9, IL-22, and IL-17. However, it is not clear whether the corresponding Th subset secreting IL-9, IL-22, and IL-17 has any function in the allergic response [42]. The main signal for Th2 differentiation is determined by the presence of IL-4 in the environment where naïve Th encounter antigens processed by antigen-presenting cells. Considering that IL-4 is produced by differentiated Th2 cells, the origin of the first (before Th differentiation) IL-4 to induce this differentia-

tion is still a matter of debate [42]. The new Th2 cells will then interact with naïve B cells and induce a class switch immunoglobulin production by two signals. First, IL-4 and IL-13 target the Cε gene for initiation switch recombination. Second, is the interaction of CD40 expressed on the B cell with its ligand (CD40L) expressed on the T cell. This interaction is required in all immune responses that induce an antibody class switching, from IgM (first antibody response) to IgG, IgA, or IgE. At the same time, V domains are subject to somatic hypermutation to provide antibody specificity (affinity) to the allergen encountered. The pathogenicity of allergen-specific IgE produced during the sensitization phase has been demonstrated by the elicitation of anaphylaxis with the passive transfer of these antibodies to naïve animals followed by challenge with the corresponding allergen [43].

Finally, IgE-specific B cells then migrate to the spleen for differentiation into long-lived plasma cells and the production of IgE antibodies. Those plasma cells may remain in the spleen, or move to bone marrow, or into inflamed tissue, in which they can survive from months to a lifetime [18, 42].

Elicitation Phase (Fig. 9.4)

Reexposure to the specific allergen induces the immune response mediated by IgE, which is consistent with an "early phase" and a "late phase." The "early phase" is induced once the IgE crosslinks to the specific allergen and its high-affinity receptor, FcεRI, expressed on mast cells. The aggregation of multiple FcεRI, induced by the crosslink of multiple IgEs with the allergen, causes degranulation of preformed mediators in mast cells (in tissue localized reactions) or basophils (in peripheral blood), along with the synthesis of lipid mediators (in minutes). The preformed mediators are histamine, heparin, serotonin, and mast cell proteases. Lipid mediators synthesized are leukotrienes, prostaglandins, and platelet-activating factors. The local effects of these pre-

formed mediators include increased vascular permeability, arteriolar dilation (which increases cutaneous blood flow), increased loss of intravascular fluid from postcapillary venules to produce erythema, and stimulation of cutaneous sensory nerves by histamines, causing pruritus. The chemokines and cytokines delivered in the "early phase" initiate the "late phase," which starts hours later (4–8 h) by inducing the gene transcription of more interleukins and chemokines. These factors induce recruitment and activation of inflammatory cells at the sensitive sites [18].

After the immediate immune response decreases, IgE induces mast cells to produce a broad set of cytokines and chemokines that will produce and activate the effector cells of allergic immune response. Chemokines such as RANTES and eotaxin recruit T cells that produce growth

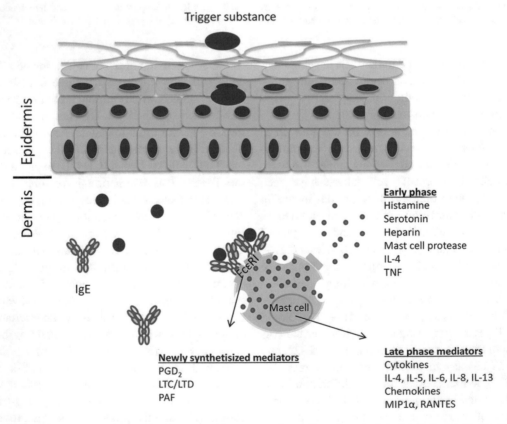

Fig. 9.4 Elicitation phase. Upon sensitization, with the following exposure to the allergen, IgE captures it and binds to its high-affinity receptor. With the aggregation of multiple receptors, the mast cell releases the preformed mediators (early phase), and initiate the synthesis of lipid mediators from the cytoplasmic membrane (lipid mediators). Finally, gene transcription of certain factors causes a late-phase reaction. *TNF* tumor necrosis factor, *PGD₂* prostaglandin 2, *LTC/LTD* leukotriene, *PAF* platelet-activating factor

factors of mast cells and eosinophils which proliferate with the presence of IL-5. Moreover, IL-4, besides the recruitment of T cells, eosinophils, basophils, and monocytes, enhances the expression of adhesion molecules, stimulates B cells to IgE synthesis to replenish IgE consumed during the allergic response, and decreases the degranulation threshold of mast cells. IL-3 enhances mast cell and basophil proliferation. This cytokine and chemokine milieu generates the perfect environment for chronic allergic responses by perpetuating and amplifying the allergic response [44–49].

Chronification of Allergic Response

In allergic patients, Langerhans cells and dendritic cells express trimeric forms of FcεRI, which uptake and process IgE-bound allergens. These cells either migrate to peripheral lymph nodes or remain in the tissue to stimulate naïve Th cells (usually when inflammation is in the mucosa or gastrointestinal tract) [50–53]. Langerhans and dendritic cells expressing FcεRI are characteristic of atopic patients, and this is suggested to critically lower the threshold to mount allergen-specific T-cell responses. It consequently perpetuates allergen-specific IgE synthesis, inducing either immediate or delayed hypersensitivity reactions [51, 53].

In addition, allergen–IgE complexes bound to CD23 expressed on activated B cells also facilitate antigen presentation to T cells [18, 54]. The interaction of CD23 with major histocompatibility complex (MHC) class II engulf the allergen–IgE–CD23 complex in endosomes to produce allergen-derived peptides that are presented to T cells [55]. Although antigen-presenting B cells through B-cell receptors are limited to their cognate T cells (T cells recognizing the same allergen), antigen-presenting B cells through CD23 to their cognate T cells overcome the B-cell specificity receptor and include unrelated allergen peptides [55]. The latter may justify the amplification of immune responses from a single allergen to unrelated allergens, a phenomenon called *epitope spreading*: this is a positive feedback mechanism that enhances allergic sensitization [18].

Antigen-Independent Effects of IgE in Allergic Response

The immediate type of hypersensitivity reaction (type I) just described is an immune response IgE-mediated and triggered by the presence of specific allergen exposure. The use of in vitro experiments as well as allergic/atopic animal models allowed demonstrating effector functions of IgE in allergic response totally independent of the exposure of a specific antigen, and therefore induced by non-allergen-specific IgE [56–58].

One of the most relevant antigen-independent roles of IgE is the effect in mast cell proliferation and survival [25]. Bone marrow-derived mast cells can be generated by culture media containing IL-3. However, in the absence of IL-3, those cells go under apoptosis. The presence of IgE in the culture media, even without IL-3, shows protection of these cells from apoptosis. This protective mechanism is still unclear, but two main theories were initially established. First, the inhibition of apoptosis could be mediated by the increased expression of FcεRI on the cell surface, which is regulated by IgE. However, the presence of IgG in the media did not prevent mast cell apoptosis [59]. The second theory considers that IgE inhibits apoptosis by maintaining antiapoptotic protein levels (i.e., Bcl-X(L)), and producing autocrine-acting cytokines [60]. Recent research results approach both previous theories, by characterizing IgE molecules with a different ability of cytokine stimulation. In this manner, highly cytokinergic IgE clones induce the production of considerable amounts of cytokines [mainly IL-6, tumor necrosis factor (TNF)-α, and IL-3], as well as FcεRI aggregation, and poorly cytokinergic IgE clones inefficiently induce those effects. Therefore, two anti-apoptotic pathways influenced by IgE have been described: (1) IL-3 dependent and (2) FcεRI aggregation [61, 62].

Besides favoring mast cell survival, IgE enhances mast cell maturation, as well as increasing its granularity and synthesis of preformed mediators promoting to maintain an inflammatory phenotype [63]. Those effects favor developing an allergic response with a lesser concentration of allergen. As the presence of IgE would increase FcεRI expression on the mast cell surface, this plus the known stable union of IgE with FcεRI may facilitate the maintenance of a pro-inflammatory status. Furthermore, the stimulation of chemokine production favors the upregulation of integrins and adhesion molecule production, leading to mast cell migration into the inflammatory tissue [56, 57, 62, 64, 65].

Some of the antigen-independent IgE effects have been described by inducing contact hypersensitivity reaction on animal models, which commonly (but not exclusively) reflect a delayed hypersensitivity reaction [56]. It has been shown that repeated epicutaneous exposure of the allergen at the same site (i.e., ear) enhances an immediate contact response. The immediate contact response was developed within a few minutes to 1 h after allergen exposure, and was followed by a late-phase reaction. Moreover, this immediate contact response was only developed when enhanced by a specific allergen, in which specific serum IgE was detected. Last, it was shown that this type of response was mast cell dependent, because mice deficient in mast cells did not developed immediate contact response. Posterior experiments showed a shift of the cytokine profile at the site of frequent application from Th1 (delayed hypersensitivity) to Th2 [66]. Further studies with different protocols of allergen frequency application demonstrated that repeated epicutaneous stimulation in a specific site with a specific allergen induced an immediate contact reaction at 1 h of exposure, followed by a delayed-type reaction that developed 24 h later without a shift of the cytokine profile. The authors justify these controversies to the different chemical properties, and the application frequency of the allergen [67]. Additionally, this group could also demonstrate the presence of allergen-specific IgE with the ability to induce disease in naïve mice when passive transfer of this IgE is followed by allergen exposure. Again, disease could not be developed in mast

cell-deficient mice. Surprisingly, this group also demonstrated that a re-challenge (antigen exposure) 3 months later did not induce an immediate-type reaction, but rather a delayed-type reaction. Although levels of allergen-specific IgE were stable from the initial response, a decreased number of mast cells in the tissue was observed, probably because of the lack of exposure of the antigen, hypothesizing that the continuous repeating exposure would enhance accumulation of mast cells in the target tissue [67]. Overall, these animal models reproduce a response similar to that observed in PCD, where immediate- and delayed-type hypersensitivity are developed with the exposure of a single allergen. Yet, as should be considered in most experimental animal models, extrapolation of these data to human pathophysiology must be performed with caution [67, 68].

By using these animal models, another antigen-independent role of IgE was observed, the enhancement of cutaneous immune sensitization. An impairment of sensitization in the absence of IgE has been shown at the first antigen exposure. Indeed, the cutaneous exposure of a sensitizer on the ear of IgE$^{-/-}$ mice did not show a cutaneous reaction compared with the wild-type mice group [56]. Moreover, the transfer of splenocytes (B cells) from sensitized IgE$^{-/-}$ mice to nonexposed wild-type mice did not show a cutaneous response, whereas the transfer of splenocytes from sensitized wild-type mice to nonexposed wild-type mice induced ear swelling. The impairment of cutaneous sensitization might be explained because cytokines such as TNFα, IL-1β, monocyte chemoattractant protein (MCP)-1, and the protease MMCP-6 (mouse mast cell protease) are commonly upregulated in antigen presentations, collaborating in antigen processing and dendritic cell migration. These cytokines are produced and released by mast cells in the presence of IgE alone. IgE$^{-/-}$ mice have low levels of TNF-α, IL-1β, MCP-1, and MMCP-6, and sensitization with cutaneous response was not developed unless local administration of these cytokines was performed [60, 63]. Furthermore, only the transfer of IgE antibodies to IgE$^{-/-}$ mice was required to restore the cytokine and protease levels [56].

Conclusions

In this chapter, we reviewed the role of IgE in immunological mechanisms of immediate contact reactions. With the presence of the specific antigen, IgE is responsible for capturing the allergen and inducing mast cell degranulation, causing the wheal or angioedema. Nonetheless, non-allergen-specific IgE favors a perfect environment for allergic response development, including antigen processing and presentation by dendritic cells (sensitization), plus mast cell maturation and survival (perpetuation and amplification of allergic response). Even though most of these functions have been demonstrated by inducing contact hypersensitivity in animals, important limitations of data interpretation are seen. Properties of the allergen and frequency of exposure protocols are different between the study groups, showing a different type of cutaneous response (immediate versus delayed hypersensitivity). Standardization of protocols and allergen properties is required to better understand, compare, and explain the controversies of the data observed.

References

1. Gimenez-Arnau A, Maurer M, De La Cuadra J, Maibach H. Immediate contact skin reactions, an update of contact urticaria, contact urticaria syndrome and protein contact dermatitis– "A Never Ending Story". Eur J Dermatol. 2010;20(5):552–62. PubMed PMID: 20732848.
2. Levin C, Warshaw E. Protein contact dermatitis: allergens, pathogenesis, and management. Dermatitis. 2008;19(5):241–51. PubMed PMID: 18845114.
3. Janssens V, Morren M, Dooms-Goossens A, Degreef H. Protein contact dermatitis: myth or reality? Br J Dermatol. 1995;132(1):1–6. PubMed PMID: 7756118.
4. Amaro C, Goossens A. Immunological occupational contact urticaria and contact dermatitis from proteins: a review. Contact Dermatitis. 2008;58(2):67–75. PubMed PMID: 18186738.
5. Hjorth N, Roed-Petersen J. Occupational protein contact dermatitis in food handlers. Contact Dermatitis. 1976;2(1):28–42. PubMed PMID: 145923.
6. Jones HE, Reinhardt JH, Rinaldi MG. Immunologic susceptibility to chronic dermatophytosis. Arch Dermatol. 1974;110(2):213–20. PubMed PMID: 4852361.
7. Conde-Salazar L, Gonzalez MA, Guimaraens D. Type I and Type IV sensitization to Anisakis simplex in 2 patients with hand eczema. Contact Dermatitis. 2002;46(6):361. PubMed PMID: 12190630.
8. Jappe U, Bonnekoh B, Hausen BM, Gollnick H. Garlic-related dermatoses: case report and review of the literature. Am J Contact Dermat. 1999;10(1):37–9. PubMed PMID: 10072338.
9. Jeannet-Peter N, Piletta-Zanin PA, Hauser C. Facial dermatitis, contact urticaria, rhinoconjunctivitis, and asthma induced by potato. Am J Contact Dermat. 1999;10(1):40–2. PubMed PMID: 10072339.
10. Kanerva L, Estlander T. Immediate and delayed skin allergy from cow dander. Am J Contact Dermat. 1997;8(3):167–9. PubMed PMID: 9249287.
11. Scharer L, Hafner J, Wuthrich B, Bucher C. Occupational protein contact dermatitis from shrimps. a new presentation of the crustacean-mite syndrome. Contact Dermatitis. 2002;46(3):181–2. PubMed PMID: 12000333.
12. Saloga J, Knop J. Does sensitization through the skin occur? Allergy. 2000;55(10):905–9. PubMed PMID: 11030369.
13. Hamilton RG. Science behind the discovery of IgE. J Allergy Clin Immunol. 2005;115(3):648–52. PubMed PMID: 15753924.
14. Stanworth DR. The discovery of IgE. Allergy. 1993;48(2):67–71. PubMed PMID: 8457034.
15. Taylor AI, Fabiane SM, Sutton BJ, Calvert RA. The crystal structure of an avian IgY-fc fragment reveals conservation with both mammalian IgG and IgE. Biochemistry. 2009;48(3):558–62. PubMed PMID: 19115948.
16. McDonnell JM, Calvert R, Beavil RL, Beavil AJ, Henry AJ, Sutton BJ, et al. The structure of the IgE Cepsilon2 domain and its role in stabilizing the complex with its high-affinity receptor FcepsilonRIalpha. Nat Struct Biol. 2001;8(5):437–41. PubMed PMID: 11323720.
17. Gergen PJ, Arbes SJ Jr, Calatroni A, Mitchell HE, Zeldin DC. Total IgE levels and asthma prevalence in the US population: results from the National Health and Nutrition Examination Survey 2005-2006. J Allergy Clin Immunol. 2009;124(3):447–53. PubMed Pubmed Central PMCID: 2758573.
18. Gould HJ, Sutton BJ. IgE in allergy and asthma today. Nat Rev Immunol. 2008;8(3):205–17. PubMed PMID: 18301424.
19. MacGlashan DW Jr, Bochner BS, Adelman DC, Jardieu PM, Togias A, Lichtenstein LM. Serum IgE level drives basophil and mast cell IgE receptor display. Int Arch Allergy Immunol. 1997;113(1–3):45–7. PubMed PMID: 9130480.
20. Saavedra MC, Sur S. Down regulation of the high-affinity IgE receptor associated with successful treatment of chronic idiopathic urticaria with omalizumab. Clin Mol Allergy. 2011;9(1):2. PubMed PMID: 21247438. Pubmed Central PMCID: 3031269.

21. Saini SS, MacGlashan DW Jr, Sterbinsky SA, Togias A, Adelman DC, Lichtenstein LM, et al. Down-regulation of human basophil IgE and FC epsilon RI alpha surface densities and mediator release by anti-IgE-infusions is reversible in vitro and in vivo. J Immunol. 1999;162(9):5624–30. PubMed PMID: 10228046.

22. Malveaux FJ, Conroy MC, Adkinson NF Jr, Lichtenstein LM. IgE receptors on human baso-phils. relationship to serum IgE concentration. J Clin Invest. 1978;62(1):176–81. PubMed PMID: 659631. Pubmed Central PMCID: 371751.

23. Jardieu P. Anti-IgE therapy. Curr Opin Immunol. 1995;7(6):779–82. PubMed PMID: 8679119.

24. Lantz CS, Yamaguchi M, Oettgen HC, Katona IM, Miyajima I, Kinet JP, et al. IgE regulates mouse basophil Fc epsilon RI expression in vivo. J Immunol. 1997;158(6):2517–21. PubMed PMID: 9058781.

25. Burton OT, Oettgen HC. Beyond immediate hyper-sensitivity: evolving roles for IgE antibodies in immune homeostasis and allergic diseases. Immunol Rev. 2011;242(1):128–43. PubMed Pubmed Central PMCID: 3122143.

26. Conrad DH, Ford JW, Sturgill JL, Gibb DR. CD23: an overlooked regulator of allergic disease. Curr Allergy Asthma Rep. 2007;7(5):331–7. PubMed PMID: 17697638.

27. Shiung YY, Chiang CY, Chen JB, Wu PC, Hung AF, Lu DC, et al. An anti-IgE monoclonal antibody that binds to IgE on CD23 but not on high-affinity IgE. Fc receptors. Immunobiology. 2012;217(7):676–83. PubMed PMID: 22226669.

28. Bonnefoy JY, Gauchat JF, Lecoanet-Henchoz S, Graber P, Aubry JP. Regulation of human IgE syn-thesis. Ann N Y Acad Sci. 1996;796:59–71. PubMed PMID: 8906212.

29. Getahun A, Hjelm F, Heyman B. IgE enhances anti-body and T cell responses in vivo via CD23+ B cells. J Immunol. 2005;175(3):1473–82. PubMed PMID: 16034084.

30. Hjelm F, Karlsson MC, Heyman B. A novel B cell-mediated transport of IgE-immune complexes to the follicle of the spleen. J Immunol. 2008;180(10):6604–10. PubMed PMID: 18453579.

31. Lemieux GA, Blumenkron F, Yeung N, Zhou P, Williams J, Grammer AC, et al. The low affinity IgE receptor (CD23) is cleaved by the metalloproteinase ADAM10. J Biol Chem. 2007;282(20):14836–44. PubMed PMID: 17389606. Pubmed Central PMCID: 2582392.

32. Marolewski AE, Buckle DR, Christie G, Earnshaw DL, Flamberg PL, Marshall LA, et al. CD23 (FcepsilonRII) release from cell membranes is medi-ated by a membrane-bound metalloprotease. Biochem J. 1998;333(Pt 3):573–9. PubMed Pubmed Central PMCID: 1219619.

33. Weskamp G, Ford JW, Sturgill J, Martin S, Docherty AJ, Swendeman S, et al. ADAM10 is a principal 'sheddase' of the low-affinity immunoglobulin E

34. Liu YJ, Zhang J, Lane PJ, Chan EY, MacLennan IC. Sites of specific B cell activation in primary and secondary responses to T cell-dependent and T cell-independent antigens. Eur J Immunol. 1991;21(12):2951–62. PubMed PMID: 1748148.

35. Frigeri LG, Liu FT. Surface expression of functional IgE binding protein, an endogenous lectin, on mast cells and macrophages. J Immunol. 1992;148(3):861–7. PubMed PMID: 1730878.

36. Frigeri LG, Zuberi RI, Liu FT. Epsilon BP, a beta-galactoside-binding animal lectin, recognizes IgE receptor (Fc epsilon RI) and activates mast cells. Biochemistry. 1993;32(30):7644–9. PubMed PMID: 8347574.

37. Hirano M, Davis RS, Fine WD, Nakamura S, Shimizu K, Yagi H, et al. IgEb immune complexes acti-vate macrophages through FcgammaRIV binding. Nat Immunol. 2007;8(7):762–71. PubMed PMID: 17558411.

38. Mancardi DA, Iannascoli B, Hoos S, England P, Daeron M, Bruhns P. FcgammaRIV is a mouse IgE receptor that resembles macrophage FcepsilonRI in humans and promotes IgE-induced lung inflamma-tion. J Clin Invest. 2008;118(11):3738–50. PubMed PMID: 18949059. Pubmed Central PMCID: 2571035.

39. Rajan TV. The Gell-Coombs classification of hyper-sensitivity reactions: a re-interpretation. Trends Immunol. 2003;24(7):376–9. PubMed PMID: 12860528.

40. Tedeschi A, Lorini M, Asero R. Anti-thyroid peroxi-dase IgE in patients with chronic urticaria. J Allergy Clin Immunol. 2001;108(3):467–8. PubMed PMID: 11544471.

41. Murphy K, Travers P, Walport M, Janeway C. Janeway's immunobiology, vol. xix. 8th ed. New York: Garland Science; 2012. p. 868.

42. van Ree R, Hummelshoj L, Plantinga M, Poulsen LK, Swindle E. Allergic sensitization: host-immune factors. Clin Transl Allergy. 2014;4(1):12. PubMed PMID: 24735802. Pubmed Central PMCID: 3989850.

43. Ovary Z. Passive cutaneous anaphylaxis. Methods Med Res. 1964;10:158–62. PubMed PMID: 14284910.

44. Feuser K, Feilhauer K, Staib L, Bischoff SC, Lorentz A. Akt cross-links IL-4 priming, stem cell factor signaling, and IgE-dependent activation in mature human mast cells. Mol Immunol. 2011;48(4):546–52. PubMed PMID: 21106245.

45. Lorentz A, Schwengberg S, Sellge G, Manns MP, Bischoff SC. Human intestinal mast cells are capa-ble of producing different cytokine profiles: role of IgE receptor cross-linking and IL-4. J Immunol. 2000;164(1):43–8. PubMed PMID: 10604991.

46. Miescher SM, Vogel M. Molecular aspects of allergy. Mol Asp Med. 2002;23(6):413–62. PubMed PMID: 12385747.

47. Pawankar R, Okuda M, Yssel H, Okumura K, Ra C. Nasal mast cells in perennial allergic rhinitics

receptor CD23. Nat Immunol. 2006;7(12):1293–8. PubMed PMID: 17072319.

exhibit increased expression of the Fc epsilonRI, CD40L, IL-4, and IL-13, and can induce IgE synthesis in B cells. J Clin Invest. 1997;99(7):1492–9. PubMed Pubmed Central PMCID: 507968.

48. Shelburne CP, Ryan JJ. The role of Th2 cytokines in mast cell homeostasis. Immunol Rev. 2001;179:82–93. PubMed PMID: 11292031.

49. Yamaguchi M, Sayama K, Yano K, Lantz CS, Noben-Trauth N, Ra C, et al. IgE enhances Fc epsilon receptor I expression and IgE-dependent release of histamine and lipid mediators from human umbilical cord blood-derived mast cells: synergistic effect of IL-4 and IgE on human mast cell Fc epsilon receptor I expression and mediator release. J Immunol. 1999;162(9):5455–65. PubMed PMID: 10228025.

50. Sutton JK, Brunso-Bechtold JK. Dendritic development in the dorsal lateral geniculate nucleus of ferrets in the postnatal absence of retinal input: a Golgi study. J Neurobiol. 1993;24(3):317–34. PubMed PMID: 8492109.

51. Novak N, Bieber T, Kraft S. Immunoglobulin E-bearing antigen-presenting cells in atopic dermatitis. Curr Allergy Asthma Rep. 2004;4(4):263–9. PubMed PMID: 15175139.

52. Bieber T. Fc epsilon RI-expressing antigen-presenting cells: new players in the atopic game. Immunol Today. 1997;18(7):311–3. PubMed PMID: 9238831.

53. Stingl G, Maurer D. IgE-mediated allergen presentation via Fc epsilon RI on antigen-presenting cells. Int Arch Allergy Immunol. 1997;113(1–3):24–9. PubMed PMID: 9130475.

54. Karagiannis SN, Warrack JK, Jennings KH, Murdock PR, Christie G, Moulder K, et al. Endocytosis and recycling of the complex between CD23 and HLA-DR in human B cells. Immunology. 2001;103(3):319–31. PubMed PMID: 11454061. Pubmed Central PMCID: 1783243.

55. Carlsson F, Hjelm F, Conrad DH, Heyman B. IgE enhances specific antibody and T-cell responses in mice overexpressing CD23. Scand J Immunol. 2007;66(2–3):261–70. PubMed PMID: 17635803.

56. Bryce PJ, Miller ML, Miyajima I, Tsai M, Galli SJ, Oettgen HC. Immune sensitization in the skin is enhanced by antigen-independent effects of IgE. Immunity. 2004;20(4):381–92. PubMed PMID: 15084268.

57. Kawakami T, Galli SJ. Regulation of mast-cell and basophil function and survival by IgE. Nat Rev Immunol. 2002;2(10):773–86. PubMed PMID: 12360215.

58. Oettgen HC, Martin TR, Wynshaw-Boris A, Deng C, Drazen JM, Leder P. Active anaphylaxis in IgE-deficient mice. Nature. 1994;370(6488):367–70. PubMed PMID: 8047141.

59. Asai K, Kitaura J, Kawakami Y, Yamagata N, Tsai M, Carbone DP, et al. Regulation of mast cell survival by IgE. Immunity. 2001;14(6):791–800. PubMed PMID: 11420048.

60. Kalesnikoff J, Huber M, Lam V, Damen JE, Zhang J, Siraganian RP, et al. Monomeric IgE stimulates signaling pathways in mast cells that lead to cytokine production and cell survival. Immunity. 2001;14(6):801–11. PubMed PMID: 11420049.

61. Bryce PJ, Oettgen HC. Antigen-independent effects of immunoglobulin E. Curr Allergy Asthma Rep. 2005;5(3):186–90. PubMed PMID: 15842955.

62. Kitaura J, Song J, Tsai M, Asai K, Maeda-Yamamoto M, Mocsai A, et al. Evidence that IgE molecules mediate a spectrum of effects on mast cell survival and activation via aggregation of the FcepsilonRI. Proc Natl Acad Sci U S A. 2003;100(22):12911–6. PubMed PMID: 14569021. Pubmed Central PMCID: 240718.

63. Kashiwakura J, Xiao W, Kitaura J, Kawakami Y, Maeda-Yamamoto M, Pfeiffer JR, et al. Pivotal advance: IgE accelerates in vitro development of mast cells and modifies their phenotype. J Leukoc Biol. 2008;84(2):357–67. PubMed Pubmed Central PMCID: 2516357.

64. Kitaura J, Kinoshita T, Matsumoto M, Chung S, Kawakami Y, Leitges M, et al. IgE- and IgE+Ag-mediated mast cell migration in an autocrine/paracrine fashion. Blood. 2005;105(8):3222–9. PubMed Pubmed Central PMCID: 1464406.

65. Lam V, Kalesnikoff J, Lee CW, Hernandez-Hansen V, Wilson BS, Oliver JM, et al. IgE alone stimulates mast cell adhesion to fibronectin via pathways similar to those used by IgE + antigen but distinct from those used by steel factor. Blood. 2003;102(4):1405–13. PubMed PMID: 12702510.

66. Kitagaki H, Ono N, Hayakawa K, Kitazawa T, Watanabe K, Shiohara T. Repeated elicitation of contact hypersensitivity induces a shift in cutaneous cytokine milieu from a T helper cell type 1 to a T helper cell type 2 profile. J Immunol. 1997;159(5):2484–91. PubMed PMID: 9278342.

67. Natsuaki M, Yano N, Yamaya K, Kitano Y. Immediate contact hypersensitivity induced by repeated hapten challenge in mice. Contact Dermatitis. 2000;43(5):267–72. PubMed PMID: 11016667.

68. Kitagaki H, Fujisawa S, Watanabe K, Hayakawa K, Shiohara T. Immediate-type hypersensitivity response followed by a late reaction is induced by repeated epicutaneous application of contact sensitizing agents in mice. J Invest Dermatol. 1995;105(6):749–55. PubMed PMID: 7490467.

Sarah H. Wakelin

Introduction

Diagnostic tests have a key role in the management of patients with immediate skin contact reactions because they provide a way of objectively evaluating the patient's history. Due to the short-lived nature of symptoms, patients with stage 1 or 2 contact urticaria syndrome (localized urticaria, generalized urticaria) typically present for medical advice after the episode has resolved and the rash has cleared. Smartphone technology allows patients to capture images, which when reviewed with a careful history of the time course of the rash, help diagnose an urticarial or eczematous process. However, the cause is often unclear.

Patients who also have severe extracutaneous symptoms such as asthma or orolaryngeal swelling (i.e., anaphylaxis) usually receive urgent medical attention, but certainty may still be lacking about the etiology of their reaction. Lack of clarity can lead to patient anxiety and the overdiagnosis of allergy. Indeed, it takes only seconds to label an itchy rash in an anxious patient who reports feeling faint with throat tightness as "allergy." Proving the case takes a little longer.

Contact urticaria can be difficult to evaluate because it often affects skin that is already inflamed by underlying atopic eczema or chronic hand eczema, and these conditions can swell and itch when flaring without exposure to an urticaria-inducing substance. It can therefore be difficult to distinguish a flare and simple irritation from a superadded contact urticarial reaction. As always in allergy diagnosis, there is no shortcut to taking a thorough and careful history, which will guide the appropriate use of diagnostic tests and enable their correct interpretation.

The main role of contact urticaria testing is to identify immediate (type 1) hypersensitivity, which is an immunological abnormality mediated by IgE that gives rise to allergic/immunological contact urticaria (ICU). Accurate identification of immediate contact allergy is essential to inform patients about allergen avoidance and to guide safe allergen substitution. Although a common phenomenon in daily life, irritant/nonimmunological contact urticaria (NICU) is seldom investigated in clinical practice because reactions are usually mild, short lived, localized, and easily overlooked.

Skin provocation tests for contact urticaria are quick, inexpensive, and simple to perform. Medical practitioners and many members of the public are familiar with the concept of skin prick testing, which is by far the most widely used in vivo test for the diagnosis of immediate-type allergy. Other less commonly performed tests

S. H. Wakelin (✉)
St. Mary's Hospital, Imperial College Healthcare
Trust, London, UK
e-mail: sarah.wakelin@nhs.net

© Springer International Publishing AG, part of Springer Nature 2018
A. M. Giménez-Arnau, H. I. Maibach (eds.), *Contact Urticaria Syndrome*, Updates in Clinical
Dermatology, https://doi.org/10.1007/978-3-319-89764-6_10

such as open tests, closed chamber, scratch, and scratch-patch tests can be useful when investigating skin reactions following contact with food, work chemicals, cosmetics, medicaments, and clothing items. These tests are not used in the investigation of systemic drug or ingested food allergy: they are nonstandardized and considerably more difficult to interpret, thus requiring specialist expertise. Positive results in these tests should be investigated further by testing asymptomatic controls, but this may not be practical and requires informed consent.

In some cases a usage/challenge test may be necessary to confirm or refute the diagnosis of contact urticaria, especially in cases of suspected immediate-type allergy to natural rubber latex examination gloves. A diagnosis of occupational contact urticaria can have considerable social, medicolegal, and financial consequences. Correct techniques should always be followed to avoid false-positive and false-negative results. Patient safety is paramount, and health professionals who undertake these tests should be trained and equipped to handle severe reactions or anaphylaxis.

Open and Closed Tests

The open test is one of the simplest tests for contact urticaria and can be used to investigate both NICU and ICU reactions, including protein contact dermatitis. The test substance, for example, a fruit, vegetable, cosmetic, or topical medicament or 0.1 ml liquid is spread gently onto a small area (3 × 3 cm) of normal skin on the upper back, the extensor aspect of the upper arm, or the forearm. The site is observed visually for up to 60 min, and evaluated at 20, 40, and 60 min for erythema and swelling (Fig. 10.1). Unlike conventional patch testing for delayed skin allergy, there is no internationally agreed scoring system for contact urticaria tests. A simple grading for erythema and edema components of + weak, ++ moderate, and +++strong has been used [1]. In experimental studies, additional noninvasive tools such as chromameters for erythema are recommended for objectivity.

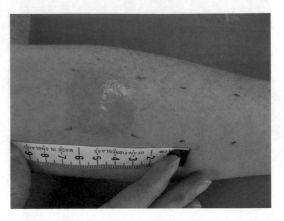

Fig. 10.1 Open test for nonimmunological contact urticaria to sorbic acid 1% in petrolatum at 60 min showing erythema and edema

The time course varies according to the underlying mechanism: ICU reactions are usually apparent after 15–20 min whereas NICU reactions evolve more slowly, over 45–60 min [2]. If the open test is negative, it may be helpful to repeat on the previously affected site, for example, the face for a cosmetic, as the results of open tests vary in sensitivity according to body site, especially for NICU.

Immediate testing can also elicit nonurticarial, vesicular reactions as described in detail by Hjorth and Roed-Petersen in 1976 in a series of food handlers. They reported that open testing of incriminated foods on areas of the hands and fingers previously affected with dermatitis caused urticarial reactions in some patients, but others developed acute eruption of vesicles within 30 min [3].

The rub test is a variation of open testing where the substance suspected of causing the symptoms is gently rubbed onto slightly affected or healthy skin. This may slightly increase sensitivity [4], but the effect of friction and dermographism need to be taken into consideration.

The closed test/chamber test involves applying the test substance on a small aluminum or plastic chamber on acrylic tape as routinely used for diagnostic patch testing for allergic contact dermatitis. For contact urticaria testing, however, the application time is reduced to 15 min and reactions are read at intervals up to 60 min.

Occlusion of the skin increases percutaneous penetration and may increase the sensitivity of the test. The advantage of the chamber test is that a smaller area of skin is needed than in the open test [5]. As for open testing, closed tests can be done on normal or previously affected skin.

The immediate skin application food test (i-SAFT) is another version of closed testing that involves applying a sample of liquid or solid piece of food to a 4 × 4 cm piece of gauze that is then fixed onto the skin of the back with acrylic tape. The test site is examined every 10 min with a maximal occlusion time of 30 min. Although this has been proposed as a reproducible and reliable way of diagnosing food allergy in young atopic children [6, 7], it is not a routine investigation. Children with suspected immediate-type food allergy (whether manifesting with localized contact urticaria or systemic symptoms) should be referred to a pediatric allergist for further assessment.

A positive open or closed test (edema and erythema) confirms that the applied substance is capable of eliciting an urticarial skin reaction in the individual, but it does not define whether the mechanism is ICU or NICU. It may be necessary to test nonstandardized substances on asymptomatic controls, especially in cases of suspected ICU when the same agent should not elicit a reaction. Chemicals capable of causing NICU such as sorbic acid, benzoic acid, and cinnamates are widely found in food, medicaments, and toiletries. Indeed they are sometimes included because they induce skin swelling, for example, methyl nicotinate in "plumping" lip gloss. It can be difficult to determine the clinical significance of a positive open test to agents that cause NICU as the majority of individuals will react when tested with sufficient concentration [8] (Table 10.1).

Skin Prick Testing (SPT)

Skin testing was first described by Charles Blackley in 1858 when he observed a wheal and flare response after applying pollen from rye grass on abraded skin. Sir Thomas Lewis, who described the "triple response" to mechanical

Table 10.1 Characteristic features of nonimmunological contact urticaria (NICU) and immunological contact urticaria (ICU) skin tests

	NICU	ICU
Peak reaction time on open testing	45–60 min	15–20 min
Variation of response according to body site	+++	+
Inhibition by oral and topical NSAIDs	Yes	No
Inhibition by H2 antihistamines	No	Yes
Inhibited by prior exposure to ultraviolet radiation	Yes	Yes

skin trauma, and the physician John Freeman introduced the skin prick test (SPT) in 1930. The test was described in greater detail by Helmtraud Ebruster in 1959 [9], and its use became widespread from the 1970s [10]. The SPT is used to demonstrate IgE-mediated sensitization to allergen, irrespective of the site of the patient's symptoms. Indeed, SPTs are used most frequently for the investigation of noncutaneous allergy, that is, rhinoconjunctivitis, respiratory allergy (pollen, house dust mites, animal dander), and food allergy. The test is also important in the diagnosis of immediate drug hypersensitivity (e.g., antibiotics, local anesthetics) and insect venom hypersensitivity.

A positive skin test to an allergen demonstrates *sensitization* but does not itself make a diagnosis of symptomatic hypersensitivity, that is, allergy; for this, the results must be considered in conjunction with the patient's history. A positive SPT does not necessarily indicate that a clinically relevant allergic reaction will occur on exposure to the allergen, which is why tests should be focused and guided by the patient's history. Unselected immediate-type allergy tests by SPT or measurement of allergen-specific IgE in asymptomatic, healthy individuals, or for non-allergic symptoms such as chronic fatigue syndrome, is not recommended and may lead to more questions than answers. This practice can be likened to throwing a trawling net into the sea and collecting a lot of weed and debris that then must be untangled before any fish can be seen.

Correctly used, the SPT has good sensitivity and specificity for detection of allergen-specific

IgE, and in some cases its sensitivity may exceed that of in vitro assays. The results are available almost immediately, and it is usually less costly than in vitro testing. However, healthcare personnel who undertake SPT require skill and expertise as correct technique is important. In addition, the results are highly dependent on the allergen extract used.

Patient Selection and Preparation

There are several limitations and contraindications to SPT (see Table 10.2). The procedure is extremely safe for aeroallergens, but for food, drug, and latex allergy there is a small but not insignificant risk of inducing systemic reactions, so that facilities for emergency treatment must always be available, including injectable adrenaline. For further guidance on the diagnosis and management of anaphylaxis see the latest publication of the Resuscitation Council UK [11].

The results of SPT are often diminished in young children and the elderly. Testing young children requires special expertise and should therefore be done in a hospital setting. Several drugs can inhibit the results of SPTs and should therefore be discontinued if possible before testing. Second-generation H1-antihistamines should be stopped 3 days before SPT. Certain antidepressants (tricyclic and mirtazapine) and benzodiazepines may also impair the response to histamine and allergens, but it is often not practical to discontinue them before testing [12]. Informed consent should be obtained before proceeding with the tests.

Reagents

Standardized glycerol-based allergen extracts are usually highly specific and accurate but can vary considerably in antigen content, and therefore in sensitivity, between manufacturers. In some cases,

Table 10.2 Comparison of skin prick tests and in vitro tests for immediate-type allergy

	Skin prick tests (SPT)	In vitro tests
Cost and facilities	Reagents usually inexpensive; wide range but limited to practitioner's current stock Special expertise to perform Need facilities for emergency treatment of anaphylaxis	Variable cost Extensive range + rarer allergens Venesection –
Results	Within 15–20 min Potential observer variability	Days–weeks Standardized
Risk	Very small risk of systemic reactions	No risk to patient
Contraindications and patient factors that reduce reliability of results	Pregnancy (potential risk to fetus from anaphylaxis) Severe anaphylaxis (risk of recurrence) H1 antihistamines, tricyclic antidepressants, mirtazapine, benzodiazepines, omalizumab (false-negative results) Recent phototherapy/UV exposure, topical glucocorticoids (false-negative results) Elevated baseline tryptase (risk of anaphylaxis) Beta-blocker or angiotensin-converting enzyme inhibitor therapy (impaired response to adrenaline) Uncontrolled, severe asthma (risk of bronchospasm) Severe dermographism (false-positive results) Widespread eczema (difficult to evaluate)	None
Test of choice for	Oral allergy syndrome: use fresh fruits and vegetables	Respiratory allergy

for example, wheat flour and soy, SPT solutions have shown low sensitivities for occupational asthma [13], and testing with multiple SPT solutions from different manufacturers in parallel is recommended to avoid false-negative results. In the future, use of recombinant allergen molecules for SPT should improve sensitivity and standardization [14]. Allergens should be stored between +2° and +8°C and not used beyond their expiry date. Stable reliable commercial allergen extracts exist for many food and aeroallergens and latex, but for certain fruit and vegetables it is more reliable to test with fresh food using a prick–prick method [15]. However, the allergen content may vary according to the variety, ripeness, and prior storage conditions. The skin/peel of apple contains a higher allergen content than the pulp and this may even vary at different locations within the peel of the same fruit [16]. SPTs with prawn and sesame extracts are often unreliable, and fresh food must be tested if commercial reagents are negative and there is a suspicion of food allergy. Histamine (10 mg/ml) and glycerol/saline solutions are used as positive and negative controls, respectively.

SPT Procedure

- Apply drops of allergen solution to normal skin on the flexor aspect of the forearm(s) at least 2–3 cm from the wrist and elbow fold (or the back in young children).
- Drops should be spaced apart by at least 2–3 cm to prevent merging of wheals. Skin should be free of moisturizing cream as this makes the droplets trickle.
- Mark the allergen sites with a water-resistant pen or allergen grid.
- Prick the skin through the allergen extract with a vertically held single-head metal SPT lancet [14] with moderate pressure (depressing the skin about 2–3 mm). A new lancet should be used for each allergen to avoid cross-contamination and the risk of sharps injury to the practitioner. Use similar pressure for all pricks to ensure even allergen placement.
- A prick-to-prick test is used for uncooked fruit and vegetables, first pricking the fruit (peel and/or flesh), then piercing the skin, through a small sample of peel/flesh. This technique can also be used for dry foods, for example, cereals crushed/ground and made into a paste with sterile saline.
- Avoid testing over prominent veins and drawing blood as this can cause a false-positive reaction.
- Test the negative (saline) control and positive (histamine) controls at the end of the tests.
- Blot away excess allergen and control solution with a large tissue.
- Use a stop watch or clock to record the test timing.

Note that the histamine-positive control reaches its maximum size after approximately 10 min whereas allergen reactions peak after 15–20 min. See Fig. 10.2.

SPT Assessment

- Record the reactions after 15 min.
- The maximum wheal diameter, not the associated erythema, is recorded and used for evaluation.
- Measure the positive and negative controls first; the histamine control should have a wheal diameter >3 mm to ensure that there are no factors inhibiting the subject's response to SPT allergens such as medication (see Table 10.2).
- The wheal induced by trauma of the lancet and negative control solution is usually zero, but may be up to 2.5 mm diameter in patients without dermographism.
- In general, only wheals >3 mm diameter are considered positive.
- The results should be documented in the medical records and discussed with the patient.
- Patients at risk of anaphylaxis should be observed for an additional 20 min in case they have a slow-onset systemic reaction.
- The prick test swellings usually flatten within an hour. Late-phase reactions may develop 6–12 h later. Their clinical significance is unclear.

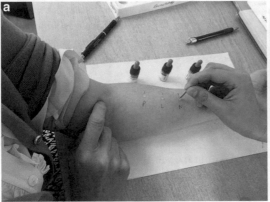

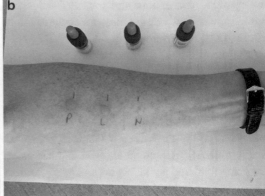

Fig. 10.2 Skin prick testing with commercial reagents. (**a**) Droplets of commercial allergen are pierced with a vertically held lancet. (**b**) Reactions are read after 15 min.

P positive control (histamine), *L* natural rubber latex extract, *N* negative control (glycerol/saline)

For further information see the British Society for Allergy and Clinical Immunology standard operating procedure at www.bsaci.org

Scratch Testing

Scratch tests were once widely used for immediate allergy diagnosis, but they are not recommended in current allergy guidelines, having been replaced by skin prick testing, which is more reliable and easier to interpret. Scratch tests have been used to investigate contact urticaria to nonstandardized allergens such as flour, root vegetables, and fruit. These tests may be more sensitive than open testing [17], but carry a risk of causing minor bleeding, irritation, and skin infection. The test involves making a 5-mm-long scratch in the skin of the arm or back with a blood lancet or intravenous needle, without drawing blood, and applying the test substance for 15–20 min before reading. Histamine and saline solutions are used as positive and negative controls, respectively, on similar-size scratches. Reactions equal to or greater than the histamine are usually clinically significant. Test substances that dry out quickly can be covered with a chamber: the *scratch-chamber test* [14] (see Fig. 10.3). Because of the current extensive availability of commercial allergen extracts and sophisticated

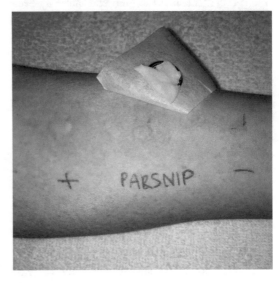

Fig. 10.3 Scratch chamber test results showing positive wheal to test substance

in vitro tests, these tests are now rarely performed.

Challenge/Usage Tests

If SPTs and the above tests are negative, a challenge or usage test may be needed to confirm or exclude a diagnosis of contact urticaria. This can be very helpful in the investigation of immediate symptoms from disposable gloves, particularly those made of natural rubber latex (NRL). Usage tests with high-protein NRL gloves can elicit contact urticaria in people with NRL allergy and even carry a risk of anaphylaxis in patients with severe hand eczema. A graded challenge is therefore recommended, as described by Turjanmaa in 1995 [18]. As for SPTs, facilities for treatment of severe allergic reactions must be available. In practice, because of improved standards for glove quality it is now difficult to source high-protein NRL gloves. Modern medical examination gloves have low residual protein content and greatly reduced allergenicity.

The "graded glove challenge" involves first wearing a finger of the offending glove on a damp finger and observing for 20 min. If negative, a whole glove can be applied to a dampened hand. A similarly sized non-latex glove should be used as the negative control on the other hand. The patient should be observed closely and should not rub the gloved skin as this can cause a false-positive dermographic reaction. Although contact urticaria (hives) should be evident within 20 min, it has been reported that prolonged wearing for several hours was needed to provoke symptoms in a few people with intact skin [18]. Puncturing the skin before putting the glove on has been recommended to improve the sensitivity of the test [19]. This method may be important for patients who do not have hand eczema and whose epidermal barrier is therefore intact and poorly penetrated by NRL proteins.

A modified glove challenge test, applying a 5 × 5 cm square of glove material to the forearm, has been advocated as a test in patients with symptoms of immediate irritation from examination gloves to distinguish between genuine contact urticaria and a dermographic response from friction and pressure of the garment [20]. However, none of these tests has been standardized and there are no formally agreed protocols for NRL glove challenge tests.

Conclusion

In vivo tests are a quick and simple way of investigating contact urticaria reactions. The choice of test substance is critical, and the tests must be performed correctly. Results must be interpreted in context to confirm or refute a suspected diagnosis of contact urticaria. Facilities for treating severe hypersensitivity reactions including anaphylaxis should always be available when testing substances that can cause systemic symptoms.

Acknowledgments I am grateful to Dr Sophie Farooque, Consultant Allergist, for her helpful comments on this manuscript.

References

1. Ylipieti S, Lahti A. Effect of the vehicle on nonimmunologic immediate contact reactions. Contact Dermatitis. 1989;21:105.
2. Amin S, Maibach HI. Immunologic contact urticaria definition. Chapter 2. In: Amin S, Lahti A, Maibach HI, editors. Contact urticaria syndrome. Boca Raton: CRC Press; 1997. p. 11–26.
3. Hjorth N, Roed-Petersen J. Occupational protein contact dermatitis in food handlers. Contact Dermatitis. 1976;2:28–42.
4. Hannuksela M. Skin tests for immediate hypersensitivity. Chapter 26. In: Rycroft RJG, Menne T, Freosch PJ, Lepoittevin J-P, editors. Textbook of contact dermatitis. 3rd ed: Berlin, Heidelberg, Germany: Springer; 2001. p. 521–6.
5. Lahti A. Nonimmunologic contact urticaria. Chapter 1. In: Amin S, Lahti A, Maibach HI, editors. Contact urticaria syndromee. Boca Raton: CRC Press; 1997. p. 5–10.
6. Oranje AP, Van Gysdel D, Mulder PG, Dieges PH. Food induced Contact Urticaria Syndrome (CUS) in atopic dermatitis: reproducibility of repeated and duplicate testing with a skin provocation test, the Skin Application Food Test (SAFT). Contact Dermatitis. 1994;31:314–8.
7. de Waard-van der Spek FB, Elst EF, Mulder PGH, Munte K, ACA D, Oranje SP. Diagnostic tests in children with atopic dermatitis and food allergy. Allergy. 1998;53:1087–91.
8. Clemmensen O, Hjorth N. Perioral contact urticaria from sorbic acid and benzoic acid in a salad dressing. Contact Dermatitis. 1982;8:1–6.

9. Ebruster H. The prick test, a recent cutaneous test for the diagnosis of allergic disorders. Wien Klin Wochenschr. 1959;71:551–4.

10. Bryden M. Skin prick testing in clinical practice. Norfolk: NADAAS; 2000.

11. Resuscitation Council UK. Emergency treatment of anaphylactic reactions; guidelines for healthcare providers. 2008. https://www.resus.org.uk/anaphylaxis/emergency-treatment-of-anaphylactic-reactions/

12. Shah KM, Rank MA, Dave SA, Lslie CL, Butterfield JH. Predicting which medication classes interfere with allergy skin testing. Allergy Asthma Proc. 2010;31:477–82.

13. vanKampen V, deBlay F, Folletti I, et al. EAACI position paper: skin prick testing in the diagnosis of occupational type 1 allergies. Allergy. 2013;68:580–4.

14. Heinzerling L, Mari A, Bergmann K-C. The skin prick test – European standards. Clin Transl Allergy. 2013;3:3–10.

15. Henzgen M, Ballmer-Weber BK, Erdmann S, et al. Skin testing with food alleergens. Guidelines of the German Society of Allergology and Clinical Immunology (DGAKI), the Physicians' Association of German Allergologists (ADA) and the Society of Pediatric Allergology (GPA)together with the Swiss Society of Allergology. J Dtsch Dermatol Ges. 2008;6:983–8.

16. Vlieg-Boerstra BJ, van de Wegg WE, van der Heide S, Dubois AE. Where to prick the apple for skin testing? Allergy. 2013;68:119608.43.

17. Niinimaki A. Scratch-chamber tests in food handler dermatitis. Contact Dermatitis. 1987;16:11–20.

18. Turjanmaa K, Makinen-Kiljunen S, Reunala T, et al. Natural rubber latex allergy. The European experience. Immunol Allergy Clin North Am. 1995;15:71–87.

19. Hamilton RG, Adkinson NF. Validation of the latex glove provocation procedure in latex-allergic subjects. Ann Allergy Asthma Immunol. 1997;79:226–72.

20. Hawkey S, Abdul Ghaffar S. Glove-related hand urticaria: an increasing occupational problem among healthcare workers. Br J Dermatol. 2016;174:1137–40.

Molecular Diagnosis in Contact Urticaria Caused by Proteins

11

Joaquin Sastre

Abbreviations

Abs   antibodies
CCD   Cross-reactive carbohydrate determinants
LTP   Lipid transfer proteins
MD   Molecular diagnosis
OAS   Oral allergy syndrome
PR 10 protein   Pathogenesis-related protein 10

Introduction

Molecular diagnosis (MD), or component-resolved diagnosis in allergy, seeks to define the allergen sensitization of a patient at the molecular level by measuring the specific IgE response to purified natural or recombinant allergens. Overall, MD can improve diagnostic accuracy (specificity), resolve cross-reactivity phenomena from true co-sensitization, discern low-risk markers from high-risk markers of disease severity (biomarkers), and improve the

J. Sastre (✉)
Allergy Department Fundación Jiménez Díaz, Universidad Autónoma de Madrid, and CIBER de Enfermedades Respiratorias (CIBERES, Institute Carlos III, Ministry of Economy and Competitiveness), Madrid, Spain
e-mail: jsastre@fjd.es

indication and selection of suitable allergens for specific allergen immunotherapy [1–3].

In general, MD provides specificity in the diagnosis; however, to have enough diagnostic sensitivity, the skin prick test or testing specific IgE with whole standardized extracts is required.

This review focuses exclusively on the clinical utility of allergenic molecules that are currently available in commercial tests for the diagnosis of contact urticaria induced by proteins of the vegetal and animal kingdoms.

Nomenclature and Allergen Components

It is important to know the names of the allergen components used in MD, including their scientific acronyms. Allergenic molecules are named using their Latin names (genus and species). A number is added to the name to distinguish various allergens from the same species (e.g., Hev b 5, Hev b 6; decimals are used in the case of isoforms, such as Hev b 6.01 for an isoform of Hev b 6); for example, Hev b 1 means allergen 1 from *Hevea brasiliensis*, or latex tree. This allergen nomenclature is approved by the World Health Organization and the International Union of Immunological Species Allergen Nomenclature Subcommittee. Different databases of known allergenic proteins can be accessed (the allergen nomenclature database of the International Union of Immunological Species at http://www.aller-gen.org"; or the allergen literature database "allergome," at http://www.allergome.org"; or the allergen database grouping the allergens into protein families, "allfam," at http://www.meduni-wien.ac.at/allergens/allfam/).

Every species contains species-specific aller-gen epitopes, and antibodies to these structures bind only to the allergen epitopes in that particular species. On the other hand, proteins with similar structures are often present in biologically related species, causing cross-reactivity phenomena. One of the most important clinical utilities of MD in allergy is its ability to reveal the allergens to which patients are sensitized, including primary or species-specific allergens and markers of cross-reactivity or panallergens [4]. Examples of proteins that induce cross-reactivity phenomena are profilin, polcalcins, lipid transfer proteins (LTPs), thaumatins, pathogenic-related protein 10, and vicillins in the vegetable kingdom or tropomyosins, serum albumins, parvalbumins, and lipocalins in the animal kingdom. For example, a patient who is primarily sensitized to grass pollen may also test positive for birch, olive, or latex using a skin prick test (SPT). This cross-reactivity occurs because all these extracts used in a SPT contain profilins (rBet v 2, nOle e 2, Hev b 8) that are largely similar to those in grass (e.g., Phl p 12). Sensitization to Hev b 8 (profilin) seems to be clinically irrelevant and not related to clinical latex reactions; in this case, other relevant latex allergens should be tested (Hev b 1, Hev b 5, Hev b 6).

Allergens that remain stable during heating and digestion are more likely to cause a severe clinical reaction, whereas heat- and digestion-labile allergens are more likely to be tolerated or only cause milder/local symptoms. Consequently, it is important to know the protein structure of the component and the allergen-protein family to which it belongs, as well as its stability during heating and digestion, because these features may affect tolerance to different foods and the degree of severity of clinical reactions.

Methods for Measuring Specific IgE Response to Purified or Recombinant Allergens

IgE response to purified or recombinant allergens is usually measured by a fluorescence enzyme immunoassay. At present, three products [ImmunoCAP (Thermo Fisher Scientific, Uppsala, Sweden), ImmuLite (Siemens AG, Erlander, Germany), and HyTec (Hycor Biomedical, Garden Grove, CA, USA)] offer the possibility of measuring specific IgE response to purified or recombinant allergens on singleplex platforms; of these, the catalogue for ImmunoCAP is the most extensive, containing 88 purified or recombinant allergens. Currently, Thermo Fisher Scientific offers a unique multiplex system capable of simultaneously detecting IgE to up to 112 components. This multiplex platform is a miniaturized, microarray-based assay [Immuno Solid-phase Allergen Chip (ISAC)] in which allergen components are immobilized in a microarray. Only 30 μl serum or plasma is needed, and both capillary and venous blood sampling can be used [5]. Using a standard calibration curve, results are reported within a dynamic range of 0.3 to 100 ISU-E (ISAC standardized units), giving a semiquantitative indication of IgE antibody levels. In contrast to multiplex-based methods, singleplex systems are more quantitative. Because of differences in assay and measurement technology, these ISU-E units differ from the kU/l units given in ImmunoCAP results and therefore are not interchangeable, although a certain correlation has been observed. Several studies have analyzed the reproducibility of this technique, comparing it with other methods of measuring specific IgE [6–8]. Nevertheless, there is general agreement that the reproducibility of ISAC is acceptable, although special attention is recommended for low specific IgE levels (0.3–1 ISU), as increased variability has been observed.

Allergens of Interest in Contact Urticaria: Allergens of Animal Origin

Hen's Egg (*Gallus domesticus*)

Gal d 1 (ovomucoid), *Gal d 2* (ovalbumin), *Gal d 3* (ovotransferrin/conalbumin), and *Gal d 4* (lysozyme) have been identified as the major allergens of egg white [3, 9]. Gal d 5 is present in egg yolk as a livetin protein and in chicken as serum albumin [10]. Although Gal d 1 (ovomucoid) constitutes only 10% of the total egg white protein, it has been shown to be the dominant allergen. It is very stable against heat and digestion by proteases, and can be allergenic in minute amounts. IgE abs to Gal d 1 is a risk factor for persistent egg allergy, and this indicates that neither raw nor cooked egg is tolerated [11–14].

Allergens available: egg; egg white; egg yolk; ovomucoid (Gal d1); ovalbumin (Gal d2); conalbumin (Gal d3); egg lysozyme (Gal d4).
Diagnosis: MD has been shown to be helpful in diagnosis of egg allergy, in particular to predict tolerance in children or to predict allergy to raw or partially cooked eggs.

Cow's Milk (*Bos domesticus*)

The major allergens of milk are caseins (e.g., Bos d 8), beta-lactoglobulins (e.g., Bos d 5), and alfa-lactoglobulins (e.g., Bos d 4), although allergies to other minor proteins such as bovine serum albumin (e.g., Bos d 6), bovine lactoferrin (Bos d lactoferrin), and immunoglobulins have also been reported [3, 15]. Most milk-allergic patients are sensitized to several cow's milk proteins. Conformational epitopes are largely destroyed by high temperatures, and recently it was shown that a majority of milk-allergic children tolerated heated milk [16]. Those children reacting to heated milk had initially higher casein and beta-lactoglobulin IgE levels and were at higher risk for systemic reactions.

Allergens available: cow's milk, heated cow's milk, caseins (Bos d 8), beta-lactoglobulins (Bos d 5), alfa-lactoglobulins (Bos d 4), bovine serum albumin (Bos d 6), bovine lactoferrin (Bos d lactoferrin).
Diagnosis: For standard diagnosis, skin prick test or specific IgE with whole cow's milk is recommended. The role of MD is not yet well defined to predict.

Meat Allergy

The α-1,3-galactose(α-Gal) is a sugar structure found on glycoproteins and glycolipids of nonprimate mammals and New World monkeys, but not in humans. IgE antibodies specific for α-Gal (anti-α-Gal-IgE) are associated with severe allergic symptoms and with delayed-type anaphylaxis to red meat (beef, pork, goat, deer) [17]. α-Gal is also present on cat IgA [18], on gelatin-containing material, and in cetuximab (a cancer drug) [19]. It is assumed that sensitization to α-Gal can be induced by tick bites or certain parasite infections [20].

Bovine serum albumin (e.g., Bos d 6) is a heat-labile allergen present in both milk and beef, which may cause cross-reactivity between different mammalian meats [21].

Allergens available: bovine serum albumin (Bos d 6), α-1,3-galactose(α-Gal).
Diagnosis: Prick or prick-by-prick test with raw meats is the first option; determination of α-1,3-galactose(α-Gal) may help in diagnosis of IgE-mediated delayed reactions to meat induced by this allergen. Bovine serum albumin (Bos d 6) may have cross-reactivity to meats. Cat albumins (Fel d 2) has been related to systemic rapid reactions to pork.

Shrimp (*Penaeus aztecus, Penaeus indicus, Penaeus monodon, Pandaluseous,* and Others)

Tropomyosin has been considered to be responsible for cross-reactivity between crustaceans and other arthropods such as dust mites, cockroaches, and nematodes [22]. In fact, tropomyosins from dust mites and other arthropods have a shared sequence identity of about 75% to 80%. However, recent publications have shown that sensitization to tropomyosins is a good marker of clinical sensitivity to crustaceans but not a marker of sensitization to mites [23, 24]. Nevertheless, cross-reactivity between mites and shrimp does exist, although it is caused by allergens other than tropomyosins, such as α-actinin, ubiquitin, or arginine kinase [25]. Therefore, and from a pragmatic point of view, in patients with clinical allergic reactions to crustaceans and with positive skin prick test (SPT) to mites, determination of markers of specific sensitization to mites (Der p 1, Der p2, Der p 23, Der f 1, Der f 2) is recommended [26].

Pen m 2, an, Lit v3 from European white shrimp (myosin light chain with high similarity to Bla g 8-cockroach-), and Lit v 4 (sarcoplasmic calcium-binding protein) from *Litopenaeus vannamei* are the other allergenic shrimp proteins described [27, 28].

Allergens available: shrimp, Pen a 1 (tropomyosin), *Pen m 2 (arginine kinase), *Pen a 4 (sarcoplasmic calcium-binding protein) (*only in ISAC platform).
Diagnosis: See Fig. 11.1.

Fish Parvalbumins from Cod (*Gadus morhua*) and Carp (*Cyprinus carpio*)

Cod Gad c 1 [29] and carp Cyp c 1 [30] are both major fish parvalbumin proteins and are repre-

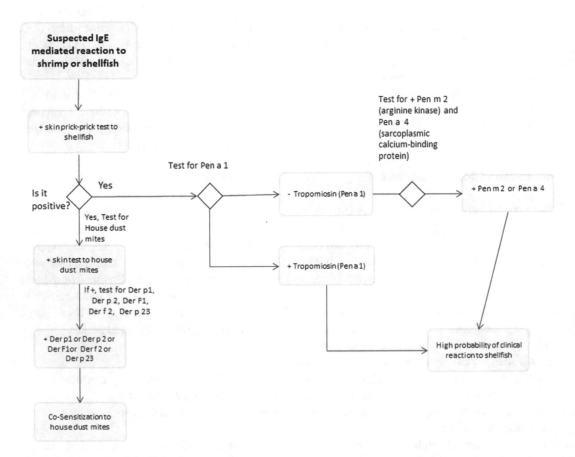

Fig. 11.1 Diagnosis of shellfish allergy

sentative markers for fish sensitization in general. As there is a high degree of cross-reactivity between parvalbumins from different species, Gad c 1 and Cyp c 1 are valuable tools in diagnosing patients with fish allergy, but selective epitope recognition in different species may occur [31]. The different expression of parvalbumins across species of fish may also explain the lack of cross-reactivity phenomena among different fish species [32, 33]. Parvalbumins have remarkable stability, which may explain why sensitization can result from ingestion even after cooking, contact, and inhalation of cooking vapor. Other important allergens other than parvalbumin have been described, such as enolases and aldolases [33].

Allergens available. prick or prick by prick test with raw fish meat species, Cod Gad c 1 [31] and carp Cyp c 1.

Diagnosis: Prick-prick test with suspected fish meat; if positive, determination of IgE to Gad c 1 [31] and carp Cyp c 1 may confirm allergy sensitization. If negative, this does not rule out sensitization because other allergens (enolase, aldolase) may be involved. Because of the lack of cross-reactivity among different fish species, clinical sensitization may require oral food challenge with each fish meat species to confirm allergy.

Pet Allergens

Salivary allergens from pets may induce contact urticaria in sensitized patients.

Dog (*Canis familiaris*)

Can f 1, Can f 2, and Can f 5 are specific allergen components indicating primary sensitization [34, 35]. Can f 1 is a lipocalin protein and is the most relevant dog allergen. Can f 2 is also a lipocalin protein. Can f 5 is a prostatic kallikrein and has been shown to cross-react with human seminal fluid [36]. Can f 5 is produced by male dogs and is responsible for sensitivity in up to 38% of dog-

allergic patients [35, 36]. This fact could explain why some patients sensitized to dog extracts may tolerate female dogs. Can f 3 is the dog serum albumin protein, a cross-reactive component indicating cross reactions to other bovine serum albumins, such as from the cat (Fel d 2 [37], pig (Sus s PSA), cow (Bos d 6), and horse (Equ c 3). Many patients are poly-sensitized to several pet allergens as shown using commercial extracts; however, the clinical history is often inconclusive, which may result in part from cross-reactivity phenomena between allergens contained in different extracts. Thus, MD may aid in clarifying the relevant sensitization when used in conjunction with clinical history.

Cat (*Felis domesticus*)

Fel d 1 (uteroglobin) is the major allergen component in cat, indicating primary sensitization. About 60% to 90% of patients with cat allergy have IgE antibodies (Abs) to Fel d 1 [35, 38]. IgE antibodies (Abs) to the cat serum albumin Fel d 2 is likely to cross-react with most other mammal albumins, such as dog Can f 3, horse Ecu c 3, pig Sus s PSA, and cow Bos d 6 [37]. It can also cause reactions when eating pork (the cat-pork syndrome) [39]. Fel d 4 is a lipocalin protein that shows cross-reactivity with major allergens from horse, dog, or cow [40].

Horse (*Equus caballus*)

Equ c 1, a lipocalin, is considered to be the major allergen of horse dander and has some cross-reactivity with mouse Mus m 1 and cat Fel d 4 [41]. Equ c 3 is a serum albumin showing cross-reactivity with other mammal serum albumins, as already mentioned.

Mouse (*Mus musculus*)

Sensitization to mouse Mus m 1 (lipocalin), as an indoor allergen, has been associated with asthma and asthma morbidity in some cities in the US

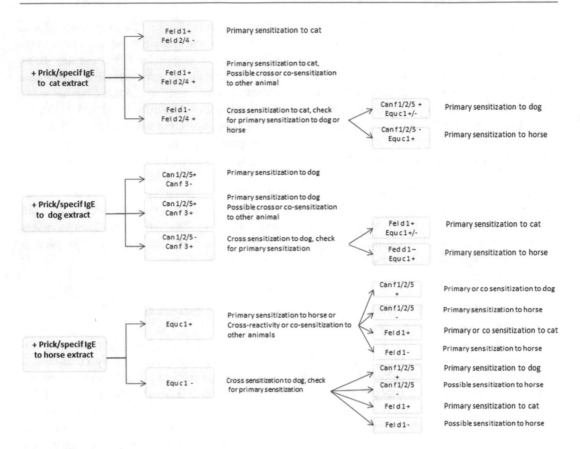

Fig. 11.2 Diagnosis of allergy to pets

[42]. Occupational allergy to the mouse is fairly common in persons handling experimental animals.

Allergens available: dog, cat, mouse, Can f 1, Can f 2, Can f 3 Can f 5, Fel d 1, Fel d 2, Fel d 4, Equ c 1, Equ c 3, Mus m 1.
Diagnosis: See Fig. 11.2.

Parasites

Anisakis (*Anisakis simplex*)

Anisakis simplex is a fish parasite that can cause severe reactions when raw infected fish is eaten or by contact [43]. Allergens Ani s 1 (serine protease inhibitor) and Ani s 4 have demonstrated their utility for diagnosing sensitization to the larvae of the

genus *Anisakis*, but seropositivity for Ani s 1 has a limited diagnostic value in clinically discriminating patients with a history consistent with gastroallergic anisakiasis [44]. Ani s 3 (tropomyosin) [45] is also a major allergen of *Anisakis simplex*, having in vitro cross-reactivity with other tropomyosins from nematodes and invertebrates. Other minor allergens are Ani s 5 and Ani s 2 (paramyosin) [46], but these are not commercially available.

Allergens available: *Anisakis simplex*, Ani s 1, 3 (both only in ISAC platform).
Diagnosis: Specific IgE to Ani s 1 has a limited diagnostic value in clinically discriminating patients with a history consistent with gastroallergic anisakiasis. Ani s 3 is a tropomyosin with limited cross-reactivity with mite or shellfish tropomyosin.

Allergens of Plant Origin

Allergens from plants may cause contact urticaria in sensitized patients.

Peanut (*Arachis hypogaea*)

IgE ab to Ara h 1, Ara h 2, Ara h 3, Ara h 6, but especially Ara h 2 and Ara h 3, is regarded as a marker for genuine sensitization to peanut [47, 48]. These proteins are stable to heat and digestion and therefore indicate an increased risk for systemic and more severe reactions to peanut. Although clinically rare, sensitization to these peanut components may also give rise to a certain degree of cross-reactivity, especially Ara h 1 to nuts and legumes such as lentil, pea, and Gly m 5 from soybean [49]; Ara h 2 to lupine and tree nuts such as almond and brazil nut [50]; and Ara h 3 to soybean, pea, and tree nuts [51].

Ara h 8 is a PR 10 protein, a Bet v 1 homologue, and thus a marker for primary sensitization through pollens such as birch and alder. Cross-reactivity with lupine and Gly m 4 from soybean has also been documented [48]. Ara h 8 is a heat-labile protein, and cooked peanuts are therefore often tolerated. Presence of Ara h 9 specific IgE Abs is often associated with systemic and more severe reactions in addition to oral allergic syndrome (OAS), especially in southern Europe [52]. Ara h 9 is a lipid transfer protein (LTP), and sensitization in most cases is probably caused by primary sensitization to peach or other LTP-containing fruits. Age may have an important influence in pattern of recognition of different peanut allergens [53].

Allergens available: peanut, Ara h 1, Ara h 2, Ara h 3, Ara h 6, ara h 8, Ara h 9.
Diagnosis: See Fig. 11.3.

Soybean (*Glycine max*)

Gly m 4 belongs to the PR-10 protein family and is a major soy allergen in birch pollen-associated, soy-allergic patients. IgE Abs to Gly m 4 is likely from primary sensitization to birch or similar tree pollens (Fagales) and is often associated with mild symptoms [54]. Gly m 4 is also cross-reactive with Ara h 8, and a relevant proportion,

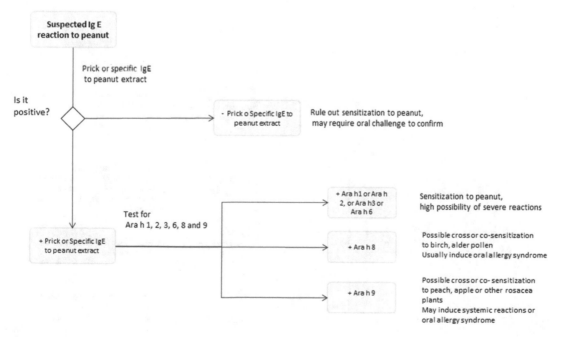

Fig. 11.3 Diagnosis of peanut allergy

about two-thirds, of soy-allergic patients in Europe are associated with peanut and soy allergy [55]. Targeted diagnostic testing with Gly m 4 is strongly recommended in pollen-sensitized patients with suspicion of soy allergy, especially if the soy extract test result is negative. Some Gly m 4-sensitized patients can show low or even negative IgE results with soy extract with a low Gly m 4 content in the extract.

IgE Abs to Gly m 5 and Gly m 6 indicates primary sensitization to soy [54]. Hence, Gly m 5 and Gly m 6 are potential diagnostic markers for severe allergic reactions to soy. Gly m 5 and Ara h1 share sequence homology and so do Gly m 6 and Ara h 3. Serological cross-reactivity between these components has also been shown.

Allergens available: soy, Gly m 4, Gly m 5, Gly m 6. *Diagnosis*: See Fig. 11.4.

Wheat (*Triticium aestivum*)

A positive result to wheat flour extract does not always correlate with clinical symptoms [56], indicating that in vitro diagnosis of allergy to wheat may be improved by using recombinant wheat seed allergens. The Tri a aA/TI (alpha-amylase/trypsin inhibitor) protein fractions of raw and cooked wheat are a relevant wheat allergen in food allergy and are also involved in wheat-dependent exercise-induced anaphylaxis [57]. Positive IgE Ab test results to Tri a gliadin indicate primary wheat sensitization with low risk of pollen cross-reactivity [58]. In children, IgE Abs to omega-5 gliadin (Tri a 19) and high molecular weight glutenin are associated with a risk of immediate reactions to wheat [59, 60].

Other important allergens are the 9-kDa wheat LTP (Tri a 14). Wheat LTP is considered a major allergen only in patients living in southern Europe [61] and also a significant allergen in baker's asthma in the same area. Sensitization to additives, such as enzymes, can also be responsible for contact urticaria in bakers.

Allergens available: wheat, other cereals, Tri a 14, Tri a 19, Gliadin, Phleum p 12 (profilin), nTri a aA/TI* (*only in ISAC platform). *Diagnosis*: See Fig. 11.5.

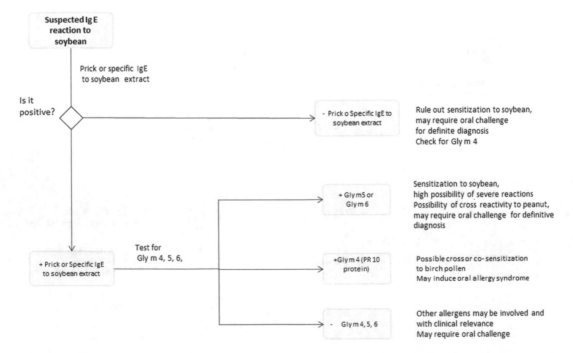

Fig. 11.4 Diagnosis of soybean allergy

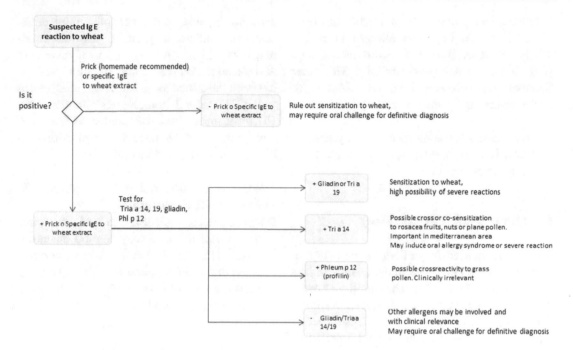

Fig. 11.5 Diagnosis of wheat allergy

Buckwheat (*Fagopyrum esculentum*)

Buckwheat, a pseudo-cereal, has been recognized as a common food allergen in Asian countries. Fag e 2 (2S albumin) is a major allergenic protein of buckwheat. Fag e 2 shows similarities with Ara h 6 from peanuts, and Ric c 1 from castor bean [62].

Allergens available: buckwheat, nFag e 2 (only in ISAC platform).

Diagnosis: If positive prick test or IgE to buckwheat, determination of IgE to nFag e 2 may help to confirm diagnosis.

Apple and Peach

Because of cross-reactivity within the botanical family Rosaceae, the Mal d 1 and Pru p 1 components are good representatives and markers for some stone fruits such as cherry and apricot, and thus not only for apple or peach [63]. Several allergy patterns were found in which the allergen families PR-10, LTP, thaumatins, and profilin

were involved. In the Western Mediterranean area, allergies to Rosaceae fruits are caused by mono-sensitization to LTP (Pru p 3), mono-sensitization to profilin, or co-sensitization to both allergens [64]. LTP sensitization is present in both pollinosis and non-pollinosis patients and is associated with peach allergy in particular. On the contrary, mono-sensitization to PR-10 and, to a lesser degree, co-sensitization to profilin and PR-10 is dominant in Northern and Central Europe, where PR-10 sensitization is primarily associated with concomitant birch pollen and apple allergy. Patients sensitized to profilin are characterized by several concomitant allergies including grass and other pollens as well as Rosaceae and non-Rosaceae fruits. IgE Abs to Pru p 3, an LTP protein, is frequently associated with severe reactions to stone fruits, but also to oral allergy syndrome (OAS) [65], whereas sensitization to PR 10 proteins Mal d1 or Pru p 1 and profilin (Pru p 4) is more often associated with OAS symptoms. LTP allergens of the Prunoideae subfamily have a similarity of about 95%, but there is also sequence homology of LTPs of botanically unrelated foods [66]. Recently, a thaumatin-like protein (Pru p 2.0201) has been described as an important allergen in peach-allergic patients from the Mediterranean area [67]. It has partial cross-reactivity with other thaumatin-like proteins from kiwi (Act c 2), apple, cherry, and plane pollen [68].

Allergens available: apple, peach, cherry, apricot, Mal d 1, Mal d 3, Pru p 1, Pru p3, Pru p 4.
Diagnosis: See Fig. 11.6.

Kiwi Fruit (*Actinidia deliciosa*)

The two main kiwi-fruit allergens are actinidin (Act d 1), a thiol protease, and a thaumatin-like protein (Act d 2) [69, 70]. The stability of Act d 1 and Act d 2 provides one explanation for the allergenic potency of kiwi fruit. Cross-reactive carbohydrate determinants and thiol-proteases that are homologous to Act d 1 are responsible for wheat-kiwi cross-reactivity in some patients [71].. In patients with allergic reactions to figs and other tropical fruits (kiwi fruit, papaya,

avocado, banana, and pineapple), thiol prote-ases can mediate, at least in part, this cross-reactivity [72]. A 40 kDa glycoprotein designated as Act d 3.02 and kiwellin (Act d 5) has been described as an important allergens as well [73]. Bet v 1-homologous allergens (PR-10) from green (Act d 8) and gold (Act c 8) kiwi fruit are recognized by birch pollen- or kiwi fruit-allergic patients [70].

Allergens available: Act c 1, 2*, 5*, and 8* (*only in ISAC platform).
Diagnosis: After prick or IgE to kiwi, determina-tion of Act d 1 or 2 may confirm diagnosis. Positive reaction to Act d 8 may show cross-reactivity to birch pollen with limited clinical significance. The sensitivity of molecular diagnosis is about 40%.

Hazelnut (*Corylus avellana*)

The main allergens are the Bet v 1 homologue Cor a 1.04, the hazelnut profilin Cor a 2, and

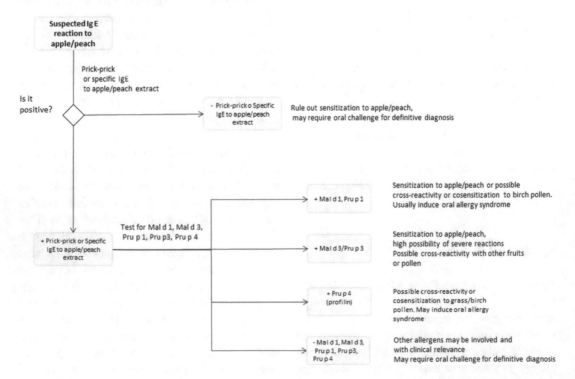

Fig. 11.6 Diagnosis of apple/peach allergy

LTP Cor a 8 [74]. Other molecules that have been investigated in connection with hazelnut allergy are the 11S globulin Cor a 9, the vicilin, Cor a 11, hazelnut oleosin, 2S albumins; and the specific carbohydrate structures, known as CCDs, for which bromelain has been used as source [75]. Sensitization to Cor a 1.04 is prevalent in the northern regions of Europe and is commonly associated with OAS, and Cor a 9 seems responsible for more severe reactions. On the other hand, sensitization to hazelnut LTP (Cor a 8) is certainly more common in patients from southern Europe [75], and these patients can develop either severe or mild allergic reactions to hazelnut. Polysensitization to hazelnut-allergen components is mostly observed in patients with severe symptoms.

Allergens available: Cor a 1.04, Cor a 8, Cor a 9, Cor a 14.

Diagnosis: See Fig. 11.7.

Celery (*Apium graveolens*)

Api g 1, the Bet v 1- PR-10, is the major celery allergen, although profilin (Api g 4) and CCD are also recognized by celery-allergic patients [76]. Api g 1 is more stable to heat than many other PR-10 proteins responsible for cross-reactivity with birch and mugwort pollen, although the structural similarity is less than that of several other PR-10 proteins.

Allergens available: Api g 1.

Diagnosis: Positivity to Api g 1 may confirm the diagnosis, but these allergens have cross-reactivity with birch pollen and other PR-10 plant allergens. An oral challenge test may be necessary to confirm diagnosis.

Sesame (*Sesamum indicum*)

The reactivity of the Ses i 1 (14 kDa, 2S albumin precursor) protein with most of the sera from

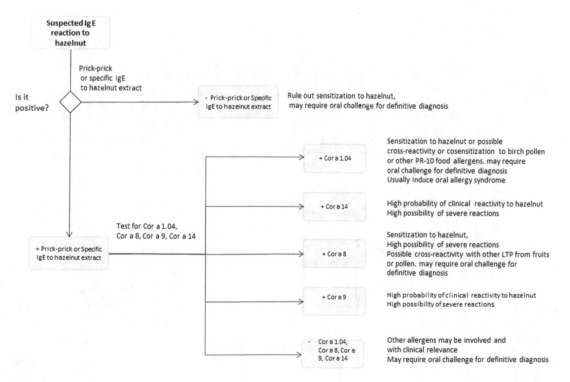

Fig. 11.7 Diagnosis of hazelnut allergy

patients allergic to sesame indicates that it is the major sesame allergen [77]. However, other allergens have been isolated, such as a 7S vicilin-type globulin; a seed storage protein of sesame and named Ses i 3, another 2S albumin, named Ses i 2 [80]; and olesins named Ses i 4 and Ses i 5 [78].

Allergens available: sesame, Ses i 1 (only in ISAC platform).

Diagnosis: Determination of Ses i 1 may confirm the diagnosis after prick or IgE to sesame. But, if negative, this may show that other allergens may be involved.

Nut Allergens [1, 3, 79]

Allergens available: cashew, brazil nut, walnut, pistachio, pecan, Ana o 2 (cashew), Ber e 1 (brazil nut), Jug r 1, 2* and 3 (walnut) (* only in ISAC platform).

Diagnosis: See Fig. 11.8.

Latex (*Hevea brasiliensis*)

Specific IgE to latex extract detected using traditional testing is common in individuals without clinical symptoms to latex. Resolving the IgE sensitization into components is a tool to distinguish genuine latex allergy from sensitization to profilin. A profilin component (Hev b 8) is included in traditional extract-based tests; however, it is usually of low clinical relevance. On the other hand, sensitization to Hev b 1, Hev b 3, Hev b 5, and Hev b 6 is associated with primary latex allergy [3, 80, 81].

Latex allergy occurs mostly among individuals exposed to latex in their occupation (e.g., healthcare workers) or in children exposed to latex early in life, such as children who have undergone multiple operations, as in those with spina bifida. Latex allergy was a major healthcare problem some decades ago, but increased knowledge and awareness has reduced both latex

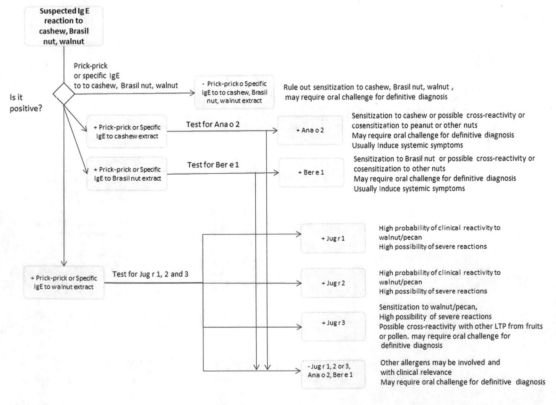

Fig. 11.8 Diagnosis of cashew/brazil nut/walnut allergy

exposure and also the number of latex-allergic patients.

Hev b 1 (rubber elongation factor) is a major latex allergen. Sensitization to Hev b 1 has a high prevalence in children who have had multiple operations and spina bifida (50–100%), and prevalence is lower among healthcare workers (10–50%) [82, 83].

Hev b 3 (small rubber particle protein) is a minor latex allergen. Hev b 3 and Hev b 1 are closely related and share stretches of sequence homology, which may explain their cross-reactivity [84].

Hev b 5 (acidic protein) is often associated with occupational latex allergy [85, 86]. Hev b 5 has a significant homology with kiwi fruit and potato, which are known to cause allergic reactions in latex-allergic patients [87].

Hev b 6 (hevein) is a major latex allergen with a prevalence of 70% to 90% among latex-allergic patients [88–92]. It is the main sensitizing allergen within healthcare workers. Hev b 6 is also associated with the so-called latex-fruit syn-

drome (latex–avocado–kiwi–banana–chestnut). Hev b 6 shares sequence homology with Hev b 11, a chitinase, which may cross-react with chitinases in some exotic fruits [91].

Hev b 8 (profilin) is not associated with primary latex allergy, and it is a panallergen belonging to the profilin family [3]. Sensitization to profilin may explain serological cross-reactivity with other allergen sources of plant origin and is usually of low clinical relevance.

Allergens available: Hev b 1, Hev b 3, Hev b 5, Hev b 6.01, Hev b 6.02, Hev b 8, Hev b 9, Hev b 11.

Diagnosis: See Fig. 11.9.

Cross-Reactive Carbohydrate Determinants (CCD): Bromelin–MUXF3; Ana c 2

Cross-reactive carbohydrate determinants (CCD) are present in plant and insect glyco-

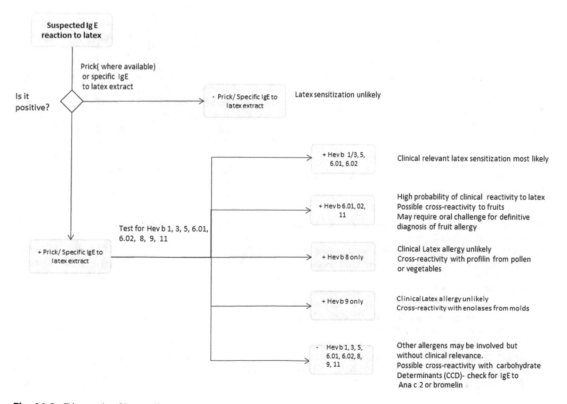

Fig. 11.9 Diagnosis of latex allergy

proteins (such as those of honeybees, wasps, and cockroaches), carrying glycans with carbohydrate determinants that do not exist in mammals. CCD is rarely associated with clinical symptoms and can be used to resolve questions on non-symptomatic sensitizations obtained when testing with allergen extract-based IgE tests [93]. A CCD test could be especially useful in four types of situations: (1) sensitization to foods of plant origin, (2) sensitization to latex in a pollen-allergic patient without occupational risk factors, (3) in subjects testing positive for both honeybee and wasp venom extracts, and (4) in subjects with perennial respiratory symptoms who test positive for cockroach in the absence of demonstrable exposure to cockroach allergens. Ana c 2 (bromelin) and MUXF3 (processed from bromelain and usually coupled to a protein backbone for IgE testing) are both markers for sensitization to CCD.

Acknowledgments I thank Oliver Shaw for editorial assistance.

Conflicts of Interest The author reports having served as a consultant to Thermo Fisher, MSD, Novartis, Genentech, Sanofi, Leti, Roche and GSK; having been paid lecture fees by Novartis, GSK, Stallergenes, LE as well as having received grant support for research from Thermo Fisher, GSK, and ALK-Abello.

References

1. Sastre J. Molecular diagnosis in allergy. Clin Exp Allergy. 2010;40:1442–60.
2. Sastre J, Sastre-Ibañez M. Molecular diagnosis and immunotherapy. Curr Opin Allergy Clin Immunol. 2016;16(6):565–70.
3. Matricardi PM, Kleine-Tebbe J, Hoffmann HJ, Valenta R, Hilger C, Hofmaier S, et al. EAACI molecular allergology user's guide. Pediatr Allergy Immunol. 2016;27(Suppl 23):1–250.
4. Radauer C, Bublin M, Wagner S, et al. Allergens are distributed into few protein families and possess a restricted number of biochemical functions. J Allergy Clin Immunol. 2008;121:847–52.
5. Canonica GW, Ansotegui IJ, Pawankar R, Schmid-Grendelmeier P, van Hage M, Baena-Cagnani CE, et al. A WAO – ARIA – GA²LEN consensus document on molecular-based allergy diagnostics. World Allergy Organ J. 2013;6(1):17.
6. Cabrera-Freitag P, Goikoetxea MJ, Beorlegui C, et al. Can component-based microarray replace fluorescent enzyme-immunoassay in the diagnosis of grass and cypress pollen allergy? Clin Exp Allergy. 2011;41(10):1440–6.
7. Cabrera-Freitag P, Goikoetxea MJ, Gamboa PM, et al. A study of the variability of the in vitro component-based microarray ISAC CDR 103 technique. J Investig Allergol Clin Immunol. 2011;21(5):414–5.
8. Lizaso MT, García BE, Tabar AI, et al. Comparison of conventional and component-resolved diagnostics by two different methods (Advia-Centaur/Microarray-ISAC) in pollen allergy. Ann Allergy Asthma Immunol. 2011;107(1):35–41.
9. Chokshi NY, Sicherer SH. Molecular diagnosis of egg allergy: an update. Expert Rev Mol Diagn. 2015;15(7):895–906.
10. Quirce S, Maranon F, Umpierrez A, et al. Chicken serum albumin (Gal d 5*) is a partially heat-labile inhalant and food allergen implicated in the bird-egg syndrome. Allergy. 2001;56:754–62.
11. Ando H, Moverare R, Kondo Y, et al. Utility of ovomucoid-specific IgE concentrations in predicting symptomatic egg allergy. J Allergy Clin Immunol. 2008;122:583–8.
12. Lemon-Mule H, Sampson HA, Sicherer SH, et al. Immunologic changes in children with egg allergy ingesting extensively heated egg. J Allergy Clin Immunol. 2008;122:977–83.
13. Urisu A, Ando H, Morita Y, et al. Allergenic activity of heated and ovomucoid-depleted egg white. J Allergy Clin Immunol. 1997;100:171–6.
14. Restani P, Ballabio C, Di Lorenzo C, et al. Molecular aspects of milk allergens and their role in clinical events. Anal Bioanal Chem. 2009;395:47–56.
15. Fiocchi A, Dahda L, Dupont C, Campoy C, Fierro V, Nieto A. Cow's milk allergy: towards an update of DRACMA guidelines. World Allergy Organ J. 2016;9(1):35.
16. Nowak-Wegrzyn A, Bloom KA, Sicherer SH, et al. Tolerance to extensively heated milk in children with cow's milk allergy. J Allergy Clin Immunol. 2008;122:342–7.
17. Mullins RJ, James H, Platts-Mills TA, Commins S. Relationship between red meat allergy and sensitization to gelatin and galactose-alpha-1,3-galactose. J Allergy Clin Immunol. 2012;129:1334–42.
18. Gronlund H, Adedoyin J, Commins SP, Platts-Mills TA, van Hage M. The carbohydrate galactose-alpha-1,3-galactose is a major IgE-binding epitope on cat IgA. J Allergy Clin Immunol. 2009;123:1189–91.
19. Chung CH, Mirakhur B, Chan E, et al. Cetuximab-induced anaphylaxis and IgE specific for galactose-alpha-1,3-galactose. N Engl J Med. 2008;358:1109–17.

20. Hamsten C, Starkhammar M, Tran TA, et al. Identification of galactose-alpha-1,3-galactose in the gastrointestinal tract of the tick Ixodes ricinus; possible relationship with red meat allergy. Allergy. 2013;68:549.

21. Restani P, Ballabio C, Tripodi S, Fiocchi A. Meat allergy. Curr Opin Allergy Clin Immunol. 2009;9:265–9.

22. Ayuso R, Reese G, Leong-Kee S, Plante M, Lehrer SB. Molecular basis of arthropod cross-reactivity: IgE-binding cross-reactive epitopes of shrimp, house dust mite and cockroach tropomyosins. Int Arch Allergy Immunol. 2002;129:38–48.

23. Gámez C, Sánchez-García S, Ibáñez MD, et al. Tropomyosin IgE-positive results are a good predictor of shrimp allergy. Allergy. 2011;66:1375–83.

24. Bronnert M, Mancini J, Birnbaum J, et al. Component-resolved diagnosis with commercially available d. Pteronyssinus der p 1, der p 2, and der p 10: relevant markers for house dust mite allergy. Clin Exp Allergy. 2012;42:1406–15.

25. Gámez C, Zafra M, Boquete M, Sanz V, Mazzeo C, Ibáñez MD, et al. New shrimp IgE-binding proteins involved in mite-seafood cross-reactivity. Mol Nutr Food Res. 2014;58(9):1915–25.

26. Pascal M, Grishina G, Yang AC, Sánchez-García S, Lin J, Towle D, Ibáñez MD, Sastre J, Sampson HA, Ayuso R. Molecular diagnosis of shrimp allergy: efficiency of several allergens to predict clinical reactivity. J Allergy Clin Immunol Pract. 2015;3(4):521–9.

27. Ayuso R, Grishina G, Bardina L, et al. Myosin light chain is a novel shrimp allergen, Lit v 3. J Allergy Clin Immunol. 2008;122:795–802.

28. Ayuso R, Grishina G, Ibanez MD, et al. Sarcoplasmic calcium-binding protein is an EF-hand-type protein identified as a new shrimp allergen. J Allergy Clin Immunol. 2009;124:114–20.

29. Van Do T, Hordvik I, Endresen C, Elsayed S. Characterization of parvalbumin, the major allergen in Alaska pollack, and comparison with codfish Allergen M. Mol Immunol. 2005;42:345–53.

30. Swoboda I, Bugajska-Schretter A, Verdino P, et al. Recombinant carp parvalbumin, the major cross-reactive fish allergen: a tool for diagnosis and therapy of fish allergy. J Immunol. 2002;168:4576–84.

31. Vázquez-Cortés S, Nuñez-Acevedo B, Jimeno-Nogales L, Ledesma A, Fernández-Rivas M. Selective allergy to the Salmonidae fish family: a selective parvalbumin epitope? Ann Allergy Asthma Immunol. 2012;108:62–3.

32. Griesmeier U, Vázquez-Cortés S, et al. Expression levels of parvalbumins determine allergenicity of fish species. Allergy. 2010;65:191–8.

33. Kuehn A, Swoboda I, Arumugam K, Hilger C, Hentges F. Fish allergens at a glance: variable allergenicity of parvalbumins, the major fish allergens. Front Immunol. 2014;5:179.

34. Saarelainen S, Taivainen A, Rytkonen-Nissinen M, et al. Assessment of recombinant dog allergens Can f 1 and Can f 2 for the diagnosis of dog allergy. Clin Exp Allergy. 2004;34:1576–82.

35. Uriarte SA, Sastre J. Clinical relevance of molecular diagnosis in pet allergy. Allergy. 2016;71(7):1066–8.

36. Mattsson L, Lundgren T, Everberg H, Larsson H, Lidholm J. Prostatic kallikrein: a new major dog allergen. J Allergy Clin Immunol. 2009;123:362–8.

37. Cabanas R, Lopez-Serrano MC, Carreira J, et al. Importance of albumin in cross-reactivity among cat, dog and horse allergens. J Investig Allergol Clin Immunol. 2000;10:71–7.

38. van Ree R, van Leeuwen WA, Bulder I, Bond J, Aalberse RC. Purified natural and recombinant Fel d 1 and cat albumin in in vitro diagnostics for cat allergy. J Allergy Clin Immunol. 1999;104:1223–30.

39. Hilger C, Kohnen M, Grigioni F, Lehners C, Hentges F. Allergic cross-reactions between cat and pig serum albumin. Study at the protein and DNA levels. Allergy. 1997;52:179–87.

40. Smith W, Butler AJ, Hazell LA, et al. Fel d 4, a cat lipocalin allergen. Clin Exp Allergy. 2004;34.1732–8.

41. Saarelainen S, Rytkonen-Nissinen M, Rouvinen J, et al. Animal-derived lipocalin allergens exhibit immunoglobulin E cross-reactivity. Clin Exp Allergy. 2008;38:374–81.

42. Phipatanakul W, Litonjua AA, Platts-Mills TA, et al. Sensitization to mouse allergen and asthma and asthma morbidity among women in Boston. J Allergy Clin Immunol. 2007;120:954–6.

43. Sastre J, Lluch-Bernal M, Quirce S, et al. A double-blind, placebo-controlled oral challenge study with lyophilized larvae and antigen of the fish parasite, Anisakis simplex. Allergy. 2000;55:560–4.

44. Caballero ML, Moneo I. Specific IgE determination to Ani s 1, a major allergen from Anisakis simplex, is a useful tool for diagnosis. Ann Allergy Asthma Immunol. 2002;89:74–7.

45. Asturias JA, Eraso E, Moneo I, Martinez A. Is tropomyosin an allergen in Anisakis? Allergy. 2000;55(9):898.

46. Perez-Perez J, Fernandez-Caldas E, Maranon F, et al. Molecular cloning of paramyosin, a new allergen of Anisakis simplex. Int Arch Allergy Immunol. 2000;123:120–9.

47. Commins SP, Kim EH, Orgel K, Kulis M. Peanut allergy: new developments and clinical implications. Curr Allergy Asthma Rep. 2016;16(5):35.

48. Klemans RJ, van Os-Medendorp H, Blankestijn M, Bruijnzeel-Koomen CA, Knol EF, Knulst AC. Diagnostic accuracy of specific IgE to components in diagnosing peanut allergy: a systematic review. Clin Exp Allergy. 2015;45(4):720–30.

49. de Leon MP, Drew AC, Glaspole IN, Suphioglu C, O'Hehir RE, Rolland JM. IgE cross-reactivity between the major peanut allergen Ara h 2 and tree nut allergens. Mol Immunol. 2007;44:463–71.

50. Barre A, Jacquet G, Sordet C, Culerrier R, Rouge P. Homology modelling and conformational analysis of IgE-binding epitopes of Ara h 3 and other legu-

min allergens with a cupin fold from tree nuts. Mol Immunol. 2007;44:3243–55.

51. Asero R. Detection and clinical characterization of patients with oral allergy syndrome caused by stable allergens in Rosaceae and nuts. Ann Allergy Asthma Immunol. 1999;83:377–83.

52. Krause S, Reese G, Randow S, et al. Lipid transfer protein (Ara h 9) as a new peanut allergen relevant for a Mediterranean allergic population. J Allergy Clin Immunol. 2009;124:771–8.

53. Ballmer-Weber BK, Lidholm J, Fernández-Rivas M, Seneviratne S, Hanschmann KM, Vogel L, et al. IgE recognition patterns in peanut allergy are age dependent: perspectives of the EuroPrevall study. Allergy. 2015;70(4):391–40.

54. Ballmer-Weber BK, Vieths S. Soy allergy in perspective. Curr Opin Allergy Clin Immunol. 2008;8(3):270–5.

55. Holzhauser T, Wackermann O, Ballmer-Weber BK, et al. Soybean (Glycine max) allergy in Europe: Gly m 5 (beta-conglycinin) and Gly m 6 (glycinin) are potential diagnostic markers for severe allergic reactions to soy. J Allergy Clin Immunol. 2009;123:452–8.

56. Jones SM, Magnolfi CF, Cooke SK, Sampson HA. Immunologic cross-reactivity among cereal grains and grasses in children with food hypersensitivity. J Allergy Clin Immunol. 1995;96:341–51.

57. Pastorello EA, Farioli L, Conti A, et al. Wheat IgE-mediated food allergy in European patients: alpha-amylase inhibitors, lipid transfer proteins and low-molecular-weight glutenins. Allergenic molecules recognized by double-blind, placebo-controlled food challenge. Int Arch Allergy Immunol. 2007;144:10–22.

58. Battais F, Pineau F, Popineau Y, et al. Food allergy to wheat: identification of immunogloglin E and immunoglobulin G-binding protcins with sequential extracts and purified proteins from wheat flour. Clin Exp Allergy. 2003;33:962–70.

59. Palosuo K, Varjonen E, Kekki OM, et al. Wheat omega-5 gliadin is a major allergen in children with immediate allergy to ingested wheat. J Allergy Clin Immunol. 2001;108:634–8.

60. Matsuo H, Kohno K, Niihara H, Morita E. Specific IgE determination to epitope peptides of omega-5 gliadin and high molecular weight glutenin subunit is a useful tool for diagnosis of wheat-dependent exercise-induced anaphylaxis. J Immunol. 2005;175:8116–22.

61. Palacin A, Quirce S, Armentia A, et al. Wheat lipid transfer protein is a major allergen associated with baker's asthma. J Allergy Clin Immunol. 2007;120:1132–8.

62. Satoh R, Koyano S, Takagi K, Nakamura R, Teshima R, Sawada J. Immunological characterization and mutational analysis of the recombinant protein BWp16, a major allergen in buckwheat. Biol Pharm Bull. 2008;31:1079–85.

63. Asero R. Plant food allergies: a suggested approach to allergen-resolved diagnosis in the clinical practice by identifying easily available sensitization markers. Int Arch Allergy Immunol. 2005;138:1–11.

64. Fernandez-Rivas M, Bolhaar S, Gonzalez-Mancebo E, et al. Apple allergy across Europe: how allergen sensitization profiles determine the clinical expression of allergies to plant foods. J Allergy Clin Immunol. 2006;118:481–8.

65. Gonzalez-Mancebo E, Fernandez-Rivas M. Outcome and safety of double-blind, placebo-controlled food challenges in 111 patients sensitized to lipid transfer proteins. J Allergy Clin Immunol. 2008;121:1507–8.

66. Asero R, Mistrello G, Roncarolo D, Amato S. Relationship between peach lipid transfer protein specific IgE levels and hypersensitivity to non-Rosaceae vegetable foods in patients allergic to lipid transfer protein. Ann Allergy Asthma Immunol. 2004;92:268–72.

67. Palacín A, Tordesillas L, Gamboa P, et al. Characterization of peach thaumatin-like proteins and their identification as major peach allergens. Clin Exp Allergy. 2010;40:1422–30.

68. Palacín A, Rivas LA, Gómez-Casado C, et al. The involvement of thaumatin-like proteins in plant food cross-reactivity: a multicenter study using a specific protein microarray. PLoS One. 2012;7(9):e44088.

69. Aleman A, Sastre J, Quirce S, et al. Allergy to kiwi: a double-blind, placebo-controlled food challenge study in patients from a birch-free area. J Allergy Clin Immunol. 2004;113:543–50.

70. Le TM, Bublin M, Breiteneder H, et al. Kiwifruit allergy across Europe: clinical manifestation and IgE recognition patterns to kiwifruit allergens. J Allergy Clin Immunol. 2013;131(1):164–71.

71. Palacin A, Quirce S, Sanchez-Monge R, et al. Allergy to kiwi in patients with baker's asthma: identification of potential cross-reactive allergens. Ann Allergy Asthma Immunol. 2008;101:200–5.

72. Hemmer W, Focke M, Gotz M, Jarisch R. Sensitization to Ficus benjamina: relationship to natural rubber latex allergy and identification of foods implicated in the Ficus-fruit syndrome. Clin Exp Allergy. 2004;34(8):1251.

73. Palacin A, Rodriguez J, Blanco C, et al. Immunoglobulin E recognition patterns to purified Kiwifruit (Actinidinia deliciosa) allergens in patients sensitized to Kiwi with different clinical symptoms. Clin Exp Allergy. 2008;38:1220–8.

74. Pastorello EA, Vieths S, Pravettoni V, et al. Identification of hazelnut major allergens in sensitive patients with positive double-blind, placebo-controlled food challenge results. J Allergy Clin Immunol. 2002;109:563.

75. Datema MR, Zuidmeer-Jongejan L, Asero R, Barreales L, Belohlavkova S, de Blay F, et al. Hazelnut allergy across Europe dissected molecularly: a EuroPrevall outpatient clinic survey. J Allergy Clin Immunol. 2015;136(2):382–91.

76. Bauermeister K, Ballmer-Weber BK, Bublin M, et al. Assessment of component-resolved in vitro

diagnosis of celeriac allergy. J Allergy Clin Immunol. 2009;124:1273–81.

77. Beyer K, Bardina L, Grishina G, Sampson HA. Identification of sesame seed allergens by 2-dimensional proteomics and Edman sequencing: seed storage proteins as common food allergens. J Allergy Clin Immunol. 2002;110:154–9.

78. Leduc V, Moneret-Vautrin DA, Tzen JT, Morisset M, Guerin L, Kanny G. Identification of oleosins as major allergens in sesame seed allergic patients. Allergy. 2006;61:349–56.

79. Byrne AM, Malka-Rais J, Burks AW, Fleischer DM. How do we know when peanut and tree nut allergy have resolved, and how do we keep it resolved? Clin Exp Allergy. 2010;40(9):1303–11.

80. Posch A, Chen Z, Raulf-Heimsoth M, Baur X. Latex allergens. Clin Exp Allergy. 1998;28:134–40.

81. Raulf-Heimsoth M, Rihs HP, Rozynek P, et al. Quantitative analysis of immunoglobulin E reactivity profiles in patients allergic or sensitized to natural rubber latex (Hevea brasiliensis). Clin Exp Allergy. 2007;37:1657–67.

82. Chen Z, Posch A, Cremer R, Raulf-Heimsoth M, Baur X. Identification of hevein (Hev b 6.02) in Hevea latex as a major cross-reacting allergen with avocado fruit in patients with latex allergy. J Allergy Clin Immunol. 1998;102:476–81.

83. Chen Z, Cremer R, Posch A, Raulf-Heimsoth M, Rihs HP, Baur X. On the allergenicity of Hev b 1 among health care workers and patients with spina bifida allergic to natural rubber latex. J Allergy Clin Immunol. 1997;100:684–93.

84. Yeang HY, Cheong KF, Sunderasan E, et al. The 14.6 kd rubber elongation factor (Hev b 1) and 24 kd (Hev b 3) rubber particle proteins are recognized by IgE from patients with spina bifida and latex allergy. J Allergy Clin Immunol. 1996;98:628–39.

85. Slater JE, Vedvick T, Arthur-Smith A, Trybul DE, Kekwick RG. Identification, cloning, and sequence of a major allergen (Hev b 5) from natural rubber latex (Hevea brasiliensis). J Biol Chem. 1996;271:25394–9.

86. Sastre J, Fernandez-Nieto M, Rico P, et al. Specific immunotherapy with a standardized latex extract in allergic workers: a double-blind, placebo-controlled study. J Allergy Clin Immunol. 2003;111:985–94.

87. Ott H, Schröder C, Raulf-Heimsoth M, Mahler V, Ocklenburg C, Merk HF, Baron JM. Microarrays of recombinant Hevea brasiliensis proteins: a novel tool for the component-resolved diagnosis of natural rubber latex allergy. J Investig Allergol Clin Immunol. 2010;20(2):129–38.

88. Drew AC, Euscbius NP, Kenins L, et al. Hypoallergenic variants of the major latex allergen Hev b 6.01 retaining human T lymphocyte reactivity. J Immunol. 2004;173(9):5872.

89. Sutherland MF, Drew A, Rolland JM, Slater JE, Suphioglu C, O'Hehir RE. Specific monoclonal antibodies and human immunoglobulin E show that Hev b 5 is an abundant allergen in high protein powdered latex gloves. Clin Exp Allergy. 2002;32:583–9.

90. Sastre J, Raulf-Heimsoth M, Rihs HP, et al. IgE reactivity to latex allergens among sensitized healthcare workers before and after immunotherapy with latex. Allergy. 2006;61:206–10.

91. Karisola P, Kotovuori A, Poikonen S, et al. Isolated hevein-like domains, but not 31-kd endochitinases, are responsible for IgE-mediated in vitro and in vivo reactions in latex-fruit syndrome. J Allergy Clin Immunol. 2005;115:598–605.

92. Pamies R, Oliver F, Raulf-Heimsoth M, et al. Patterns of latex allergen recognition in children sensitized to natural rubber latex. Pediatr Allergy Immunol. 2006;17:55–9.

93. Malandain H, Giroux F, Cano Y. The influence of carbohydrate structures present in common allergen sources on specific IgE results. Eur Ann Allergy Clin Immunol. 2007;39:216–20.

Preventive Measures for Occupationally Induced Immediate Contact Reactions

Jose Hernán Alfonso

Introduction

In clinical dermatology, prevention is often linked to early diagnosis and proper treatment. From the perspective of occupational medicine and health education, the conception of prevention is even greater, including preventive actions that can take place at an earlier point, when the main goal is not only to reduce the damage of the disease through early diagnosis, but also to maintain a healthy worker by creating safe workplaces.

In Chaps. 2 and 3 we saw that epidemiology is concerned with conducting research at the population and group levels to identify risk factors and provide evidence for whether exposures are associated with health problems and disease. After research is conducted and evidence collected, identification of exposures associated with disease constitutes the basis of preventive actions with potential impacts on public health.

Skin diseases caused or worsened by occupational exposures – work-related and occupational skin diseases – are among the most common and prevalent work-related and occupational diseases. Immediate contact reactions such as contact urticaria and protein contact dermatitis represent up to 30% of registered occupational skin diseases. Because of the negative consequences of work-related and occupational skin diseases, such as frequent use of healthcare services and high occurrence of sick leave, job loss, job change, and mental distress, they constitute a top priority health problem [1].

Work-related and occupational skin diseases have a common feature: they are highly preventable by reducing exposure to occupational hazards. Therefore, prevention strategies and measures that aim to reduce onset and a chronic and relapsing course of these conditions are presented in this chapter.

Scope of Preventive Measures

It is often claimed that prevention is better than cure, and this is the case for work-related and occupational immediate contact reactions. For instance, the ultimate goal of prevention is to keep skin healthy in safe workplaces. But how can we define prevention and preventive measures? In 1983 Gorden Jr. [2] defined prevention as

> measures adopted by or practiced on persons not currently feeling the effects of a disease, intended to decrease the risk that disease will afflict them in the future.

J. H. Alfonso (✉)
Department of Occupational Medicine and Epidemiology, National Institute of Occupational Health, Oslo, Norway
e-mail: jose.alfonso@stami.no

© Springer International Publishing AG, part of Springer Nature 2018
A. M. Giménez-Arnau, H. I. Maibach (eds.), *Contact Urticaria Syndrome*, Updates in Clinical Dermatology, https://doi.org/10.1007/978-3-319-89764-6_12

Most of us have probably heard about primary, secondary, and tertiary prevention, such classification is attractive and simple, but it does not serve to distinguish between preventive interventions, which have different epidemiological justifications and require different strategies for optimal utilization. Moreover, an unintended side effect of such a classification is the idea of a "priority ranking," whereof the terms "primary" and "secondary" and "tertiary" may be interpreted as an ordinal value, particularly among stakeholders who are responsible for decisions and priorities that bear on preventive programs.

Thus, from a public health perspective, preventive measures include these:

1. *Universal measures:* include health promotion strategies, as they involve the full population based on evidence that it is likely to provide some benefit to all. A good example of universal measure is legislation regulating the availability of skin urticariogens and allergens. For instance, a significant decline of occupational contact urticaria attributed to latex in gloves was observed in Germany, France, and the United Kingdom after legislation to reduce occupational exposure [3–5]. Germany banned the use of powdered natural rubber latex gloves in 1998, and the incidence of natural rubber latex-induced contact urticaria among healthcare workers decreased from 0.3 cases/1000 workers/year in 1996 to 0.07 cases/1000 workers/year in 2002 [3]. In France, the number of cases of occupational contact urticaria from to natural rubber latex declined significantly between 2001 and 2010 (19% per year) [4].
2. *Selective measures:* include specific preventive actions recommended to specific risk groups according to established risk factors for developing the disease. Examples include education about risk factors for developing work-related skin problems, training on skin protection such as proper use of protective equipment, provision, and training on use of moisturizers, and periodical health surveillance in risk occupations. The effectiveness of these measures to prevent work-related and

occupational skin diseases depends on the knowledge, awareness, and motivation of both employers and employees. First, employers should be aware of the risks at work to develop immediate contact reactions and provide the workers with proper skin education and protective elements. Second, workers should be motivated to carry out or seek out specific preventive measures. Occupational health professionals and health educators have an essential role to facilitate the effective design and implementation of these actions.
3. *Indicated measures:* include those preventive actions that are advisable only for persons who, on examination, are found to manifest a risk factor, condition, or abnormality that identifies them, individually, as being at sufficiently high risk to require the preventive intervention, for example, the application of specific diagnostic procedures in workers with already established skin problems. Indicated prevention is most commonly applied in the clinical setting, as the indication is ordinarily one discovered through medical examination or laboratory testing, and many of the preventive measures require professional advice or assistance for optimal results [2].

We have seen that measures to prevent immediate skin contact reactions starts at the population level and include specific actions from legislation to reduce irritants, allergens, and urticariogens, health education on skin protection, to the application of specific diagnostic procedures. Figure 12.1 summarizes the scope of prevention based on a population approach for whom the measure is advisable according to the scientific evidence and cost-benefit analysis.

Standards for Prevention

Work-related and occupational skin diseases are considered as an important emerging risk related to the exposure of chemical, physical, and biological risk factors [1]. Patients with such work-related skin diseases should be treated and assessed based on scientific evidence-based criteria.

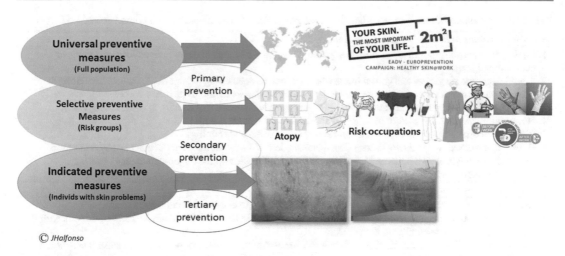

Fig. 12.1 Scope of preventive measures according to population groups. (Servier Medical Art kindly provided graphic images for the design of this figure)

By 2010, Nicholson et al. provided 36 graded statements and 10 evidence-based recommendations for the prevention, identification, and management of occupational contact dermatitis and urticaria after a systematic review of the literature (Table 12.1) [6].

By 2017, minimum standards for effective prevention, diagnosis, and treatment of work-related and occupational skin diseases have been established by a consensus-based approach by means of the Delphi method with more than 80 experts (dermatologists, occupational physicians, health educators, epidemiologists) from 31 European countries (COST Action TD 1206, STANDERM) [7]. Figure 12.2 summarizes these minimum standards.

Overall, prevention focus is on human, organizational, and technical and organizational prevention measures as well as on avoidance/limitation of exposure to allergic substances or irritants at the workplace according to legislation and the provision of a regular training in use of personal protective measures adapted to the needs of the employees [7].

In addition to legislation, a reliable surveillance system for work-related skin diseases is necessary to identify new work-related allergens, urticariogens, and irritants. Most of the current reporting systems are incomplete [7], and urgent actions are needed to improve the existing systems as they can contribute to identify targets for primary prevention. A more complete reporting system can be achievable by a specific surveillance system for work-related skin diseases. For example, in Great Britain, THOR and EPIDERM combine information from dermatologists, occupational physicians, and general practitioners [8]. The German "Dermatologist's procedure" may also serve as a model on how to identify early work-related skin problems by mandatory reporting and prevent social, psychological, and economic consequences of work-related skin diseases [9].

Primary Prevention Measures

Primary prevention measures should be implemented to avoid the development of work-related skin diseases–including immediate contact reactions–in healthy individuals [7]. The application of risk management process involving risk analysis, risk assessment, and risk control practices is the basis for primary prevention [10]. The risk management process should be reviewed and updated regularly.

The occupational risk assessment is a crucial step in the prevention process, and it is usually carried out by occupational hygienists, health and safety engineers, as well as occupational physicians in an inter-

Table 12.1 Evidence-based recommendations for the prevention of occupational contact dermatitis and urticaria

Recommendations to health and safety personnel

1. Implement programs to remove or reduce exposure to agents that cause occupational contact dermatitis or occupational contact urticaria.
2. Provide appropriate gloves and cotton liners where the risk of developing occupational contact dermatitis or occupational contact urticaria cannot be eliminated by removing exposure to its causes.
3. Make after-work creams readily available in the workplace and encourage workers to use them regularly.
4. Not promote the use of pre-work (barrier) creams as a protective measure.
5. Provide workers with appropriate health and safety information and training.
6. Ensure that workers who develop occupational contact dermatitis or occupational contact urticaria are properly assessed by a physician who has expertise in occupational skin disease for recommendations regarding appropriate workplace adjustments.

Recommendations to health practitioners

1. Ask a worker who has been offered a job that will expose them to causes of occupational contact dermatitis whether they have a personal history of dermatitis, particularly in adulthood, and advise them of their increased risk, and how to care for and protect their skin.
2. Ask the worker who has been offered a job that will expose them to causes of occupational contact urticaria whether they have a personal history of atopy and advise them of their increased risk, and how to care for and protect their skin.
3. Take a full occupational history whenever someone of working age presents with dermatitis or urticaria, asking about their job, the materials with which they work, the location of the rash, and any temporal relationship with work (Chap. 3).
4. Arrange for a diagnosis of occupational contact dermatitis or occupational contact urticaria to be confirmed objectively (patch tests and/or prick tests) and not on the basis of a compatible history alone, because of the implications for future employment.

Source: Adapted from Nicholson et al. [6]

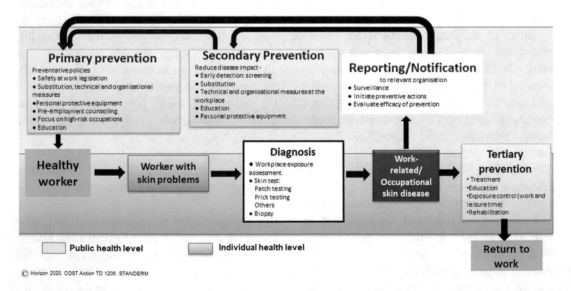

Fig. 12.2 Minimum European standards for primary, secondary, and tertiary prevention of work-related and occupational skin diseases [7]. (© Horizon 2020, COST Action TD 1206, STANDERM; used with permission)

disciplinary manner. Such an assessment will identify and measure exposure to hazardous substances (chemical, physical, and biological products) in the workplace [11]. The most appropriate preventive actions will then be defined accordingly.

Primary prevention measures aimed at maintaining a healthy skin at safe workplaces should follow the **STOP** concept (**S**ubstitution, **T**echnical measures, **O**rganizational measures, and **P**ersonal protection) [12]. Table 12.2

Table 12.2 Preventive measures for work-related/occupational hand eczema, including skin immediate contact reactions

Preventive measure	
Substitution and replacement	Regulation of exposure by legislation on threshold values. Replacement, modification, or inactivation of hazardous substance [3–5, 15, 16].
Technical measures	Proper labeling and storage of chemicals and regular maintenance of tools. Industrial measures to avoid direct skin contact with skin allergens and urticariogens [10, 11]. Technical measures such as ventilation and automatization in work practices may reduce if not eliminate the risk of respiratory and dermal sensitization [17].
Organizational measures	Reduce wet work to less than 2 h [18, 19]. Rotate work tasks to reduce wet work. Skin protection programs providing information on healthy and diseased skin and skin care to facilitate a behavioral change regarding skin protection and decrease the occurrence of work-related skin problems. Such recommendations should be evidence-based [20]. They should be implemented in the curriculum of vocational schools and provided regularly at the workplaces, as some studies have shown that protective measures are applied insufficiently. These programs have been shown to be effective not only in primary prevention, but also in secondary and tertiary prevention [21–23].

Personal protection	*Good hand hygiene regimes* should include:
	  Alcohol hand rubs, or
	  Hand washing with lukewarm water, rinsing the liquid soap thoroughly, and drying hands carefully with single-use paper towels.
	Protective gloves (powder- and accelerator-free):
	  Should be worn on dry and clean hands for wet work and work with hazardous substances for as short a time as possible;
	  Cotton glove liners should be used if gloves have to be worn longer than 10 min;
	  Single-use gloves should be worn only once;
	  Defective gloves must be removed immediately.
	Moisturizers:
	  Should be used to prevent and support the treatment of irritant hand dermatitis;
	  Should be applied all over the hands including the finger webs, fingertips, and back of the hand;
	  Should not contain fragrances, coloring agents, and preservatives [24–29].

Source: Adapted from Alfonso et al. [7]

shows examples of primary preventive measures.

When substitution, technical, and organizational prevention measures are not sufficient, personal protective equipment (e.g., gloves, moisturizers) must be provided and the correct application/use must be trained regularly. Several studies have shown that protective strategies are applied insufficiently; therefore, regular instructions on use and application are necessary [13]. In the planning and implementation of primary prevention measures, the focus should be on high-risk occupations (Chap. 3) and the most common occupational exposures.

Knowledge dissemination in the general population in terms of health promotion and health education is also needed. For example, the German Social Accident Insurance (DGUV) launched in 2008 a massive awareness campaign, **"Your skin: the most important 2m^{2}of your life,"** which had good success [14]. Since 2009, a pan-European awareness campaign has been supported by the Academy of Dermatology and Venereology (JEADV) and successfully used in several European countries. The same logo is now available in 12 languages (Fig. 12.3). Further use of this logo is encouraged to raise awareness on the importance of keeping a healthy skin at work and on the prevention of work-related and occupational skin diseases.

The design and implementation of the preventive measures described here require knowledge dissemination from research to stakeholders. A successful knowledge dissemination strategy

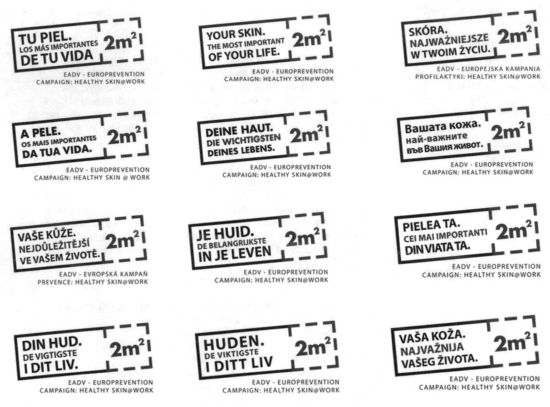

Fig. 12.3 Logo "your skin the most important 2m² of your life" in different languages. (Courtesy from the German Social Accident Insurance (DGUV) and JEADV)

requires building linkages among stakeholders, building partnership to gain support in the design and implementation of health promotion and preventive measures [30].

Recommendations for the Use of Protective Gloves

Accelerators-Free Gloves

We have seen in Chap. 3 that protective gloves can lead to skin problems, not only because of the presence of allergens and urticariogens but also because of the effect of occlusion. For instance, although an effective reduction in the occurrence of occupational contact urticaria caused by natural rubber latex has been registered [3–5], rubber additives are still causing occupational contact dermatitis and urticaria [31]. Fortunately, new

technologies have developed low-protein rubber gloves, vulcanization accelerator-free, or gloves containing antimicrobial agents or moisturizers [31]. These gloves are useful not only for primary prevention among healthy workers employed in risk occupations, but also in secondary prevention among workers with already established skin problems. It must be highlighted that these gloves may be more expensive than regular non-accelerator-free gloves as less expensive gloves are usually not tested for allergy and may still contain both allergens and urticariogens. Table 12.3 displays an overview of some available accelerator-free gloves to be recommended in risk occupations.

It is highly recommended that food handlers do not use natural rubber latex gloves, as latex proteins can be transferred to food [32, 33]. Latex-allergic subjects may have severe allergic reactions to foods handled by latex gloves [34],

Table 12.3 Accelerator-free gloves to prevent the development of immediate contact reactions

Occupational group	Material	Manufacturer
Health workers Veterinarians	Low-protein latex gloves: use of desproteinized and purified natural rubber latex are obtained by adding proteolytic enzymes and/or surfactants, chlorination, and high-temperature post-washing [31].	Ansell http://medical. ansell.eu/
	Non-latex surgical gloves. MEDI-GRIP Made from synthetic neoprene and free from latex proteins and chemical accelerators.	
	GAMMEX® Non-Latex PI. Made of 100% synthetic polyisoprene. Safe for latex-sensitive (type I)	
	MICRO-TOUCH Nitrile accelerator-free	
Surgical personnel (surgical gloves)	Biogel NeoDerm made of polychloroprene, without accelerators.	Mölnlycke http://www. molnlycke.us/
	Sempermed Syntegra UV Polyisoprene photo-crosslinked (powder free, natural latex free, accelerator free)	Sempermed https://www. sempermed.com/ en/
	Finessis Corium Styrene elastomer (SEBS) (powder free, natural latex free, accelerator free)	Finessis http://finessis. com/
Food handlers, catering, cleaners, hairdressers	Accelerators-free, powder free, nitrile gloves	Granberg http://www. granberg.no/

Table 12.4 Websites with information on allergens content in gloves

Website	Information
German website of BG BAU http://www.bgbau.de/gisbau/ service/allergene/ allergeneliste-nach-hersteller-1	List of gloves sorted by manufacturer and indicates the presence of the following allergens: thiurams, dithiocarbamates, thioureas, mercaptobenzothiazoles, and their derivatives. Additional allergens may be mentioned, such as 1,3-diphenylguanidine, N,N'-diphenyl-p-phenylenediamine (an antioxidant found in rubber formulations such as bromobutyl), p-phenylenediamine in butyl rubber, hexahydro-1,3,5-triethyl-s-triazine (a formaldehyde releaser found in protection gloves), colophony, nickel, and hexavalent chromium.
Ann Goossens's website http://contactallergy. uzleuven.be	Detailed bibliographic information on glove manufacturers based on allergens, as well as retailers' contact information.
http://www.2mains.ch/fr/ professions/by_field	Information on how to choose gloves based on the occupation of the person involved.

even when cross-reactivity is not an issue. Highly sensitive patients may still be able to react to food handled by low-protein gloves. The website of the American Latex Allergy Association provides with an extensive list of alternative latex-free products at http://latexallergyresources.org/latex-free-products.

Overall proper use of protective gloves is not intended to be a substitute for the other preventive measures already presented, such as elimination, substitution, and reduction of hazardous skin exposures through legislation, and risk assessment.

Several websites provide with useful information on allergens found in gloves as well as avoidance lists (Table 12.4) [31].

Tips on Proper Glove Use

To prevent skin barrier disruption and further development of work-related and occupational skin diseases, not only the glove material, but also the way in which gloves are handled, is important [34–36]. Table 12.5 summarizes good advice for proper glove use.

Table 12.5 Tips on proper glove use

1. Use the recommended gloves by the data safety material sheet of the chemical products you are handling. In case of doubt, contact the producer or ask for advice to occupational hygienists or safety engineers.
2. Use accelerator-free gloves as shown in Table 12.3 (Fig. 12.4)
3. Always choose gloves that are CE marked.
4. Protective gloves should be used when necessary, but for as short a time as possible.
5. Protective gloves should be intact and clean and dry inside.
6. Use gloves with long cuffs to avoid water and chemical products coming inside the glove.
7. Hands must be washed after glove removal. Gloves have an imperfect barrier to infectious material.
8. Avoid finger rings and long fingernails when using gloves
9. Use gloves made of cotton or bamboo viscose fiber, which will absorb moisture and sweat, under the protective glove (Fig. 12.5). Gloves made of bamboo viscose fiber are softer and more comfortable. The fingertips of the glove can be cut off to keep good finger sensation (Fig. 12.6).
10. Disposable gloves are gloves for a single use. They should not be cleaned and reused.
11. Choose the right glove size.
12. Remove the gloves without touching the outer surface of the glove to avoid contact with substances that may cause allergy or irritation on the skin.
13. Use protective gloves when performing wet work during domestic or free-time activities.

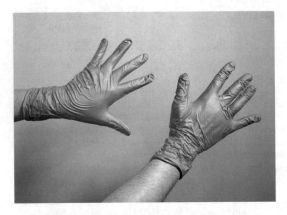

Fig. 12.4 Nitrile accelerator-free gloves. (Photo: Andreas Hvid Ramsdal. National Institute of Occupational Health, STAMI)

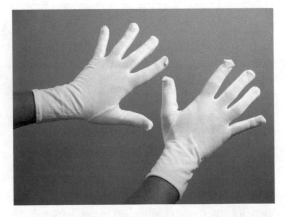

Fig. 12.5 Gloves made of bamboo viscose fiber. (Photo: Andreas Hvid Ramsdal. National Institute of Occupational Health, STAMI)

Moisturizers

A healthy skin assures protection against physical agents, chemicals, mechanical injuries, impact, light, UV radiation, cold, and heat. Extrinsic factors such as occupational exposure to chemical, physical, and mechanical factors may threaten skin integrity and proper restoration, leading to skin barrier disruption.

Skin barrier disruption may lead to irritant contact dermatitis, facilitate the penetration of skin urticariogens, allergens with further sensitization, and is a prerequisite for the development of protein contact dermatitis. Moisturizers have been shown to promote regeneration and reparation of a disrupted skin barrier [37, 38]. A lipid-rich moisturizer free from fragrances and with preservatives and the lowest allergen potential is highly recommended [20]. First, lipid-rich moisturizers promote a fast regeneration [39]. Second, fragrances and preservatives may lead to sensitization and allergic contact dermatitis [40].

According to the evidence-based statements developed by Nicholson et al. [6], there is moderate evidence available on the regular application of moisturizers contributing to prevent the development of occupational contact dermatitis [41, 42].

Moreover, strong evidence, from independent studies of high quality, support that some pre-work moisturizers may help to prevent the development of occupational contact dermatitis, but pre-work creams are not generally effective as a protective measure alone [6, 41, 43]. Therefore, the denomination "barrier cream" is highly discouraged as it may provide a false feeling of full skin protection.

After a literature review focusing on primary prevention through the use of skin creams in healthy populations, an expert panel suggested three moments for skin cream application to prevent irritant contact dermatitis in the workplace: before work; during work after hand washing; and after work [29] (Fig. 12.7). This suggestion can be applied to all industrial sectors, with evidence drawn from different workplace scenarios such as hairdressers, food handlers, timber, the building trade, machinists, and metalworkers [29]).

More randomized controlled trials including long-term controlled observations as well as interventions studies in risk occupations are needed to confirm the effectiveness of this proposal. To our knowledge, no studies have specifically assessed the role of moisturizers in the prevention of immediate contact reactions, but the correct use of moisturizers will contribute to maintaining a healthy skin barrier and to restoring it when occupational factors do not allow its physiological recovery.

Proper use of moisturizers should not be a substitute for the other preventive measures presented here, such as elimination, substitution and reduction of hazardous skin exposures through legislation, risk assessment, and proper use of personal protective equipment use according to worksite requirements.

Secondary Prevention Measures

The aim of secondary prevention is to avoid disease progression by early diagnosis and intervention. Thus, secondary prevention measures are implemented to detect and treat early stages of the disease, to prevent relapses or chronicity by improvement of hazardous workplace situations, behavioral change, and proper skin protection during both work and free time. Psychological support is also of great importance as severe cases may impair life quality with serious consequences on working life (Chap. 3).

As Fig. 12.2 shows, notification systems for work-related and occupational skin diseases are of vital relevance for early intervention, as they may be necessary to initiate diagnostic, treatment, and interventions in the workplace.

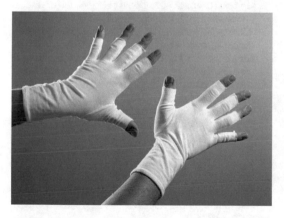

Fig. 12.6 Customized gloves made of bamboo viscose fiber to keep good sensation in the fingertips. (Photo: Andreas Hvid Ramsdal, National Institute of Occupational Health, STAMI)

Fig. 12.7 Three moments of skin cream application (before work, after wet work exposure, and after work) [29]

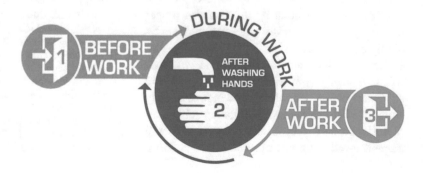

Tertiary Prevention Measures

The aim of tertiary prevention is medical, occupational, and psychosocial rehabilitation of workers with an established disease. These measures aim to facilitate social rehabilitation and quality of life of workers who are at risk of losing their jobs or even have already suffered job loss. Experiences from Germany suggest that tertiary individual programs including psychological interventions contribute to improved mental health in patients with severe occupational hand eczema [44].

Currently there is a lack of evidence-based guidelines addressing secondary and tertiary prevention of immediate contact reactions. Hence, we suggest following recommendations from the evidence-based standards for the prevention and management of work-related and occupational skin diseases [6, 7].

Interdisciplinary teams composed of dermatologists, occupational physicians, allergists, safety engineers, and health educators are necessary for effective measures in all levels of prevention.

Conclusion

The most effective preventive measures to prevent immediate contact reactions at work include legislation, elimination, substitution, and reduction of exposure to skin hazardous substances. For instance, a significant reduction in the incidence of occupational cases of contact urticaria from natural rubber latex has been well documented in several countries. When substitution, technical, and organizational measures are not feasible, skin protection by the terms of proper use of protective gloves and moisturizers is highly encouraged.

Continuous training and education will contribute not only to maintaining a healthy skin in safe workplaces, but also to recognizing early signs of skin disease and facilitating rehabilitation. Hence, early diagnosis and intervention will prevent a relapsing and chronic disease course.

When an occupational disease is already established, measures aimed to facilitate medical, occupational, social, economic compensation, and psychological rehabilitation should be available.

Standards for prevention of work-related and occupational skin diseases have been developed, although most of these focus on the prevention and management of occupational hand eczema. Future studies should specifically focus on immediate contact reactions.

References

1. European Agency for Safety and Health at Work. Occupational skin diseases diseases and dermal exposure in the European Union (EU-25): Policy and practice review. 2008. Available at: https://osha.europa.eu/en/publications/reports/TE7007049ENC_skin_diseases. Accessed 20 Nov 2017.
2. Gordon RS Jr. An operational classification of disease prevention. Public Health Rep. 1983;98:107–9.
3. Allmers H, Schmengler J, John SM. Decreasing incidence of occupational contact urticaria caused by natural rubber latex allergy in German health care workers. J Allergy Clin Immunol. 2004;114:347–51.
4. Bensefa-Colas L, Telle-Lamberton M, Faye S, Bourrain JL, Crépy MN, Lasfargues G, et al. Occupational contact urticaria: lessons from the French National Network for Occupational Disease Vigilance and Prevention (RNV3P). Br J Dermatol. 2015;173:1453–61.
5. Turner S, McNamee R, Agius R, Wilkinson SM, Carder M, Stocks SJ. Evaluating interventions aimed at reducing occupational exposure to latex and rubber glove allergens. Occup Environ Med. 2012;69:925–31.
6. Nicholson PJ, Llewellyn D, English JS, On behalf of the Guidelines Development Group. Evidence-based guidelines for the prevention, identification and management of occupational contact dermatitis and urticaria. Contact Dermatitis. 2010;63:177–86.
7. Alfonso JH, Bauer A, Bensefa-Colas L, Boman A, Bubas M, Constandt L, Crepy MN, Goncalo M, Macan J, Mahler V, Mijakoski D, Ramada Rodilla JM, Rustemeyer T, Spring P, John SM, Uter W, Wilkinson M, Giménez-Arnau AM. Minimum standards on prevention, diagnosis and treatment of occupational and work-related skin diseases in Europe – position paper of the COST Action StanDerm (TD 1206). J Eur Acad Dermatol Venereol. 2017;31(Suppl. 4):31–43.
8. Health and Safety Executive. Work-related skin disease in Great Britain 2014. 2016. www.hse.gov.uk/statistics/. Accessed 25 Nov 2017.

9. Voß H, Gediga G, Gediga K, Maier B, Mentzel F, Skudlik C, et al. Secondary prevention of occupational dermatoses: first systematic evaluation of optimized dermatologist's procedure and hierarchical multi-step intervention. J Dtsch Dermatol Ges J Ger Soc Dermatol. 2013;11:662–71.

10. OSHA. https://oshwiki.eu/wiki/Occupational_safety_and_health_risk_assessment_methodologies.

11. Council Directive 89/391/EEC of 12 June 1989 on the introduction of measures to encourage improvements in the safety and health of workers at work.

12. Wulfhorts R, John SM, Strunk M. Worker's protection: gloves and cream. In: Duus Johansen J, Lepoittevin JP, Thyssen JP, editors. Quick guide to contact dermatitis. Berlin: Springer; 2016. p. 275–87.

13. Diepgen TL, Andersen KE, Chosidow O, Coenraads PJ, Elsner P, English J, et al. guidelines for diagnosis, prevention and treatment of hand eczema--short version. J Dtsch Dermatol Ges J Ger Soc Dermatol JDDG. 2015;13:77–85.

14. DGUV. Healthy skin Campaign. Available at: http://www.dguv.de/en/prevention/campaigns/prev_campaigns/kampagne_haut/index.jsp. Accessed 27 Nov 2017.

15. Geier J, Krautheim A, Uter W, Lessmann H, Schnuch A. Occupational contact allergy in the building trade in Germany: influence of preventive measures and changing exposure. Int Arch Occup Environ Health. 2001;84:403–11.

16. Uter W, Geier J, Lessmann H, Schnuch A. Is contact allergy to glyceryl monothioglycolate still a problem in Germany? Contact Dermatitis. 2006;55:54–6.

17. Douglas JD, McSharry C, Blaikie L, Morrow T, Miles S, Franklin D. Occupational asthma caused by automated salmon processing. Lancet. 1995;346:737–40.

18. Uter W, Pfahlberg A, Gefeller O, Schwanitz HJ. Hand dermatitis in a prospectively followed cohort of hairdressing apprentices: final results of the POSH study. Prevention of occupational skin disease in hairdressers. Contact Dermatitis. 1999;41:280–6.

19. Bundesanstalt für Arbeitsschutz und Arbeitsmedizin. [TRGS 401: risks resulting from skin contact – determination, evaluation, measures]. 2008. Available at: http://www.baua.de/cln_135/en/Topicsfrom-A-to-Z/Hazardous-Substances/TRGS/TRGS.html. Accessed 26 Jan 2016.

20. Agner T, Held E. Skin protection programmes. Contact Dermatitis. 2002;47:253–6.

21. Brown T. Strategies for prevention: occupational contact dermatitis. Occup Med (London). 2004;54:450–7.

22. English J, Aldridge R, Gawkrodger DJ, Kowancki S, Statham B, White JML, et al. Consensus statement on the management of chronic hand eczema. Clin Exp Dermatol. 2009;34:761–9.

23. Held E, Mygind K, Wolff C, Gyntelberg F, Agner T. Prevention of work related skin problems: an intervention study in wet work employees. Occup Environ Med. 2002;59:556–61.

24. BAuA – Hazardous Substances/Topics from A to Z/Federal Institute forOccupational Safety and Health. http://www.baua.de/en/Topics-from-A-to-Z/Hazardous-Su bstances/Hazardous-Substances.html. Last accessed 20 Nov 2017.

25. Microsoft Word - 013-056l_S1_Berufliche_Hautmittel_2014-10.docx -013-056l_S1_Berufliche_Hautmittel_2014-10.pdf. http://www.awmf.org/uploads/tx_szleitlinien/013-056l_S1_Berufliche_Hautmittel_2014-10.pdf. Last accessed 20 Nov 2017.

26. Korinth G, Geh S, Schaller KH, Drexler H. In vitro evaluation of the efficacy of skin barrier creams and protective gloves on percutaneous absorption of industrial solvents. Int Arch Occup Environ Health. 2003;76:382–6.

27. Korinth G, Lüersen L, Schaller KH, Angerer J, Drexler H. Enhancement of percutaneous penetration of aniline and o-toluidine in vitro using skin barrier creams. Toxicol Vitro Int J Publ Assoc BIBRA. 2008;22:812–8.

28. Korinth G, Weiss T, Penkert S, Schaller KH, Angerer J, Drexler H. Percutaneous absorption of aromatic amines in rubber industry workers: impact of impaired skin and skin barrier creams. Occup Environ Med. 2007;64:366–72.

29. Hines J, Wilkinson SM, John SM, Diepgen T, English J, Rustemeyer T, et al. The three moments of skin cream application: an evidence-based proposal for use of skin creams in the prevention of irritant contact dermatitis in the workplace. J Eur Acad Dermatol Venereol. 2017;31:53–64.

30. Wilke A, Bollmann U, Cazzaniga S, Hubner A, John SM, Karadzinska-Bislimovska J, et al. The implementation of knowledge dissemination in the prevention of occupational skin diseases. J Eur Acad Dermatol Venereol. 2018;3:449–458. https://doi.org/10.1111/jdv.14653. [Epub ahead of print].

31. Crepy MN. Rubber: new allergens and preventive measures. Eur J Dermatol. 2016;26:523–30.

32. Beezhold DH, Kostyal DA, Wiseman JS. The transfer of protein allergens from latex gloves. A study of influencing factors. AORN. 1994;59:605–14.

33. Palosuo T, Antoniadou I, Gottrup F, Phillips P. Latex medical gloves: time for a reappraisal. Int Arch Allergy Immunol. 2011;156:234–46.

34. Bernardini R, Novembre E, Lombardi E, Pucci N, Marcucci F, Vierucci A. Anaphylaxis to latex after ingestion of a cream-filled doughnut contaminated with latex. J Allergy Clin Immunol. 2002;110:534–5.

35. Lind ML, Boman A, Sollenberg J, Johnsson S, Hagelthorn G, Meding B. Occupational dermal exposure to permanent hair dyes among hairdressers. Ann Occup Hyg. 2005;49:473–80.

36. Oreskov KW, Søsted H, Johansen JD. Glove use among hairdressers: difficulties in the correct use of gloves among hairdressers and the effect of education. Contact Dermatitis. 2015;72:362–6.

37. Loden M, Andersson AC. Effect of topically applied lipidson surfactant-irritated skin. Br J Dermatol. 1996;134:215–20.

38. Held E, Agner T. Comparison between 2 test models inevaluating the effect of a moisturizer on irritated human skin. Contact Dermatitis. 1999;40:261–8.

39. Held E, Agner T. Effect of moisturizers on skin susceptibility to irritants. Acta Derm Venereol. 2001;81:104–7.

40. Held E, Johansen JD, Agner T, Menne T. Contact allergyto cosmetics: testing with patients' own products. Contact Dermatitis. 1999;40:310–5.

41. Saary J, Qureshi R, Palda V, DeKoven J, Pratt M, Skotnicki-Grant S, Holness L. A systematic review of contact dermatitis treatment and prevention. J Am Acad Dermatol. 2005;53:845–855.75.

42. Arbogast JW, Fendler EJ, Hammond BS, Cartner TJ, Dolan MD, Ali Y, Maibach HI. Effectiveness of a hand care regimen with moisturizer in manufacturing facilities where workers are prone to occupational irritant dermatitis. Dermatitis. 2004;15:10–7.

43. Winker R, Salameh B, Stolkovich S, Nikl M, Barth A, Ponocny E, et al. Effectiveness of skin protection creams in the prevention of occupational dermatitis: results of a randomized, controlled trial. Int Arch Occup Environ Health. 2009;82:653–62.

44. Breuer K, John SM, Finkeldey F, Boehm D, Skudlik C, Wulfhorst B, et al. Tertiary individual prevention improves mental health in patients with severe occupational hand eczema. J Eur Acad Dermatol Venereol. 2015;29:1724–31.

Management and Treatment of Contact Urticaria Syndrome

13

Gustavo Deza and Ana M. Giménez-Arnau

Key Messages

- Contact urticaria syndrome (CUS) represents nowadays a worldwide health problem that needs a global approach.
- A high index of suspicion is needed to elicit the clinical history that would suggest this condition.
- CUS is treated mainly by prevention.
- Prognosis of CUS is entirely dependent on the ability of the patient to avoid the etiological substances.
- No standard recommendations on the use or consensus on the efficacy of pharmacological therapies for CUS currently exist.

Introduction

Contact urticaria syndrome (CUS), contact urticaria (CoU), and protein contact dermatitis (PCD) are conditions characterized by the immediate development of contact inflammatory skin reactions [1–5]. These reactions usually appear within minutes after contact with eliciting substances, and their signs and symptoms are determined by a wide range of factors, such as the route, duration, and extent of exposure; the sensitizing properties of the allergen; and the individual's inherited and/or acquired susceptibility [2]. Initial presentation of the reaction mainly manifests as wheals and/or dermatitis/eczema, and usually remains in the contact area. However, symptoms connected with CUS (particularly the immunological type) may occasionally spread beyond the initial site of contact and progress to generalized urticaria, and/or systemic symptoms may develop that are similar to those found in angioedema, asthma, or anaphylactic shock [1, 2, 6–8] (Table 13.1).

The clinical importance of immediate contact skin reactions, which can be commonly seen in dermatology practice [9], is not only because of the aforementioned risk of developing life-threatening reactions, but also because of their relevance in the occupational setting [10, 11]. Thus, occupational CoU can account for 5% to 10% of reported cases of occupational skin diseases and can have a significant impact on the quality of life of workers, resulting in physical, psychological, and financial hardships [10, 12]. For these reasons, early and proper diagnosis, and appropriate management of patients when they have been correctly diagnosed, is mandatory to avoid such undesirable consequences.

The purpose of this chapter is to discuss the different therapeutic options available for the management of CUS, review the mechanisms by which these treatments might achieve their

G. Deza · A. M. Giménez-Arnau (✉)
Hospital del Mar - Institut Mar d'Investigacions
Mediques, Universitat Autònoma de Barcelona (UAB),
Department of Dermatology, Barcelona, Spain
e-mail: 22505aga@comb.cat

Table 13.1 Stages of contact urticaria syndrome

Stage 1	Localized urticaria Nonspecific symptoms (itching, tingling, burning sensation) immediate contact dermatitis (eczema: protein contact dermatitis)
Stage 2	Generalized urticaria
Stage 3	Extracutaneous involvement (rhinoconjunctivitis, bronchospasm, orolaryngeal, gastrointestinal)
Stage 4	Anaphylactic or anaphylactoid reaction (shock)

Source: Von Krogh and Maibach [7]

therapeutic effects on patients with CUS, and propose a simple and effective algorithm for the management and treatment of this condition.

Pathogenic Mechanisms in CUS

To understand the beneficial effects of the treatments available for the management of immediate contact skin reactions, knowledge of the mechanisms involved in the pathogenesis of the disease is of utmost importance. Although such mechanisms are not yet fully understood, the general classification distinguishes these types [7].

1. Immunological contact urticaria (ICoU). ICoU is a type I immunoglobulin E (IgE)-mediated hypersensitivity reaction in which the patient's immune system has been previously sensitized to the eliciting substance [1, 9, 13, 14]. Thus, after the initial binding of allergen-bound IgE to mast cells and basophils, histamine (mainly) and other inflammatory mediators are released, causing the itch, inflammation, and swelling in the skin [1, 5, 8]. Therefore, the release of histamine is the central mechanism in the pathogenesis of this type of CoU.
2. Nonimmunological contact urticaria (NICoU). NICoU is probably the most common form of the disease, does not require presensitization to an allergen, and causes the skin reaction without the involvement of immunological

processes [12]. In these cases, it is presumed that some urticants may cause the epidermal release of vasoactive substances, such as prostaglandins and leukotrienes, and a non-IgE-mediated histamine release from mast cells after a direct insult to the local blood vessels [1, 12, 15, 16]. Because of the lack of response to antihistamines, histamine is not considered the main inflammatory mediator involved in this type of CoU [5, 17]. Instead, because oral and topical nonsteroidal antiinflammatory drugs (NSAIDs) can provide a satisfactory clinical response, prostaglandins and leukotrienes are considered the main agents in NICoU [18–21].
3. Idiopathic or CoU of unknown origin. A third category of CoU reactions also exists for substances that elicit mixed features of both NICoU and ICoU, or where the mechanism remains uncertain [9, 15].

Furthermore, in cases of PCD, which is a particular type of immediate skin reaction caused by the recurrent exposure to high molecular weight proteins [22], a different molecular mechanism could be identified. Although its pathogenesis remains unclear, it may involve a type I hypersensitivity reaction, type IV (cell-mediated delayed) hypersensitivity reaction, and/or a delayed reaction from IgE-bearing Langerhans cells, similar to that which is observed in atopic dermatitis [22–24]. Such mechanisms could explain the clinical features observed in PCD (typically presents with hand and fingertip eczematous dermatitis) and the symptomatic relief achieved with topical corticosteroids or nonsteroidal topical immunomodulators [22, 25]. Finally, it should be also noted that PCD and CoU can be induced by the same allergen through immunological processes and can occasionally be present in the same patient [2].

Management and Treatment of Contact Urticaria Syndrome

Management of CUS is similar to that of other diseases caused by hypersensitivity reactions. Thus, the safest and most effective measure is the complete avoidance of the particular allergen. In other words, CUS is mainly treated by prevention [26]. Therefore, once the culprit substance is identified, the patient should be advised to avoid that substance and potential cross-reacting substances. Complete avoidance of the allergen is not always feasible, however, especially in the occupational setting. In those cases where prevention has failed and the symptoms interfere with the patient's career and/or quality of life, pharmacological agents could be used to provide symptomatic relief [4]. Importantly, the first-line medications depend on the type of immediate contact skin reaction, but the overall goal is to inhibit the release of the inflammatory mediators involved in the pathogenesis of the disease.

Because preventive measures solve most cases of CUS, there is a lack of published experience regarding the management of this condition with topical or systemic drugs. These therapeutic options, which are discussed next, are similar to those used for chronic urticaria (in cases of CoU) or chronic eczema (in cases of PCD) (Table 13.2). However, no standard recommendations on the use or consensus on the efficacy of these thera-pies currently exist for CUS. A simple and practical algorithm for the management of CUS is proposed in Fig. 13.1.

Prevention

As previously mentioned, emphasis for treatment of CUS should be placed on prevention, which remains the desideratum of therapy [26]. A thorough history and appropriate clinical testing will help determine the responsible substances. Afterward, patients must be educated on their disorder, understand its possible evolution over time, and be aware of the therapeutic options available. Furthermore, in cases of ICoU, it is also important to stress that recurrent exposures to the eliciting substances can precipitate the progression to subsequent stages of the disease and therefore a greater risk of development systemic symptoms and/or life-threatening reactions [6, 8].

Primary prevention (which aim is to avert the onset of disease, for example, by the replacement of the responsible substances with

Table 13.2 Treatment options for contact urticaria syndrome

Therapeutic alternative	Indications	Adverse side effects
Prevention	NICoU, ICoU, PCD	None
H1 antihistamines	ICoU, PCD	Drowsiness, psychomotor impairment or anticholinergic effects (lower side effects with second-generation H1 antihistamines)
Topical corticosteroids	PCD	Skin atrophy, purpura, stretch marks, and possible alteration of intrinsic adrenocortical production
Topical calcineurin inhibitors	PCD	Stinging, burning, soreness, or itching in the area of treated skin during the first few days of treatment
Nonsteroidal antiinflammatory drugs (NSAIDs)	NICoU	Nausea, vomiting, headache, dizziness, reduced appetite. The most serious side effects are ulcers, bleeding, kidney failure, and, rarely, liver failure
Systemic corticosteroids	NICoU, ICoU, PCD	If long-term therapy: weight gain, hyperglycemia, hypertension, osteoporosis, cataracts, gastrointestinal bleeding
Phototherapy	NICoU, ICoU, PCD	Erythema, hyperpigmentation, polymorphic light eruption, fatigue and premature aging of the skin
Leukotriene receptor antagonists	NICoU, ICoU	Hypersensitivity, gastrointestinal disturbances, bleeding
Immunosuppressive agents (cyclosporine, methotrexate…)	NICoU, ICoU, PCD	Cyclosporine: hypertension and renal toxicity; methotrexate: bone marrow suppression and hepatitis
Anti-IgE therapy	ICoU	Local symptoms at the site of injection, headache, nasopharyngitis, sinusitis, nausea, diarrhea

NICoU nonimmunological contact urticaria, *ICoU* immunological contact urticaria, *PCD* protein contact dermatitis, *IgE* immunoglobulin E

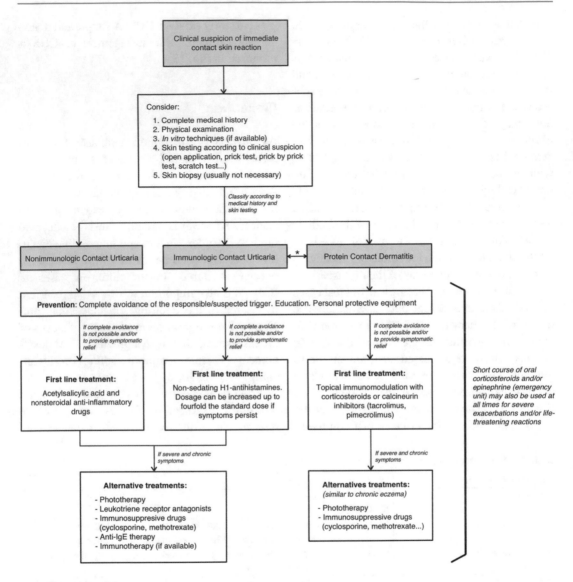

Fig. 13.1 Proposed algorithm for the management of contact urticaria syndrome

less harmful materials) and secondary prevention (which aim is to detect and treat early stages of the disease, to prevent relapses or chronicity, and/or to induce behavioral change) are highly recommended for occupational CUS [10, 11, 27]. If the responsible substance cannot be replaced or eliminated, then an adequate control must be implemented to prevent worker exposure to the allergen. Other recommended measures may include providing personal pro-

tective equipment to the workers to reduce allergen exposure (e.g., in cases of latex-induced CoU, the use of polyvinyl or nitrile gloves could be a useful alternative if rubber hypersensitivity has been appropriately detected among these patients) and making after-work creams readily available in the workplace and encouraging workers to use them regularly, ensuring physician assessment when appropriate [10, 11].

Table 13.3 H1 antihistamines commonly used in urticaria

Chemical class	Active substance	Dosage	Mechanism of action
Alkylamines	Dexchlorpheniramine[a]	2 mg/4–6 h	H1-receptor inverse agonist
	Chlorpheniramine[a]	4–8 mg/6 h	H1-receptor inverse agonist
	Brompheniramine[a]	4–8 mg/6 h	H1-receptor inverse agonist
	Acrivastine[b]	16–24 mg/24 h	H1-receptor inverse agonist
Ethanolamines	Diphenhydramine[a]	25–50 mg/4–6 h	H1-receptor inverse agonist, anticholinergic
Ethylenediamines	Tripelennamine[a]	25–50 mg/4 h	H1-receptor inverse agonist
Phenothiazines	Promethazine[a]	25 mg/8 h	H1-receptor inverse agonist
	Methdilazine[a]	8 mg/6–12 h	H1-receptor inverse agonist
Piperazines	Hydroxyzine[a]	25 mg/6–8 h	H1-receptor inverse agonist, antiadrenergic, bronchodilator, antiemetic
	Cetirizine[b]	10 mg/24 h	H1-receptor inverse agonist, inhibits eosinophil adhesion, eosinophil and neutrophil chemotaxis, T-cell and monocyte chemotaxis, IL-8, MCP1/RANTES, NF-κB 19, ICAM-1, LTC4
	Levocetirizine[b]	5 mg/24 h	H1-receptor inverse agonist, inhibits eosinophil adhesion eosinophil and neutrophil chemotaxis, T-cell and monocyte chemotaxis
Piperidines	Cyproheptadine[a]	4 mg/8 h	H1-receptor inverse agonist, anticholinergic, antiserotonergic
	Mizolastine[b]	10 mg/24 h	H1-receptor inverse agonist, neutrophil recruitment, VEGF, TNF, 5-lipoxygenase
	Terfenadine[b]	60–120 mg/24	H1-receptor inverse agonist, inhibits eosinophil chemotaxis, eosinophil adherence, superoxide synthesis, IL-6, IL-8, TNF, GM-CSF
	Fexofenadine[b]	180 mg/24 h	H1-receptor inverse agonist
	Loratadine[b]	10 mg/24 h	H1-receptor inverse agonist, inhibits eosinophil chemotaxis, IL-8, RANTES, ICAM-1
	Desloratadine[b]	5 mg/24 h	H1-receptor inverse agonist, inhibits eosinophil chemotaxis, superoxide production, TNF, IL-1, IL-6, IL-8, IL-13, P-selectin, ICAM-1, eosinophil apoptosis
	Rupatadine[b]	10 mg/24 h	H1-receptor inverse agonist, anti PAF, inhibits mast cell degranulation, TNF, Il-6, IL-8
	Ebastine[b]	10–20 mg/24 h	H1-receptor inverse agonist
	Bilastine[b]	20 mg/24 h	H1-receptor inverse agonist

Source: Deza and Giménez-Arnau [31]

IL interleukin, *MCP1* monocyte chemoattractant protein-1, *RANTES* regulated and normal T-cell expressed and secreted, *NF-κB* nuclear factor-kappa B, *ICAM* intercellular adhesion molecule, *LTC4* leukotriene C4, *VEGF* vascular endothelial growth factor, *TNF* tumor necrosis factor, *PAF* platelet activation factor

[a]Classical or first-generation H1 antihistamines

[b]Modern second-generation H1 antihistamines

Importantly, the prognosis of CUS is entirely dependent on the ability of the patient to avoid etiological substances [28]. Thus, even in cases of severe ICoU, the long-term prognosis can be good if patients take an active role in controlling their environment and taking all proper precautions.

Antihistamines

Because histamine release has a key role in the pathogenesis of ICoU, antihistamines are considered the first-line therapy for this disorder, as for chronic urticaria [2, 4, 6, 29–31] (Table 13.3). These agents can also provide symptomatic relief in cases of PCD, reducing the itch and burning sensation of the eczematous dermatitis. Antihistamines act as inverse agonists of the histamine receptor, modifying the balance that normally exists between the active and inactive state of the receptor, stabilizing the inactive conformation [32]. Thereby, the local and systemic effects of histamine on target organs are blocked. Some of the antihistamines have additional antiinflammatory properties, reducing the expression of cell adhesion molecules, interfering in the recruitment of inflammatory cells such as neutrophils and eosinophils, and/or inhibiting the secretion of other inflammatory mediators, such as eicosanoids and leukotrienes [33, 34].

Second-generation H1 antihistamines are currently preferred to their predecessors as these have a better safety profile (fewer side effects such as drowsiness, psychomotor impairment, or anticholinergic effects), greater receptor specificity, greater efficacy, and longer duration of action [35]. It should be noted that the dose of H1 antihistamines should be increased (up to fourfold the standard dose) for maximum symptom control before considering alternative therapies, so long as no adverse effects are intolerable [29]. On the other hand, because 15% of histamine receptors in the skin are H2 type, H2 antihistamines may also have some effect on the symptoms of CoU [5, 36]. However, these drugs should not be used as monotherapy because they have only minimal effects on pruritus [33, 37], and current guidelines do not recommend H2 antihistamines as an evidence-based treatment in urticaria [29].

Topical Immunomodulation: Corticosteroids and Calcineurin Inhibitors

Considering that the hands are the site most frequently affected in cases of PCD, current guidelines for the management and treatment of hand eczema could be also used for this condition [38]. Thus, topical immunomodulation with high-potency corticosteroids should be considered the first-line therapy for PCD, as this method may decrease inflammation, accelerate the healing process, and inhibit the nuclear expression of genes that promote the synthesis of proinflammatory interleukins and cytokines [22, 39]. However, the likelihood of developing numerous side effects (such as skin atrophy, purpura, stretch marks, and possible alteration of intrinsic adrenocortical production) make these agents a poor long-term option. In cases of PCD with no satisfactory clinical response to topical steroids and/or with chronic cutaneous symptoms, topical calcineurin inhibitors (TCI) have been also reported as a useful therapeutic alternative [25]. TCI, such as tacrolimus and pimecrolimus, may inhibit the phosphorylase activity of the calcium-dependent serine/threonine phosphatase calcineurin and the dephosphorylation of the nuclear factor of activated T-cell protein necessary for the expression of IL-2, IL-4, IL-5, granulocyte macrophage colony-stimulating factor (GM- CSF), and tumor necrosis factor (TNF)-α [40], thus decreasing the local inflammation seen in such cases as atopic dermatitis. Furthermore, their mechanism of action in PCD has been also attributed to a decreased expression of the high-affinity Langerhans cells and epidermic dendritic inflammatory cells and to an inhibition of the stimulatory function of these Langerhans cells [25]. Local side effects derived from their use may include stinging, burning, soreness, or itching in the area of treated skin during the first few days of treatment. Headache, acne, folliculitis, flu-like symptoms (e.g., fever, chills, runny nose, sore throat, muscle aches), or increased sensitivity of the skin may also occur.

Nonsteroidal Antiinflammatory Drugs

Some of the most commonly reported causes of NICoU include ingredients of cosmetics and medicaments (e.g., balsam of Peru, benzoic acid, cinnamic alcohol, cinnamic aldehyde), sorbic acid (a preservative used in many foods), dimethyl sulfoxide, metals (cobalt chloride, nickel sulfate, palladium), raw meat, and fish and vegetables [1]. First-line therapies in these cases should include aspirin and NSAIDs, given the important role of prostaglandins (mainly) and leukotrienes in the pathophysiology of this type of CoU [4, 5, 26]. These agents act by blocking the cyclooxygenase enzymes, thus reducing the production of prostaglandins and thromboxanes throughout the body. As noted earlier, antihistamines are unable to inhibit the reactions caused by nonimmunological pathways.

Systemic Corticosteroids

Systemic corticosteroids should be considered when a rapid and complete disease control is necessary. Thus, a short course of oral steroids is recommended for severe cases/exacerbations of CoU [2, 4, 29, 30], generally for a maximum of 10 days, similar to its use in chronic urticaria [29]. They can be also used briefly (for a maximum of 3 weeks) to treat severe cases/exacerbations of eczematous dermatitis in cases of PCD [38]. Long-term therapy should be avoided because of their frequent side effects, such as weight gain, hyperglycemia, hypertension, osteoporosis, cataracts, and gastrointestinal bleeding.

Epinephrine

Rescue therapy, in addition to systemic corticosteroids, may include epinephrine injection, which is considered the first-line treatment in cases of anaphylaxis. For this reason, it is recommended that patients with ICoU always, in addition to medic alert tags detailing their allergens, carry an injectable epinephrine with them and receive appropriate education for its self-administration in cases of life-threatening reactions [4, 5].

Alternative Therapies

Alternative therapies such as phototherapy, leukotriene receptor antagonists, or immunosuppressive drugs, which are used for chronic idiopathic/spontaneous urticaria, have not been extensively studied for CUS. However, they could be used when first-line treatments are not sufficient to ameliorate the symptoms of CUS and these interfere too greatly with the patient's quality of life [5]. These alternative therapies may include the following options.

• Phototherapy

Ultraviolet (UV) radiation, which has been successfully used in chronic urticaria, may also be effective in CUS if extensive and/or chronic symptoms are present [41, 42]. Although the mechanism of action by which phototherapy exerts its therapeutic effects in patients with urticaria is not entirely understood, it has been proposed that UVA (long wave, above 340 nm) and UVB (short wave, above 300 nm) radiation may induce T-lymphocyte apoptosis, reduce mast cells and Langerhans cells in the dermis, and also inhibit the release of histamine from mast cells and basophils [43]. Adverse effects may include erythema, hyperpigmentation, polymorphic light eruption, fatigue, and premature aging of the skin.

• Leukotriene receptor antagonists

Leukotrienes are potent mediators in urticaria that act by intensifying the inflammatory response and recruiting cells to sites of inflammation [44]. Because these mediators are allegedly involved in the pathogenesis of both NICoU and ICoU, leukotriene receptor antagonists such as montelukast and zafirlukast may in part control the symptoms of CUS with relatively few side effects [5, 45]. However, the level of evidence for recommending the use of this treatment is weak [29].

• Immunosuppressive drugs

For patients with severe and chronic symptoms of CUS in which complete avoidance of the responsible allergens is not possible and prolonged use of systemic corticosteroids is essential, corticosteroid-sparing immunosuppressive modalities could be considered as therapeutic alternatives to ameliorate the symptoms. These agents, such as cyclosporine (3–5 mg/kg/day) and methotrexate (5–20 mg per week), may act by modulating the mast cell response or preventing the initial mast cell activation [31]. For example, it has been demonstrated that cyclosporine can downregulate type 1 helper T cells and inhibit anti-IgE-stimulated histamine release from mast cells and basophils, thereby achieving disease control in patients with chronic urticaria [46, 47]. However, long-term corticosteroid therapy is limited by the adverse side effects, which include hypertension and renal toxicity secondary to cyclosporine and bone marrow suppression and hepatitis secondary to methotrexate [29, 31].

• Anti-IgE therapy

Omalizumab is a humanized recombinant monoclonal antibody that specifically binds to the Cε3 domain of the IgE heavy chain. This domain is the site at which IgE binds to the high-affinity IgE receptor (FcεRI) on the surface of target cells (mast cells and basophils). Thereby, omalizumab reduces the levels of free IgE and the density of the FcεRI receptor, both of which are essential in the activation (and consequently degranulation) of mast cells and basophils [48, 49]. Omalizumab was approved in 2014 to be administered subcutaneously every 4 weeks for the treatment of chronic spontaneous urticaria refractory to H1 antihistamines. During the past years, its efficacy has been also demonstrated for patients suffering from different types of chronic inducible urticarias, such as symptomatic dermographism, cold urticaria, and solar urticaria [50–52]. Similarly, and although there is no current evidence available on CUS, omalizumab may be a potentially interesting treatment for a certain subset of patients with severe and refractory ICoU because IgE has a key role in the pathophysiology of this condition. Side effects derived from its use are usually mild or moderate, including headache, nasopharyngitis, sinusitis, nausea, diarrhea, and local symptoms at the site of injection [49].

• Immunotherapy

Finally, another alternative treatment that shows promise in controlling symptoms of CUS when complete avoidance of the responsible allergens is not possible is the induction of tolerance through immunotherapy. In this sense, an Italian group reported a satisfactory clinical improvement among bakers and pastry makers with occupational disease from wheat flour sensitization by using specific immunotherapy: 83% of the patients were still at work and 70% claimed only weak or no symptoms during work years after this treatment [53]. Regarding its safety profile, Nettis et al. evaluated the tolerability of sublingual immunotherapy with latex extract among patients with latex-induced CoU in a double-blind, placebo-controlled study [54]. Their results supported the safety of this specific immunotherapy as no statistically significant differences were found between the proportions of adverse events in both the latex-induced CoU group and the placebo group. Nevertheless, these experimental immunotherapies for select urticants are undergoing evaluation and they are not currently available for widespread use.

Conclusions

The avoidance of the responsible/suspected allergen whenever possible is considered the mainstay of the treatment of CUS. First-line medications used to provide symptomatic relief depend on the type of immediate contact skin reaction and its pathophysiology. Thus, antihistamines are considered the best treatment for CoU in which an immunological mechanism is suggested, whereas acetylsalicylic acid and NSAIDs are reserved for cases of NICoU. Topical immunomodulation should be used in cases of CUS presented with eczematous dermatitis (PCD). Alternative systemic therapies, such as phototherapy, leukotriene receptor antagonists, immunosuppressive drugs, and omalizumab, can be considered in cases of severe or chronic CUS; however, the level of evidence for recommending the use of these agents in CUS is weak. Further biochemical research is certainly required to definitively illustrate the immunologic signaling and cellular mechanisms activated by contact urticants.

References

1. Wakelin SH. Contact urticaria. Clin Exp Dermatol. 2001;26(2):132–6.
2. Gimenez-Arnau A, Maurer M, De La Cuadra J, Maibach H. Immediate contact skin reactions, an update of contact urticaria, contact urticaria syndrome and protein contact dermatitis – "A never ending story". Eur J Dermatol. 2010;20(5):552–62.
3. Maibach HI, Johnson HL. Contact urticaria syndrome. Contact urticaria to diethyltoluamide (immediate-type hypersensitivity). Arch Dermatol. 1975;111(6):726–30.
4. Aquino M, Mawhirt S, Fonacier L. Review of contact urticaria syndrome- evaluation to treatment. Curr Treat Options Allergy. 2015;2(4):365–80.
5. Bhatia R, Alikhan A, Maibach HI. Contact urticaria: present scenario. Indian J Dermatol. 2009;54(3):264–8.
6. Wang CY, Maibach HI. Immunologic contact urticaria- the human touch. Cutan Ocul Toxicol. 2013;32(2):154–60.
7. Von Krogh G, Maibach HI. The contact urticaria syndrome- an updated review. J Am Acad Dermatol. 1981;5(3):328–42.
8. McFadden J. Immunologic contact urticaria. Immunol Allergy Clin N Am. 2014;34(1):157–67.
9. Verhulst L, Goossens A. Cosmetic components causing contact urticaria: a review and update. Contact Dermatitis. 2016;75(6):333–44.
10. Nicholson PJ, Llewellyn D, English JS, Guidelines Development Group. Evidence-based guidelines for the prevention, identification and management of occupational contact dermatitis and urticaria. Contact Dermatitis. 2010;63(4):177–86.
11. Adisesh A, Robinson E, Nicholson PJ, Sen D, Wilkinson M, Standards of Care Working Group. U.K. standards of care for occupational contact dermatitis and occupational contact urticaria. Br J Dermatol. 2013;168(6):1167–75.
12. Chowdhury MMU. Occupational contact urticaria: a diagnosis not to be missed. Br J Dermatol. 2015;173(6):1364–5.
13. Amaro C, Goossens A. Immunological occupational contact urticaria and contact dermatitis from proteins: a review. Contact Dermatitis. 2008;58(2):67–75.
14. Dean AM, Secrest AM, Powell DL. Contact urticaria from occupational exposure to formaldehyde. Dermatitis. 2016;27(4):232.
15. Saluja SS, Davis CL, Chong TA, Powell DL. Contact urticaria to nickel: a series of 11 patients who were prick test positive and patch test negative to nickel sulfate 2.5% and 5.0%. Dermatitis. 2016;27(5):282–7.
16. Gomułka K, Panaszek B. Contact urticaria syndrome caused by haptens. Postepy Dermatol Alergol. 2014;31(2):108–12.
17. Venarske D, deShazo RD. Molecular mechanisms of allergic disease. South Med J. 2003;96(11):1049–54.
18. Lahti A, Oikarinen A, Viinikka L, Ylikorkala O, Hannuksela M. Prostaglandins in contact urticaria induced by benzoic acid. Acta Derm Venereol. 1983;63(5):425–7.
19. Lahti A, Väänänen A, Kokkonen EL, Hannuksela M. Acetylsalicylic acid inhibits non-immunologic contact urticaria. Contact Dermatitis. 1987;16(3):133–5.
20. Johansson J, Lahti A. Topical non-steroidal anti-inflammatory drugs inhibit non-immunologic immediate contact reactions. Contact Dermatitis. 1988;19(3):161–5.
21. Morrow JD, Minton TA, Awad JA, Roberts LJ. Release of markedly increased quantities of prostaglandin D2 from the skin in vivo in humans following the application of sorbic acid. Arch Dermatol. 1994;130(11):1408–12.
22. Levin C, Warshaw E. Protein contact dermatitis: allergens, pathogenesis, and management. Dermatitis. 2008;19(5):241–51.
23. Kanerva L, Estlander T. Immediate and delayed skin allergy from cow dander. Am J Contact Dermat. 1997;8(3):167–9.
24. Conde-Salazar L, González MA, Guimaraens D. Type I and Type IV sensitization to Anisakis simplex in 2 patients with hand eczema. Contact Dermatitis. 2002;46(6):361.
25. Mercader P, de la Cuadra-Oyanguren J, Rodríguez-Serna M, Pitarch-Bort G, Fortea-Baixauli JM. Treatment of protein contact dermatitis with topical tacrolimus. Acta Derm Venereol. 2005;85(6):555–6.
26. Giménez-Arnau A. Contact urticaria and the environment. Rev Env Health. 2014;29(3):207–15.
27. Alfonso JH, Bauer A, Bensefa-Colas L, Boman A, Bubas M, Constandt L, et al. Minimum standards on prevention, diagnosis and treatment of occupational and work-related skin diseases in Europe - position

paper of the COST Action StanDerm (TD 1206). J Eur Acad Dermatol Venereol. 2017;31(Suppl 4):31–43.

28. Mälkönen T, Jolanki R, Alanko K, Luukkonen R, Aalto-Korte K, Lauerma A, et al. A 6-month follow-up study of 1048 patients diagnosed with an occupational skin disease. Contact Dermatitis. 2009;61(5):261–8.

29. Zuberbier T, Aberer W, Asero R, Bindslev-Jensen C, Brzoza Z, Canonica GW, et al. The EAACI/GA(2) LEN/EDF/WAO Guideline for the definition, classification, diagnosis, and management of urticaria: the 2013 revision and update. Allergy. 2014;69(7):868–87.

30. Magerl M, Altrichter S, Borzova E, Giménez-Arnau A, Grattan CE, Lawlor F, et al. The definition, diagnostic testing and management of chronic inducible urticarias – The EAACI/GA(2) LEN/EDF/UNEV consensus recommendations 2016 update and revision. Allergy. 2016;71(6):780–802.

31. Deza G, Giménez-Arnau AM. Itch in urticaria management. Curr Probl Dermatol. 2016;50:77–85.

32. Leurs R, Church MK, Taglialatela M. H1-antihistamines: inverse agonism, anti-inflammatory actions and cardiac effects. Clin Exp Allergy. 2002;32(4):489–98.

33. Jáuregui I, Ferrer M, Montoro J, Dávila I, Bartra J, del Cuvillo A, et al. Antihistamines in the treatment of chronic urticaria. J Investig Allergol Clin Immunol. 2007;17(2):41–52.

34. Khalaf AT, Li W, Jinquan T. Current advances in the management of urticaria. Arch Immunol Ther Exp. 2008;56(2):103–14.

35. Simons FE. Advances in H1-antihistamines. N Engl J Med. 2004;351(21):2203–17.

36. Thurmond RL, Kazerouni K, Chaplan SR, Greenspan AJ. Antihistamines and itch. Handb Exp Pharmacol. 2015;226:257–90.

37. Lee EE, Maibach HI. Treatment of urticaria. An evidence-based evaluation of antihistamines. Am J Clin Dermatol. 2001;2(1):27–32.

38. Diepgen TL, Andersen KE, Chosidow O, Coenraads PJ, Elsner P, English J, et al. Guidelines for diagnosis, prevention and treatment of hand eczema. J Dtsch Dermatol Ges. 2015;13(1):e1–22.

39. Kaplan AP. Treatment of chronic urticaria: approaches other than antihistamines. In: Kaplan A, Greaves M, editors. Urticaria and angioedema. New York: Informa Healthcare; 2009. p. 365–72.

40. Lebwohl MG, Del Rosso JQ, Abramovits W, Berman B, Cohen DE, Guttman E, et al. Pathways to managing atopic dermatitis: consensus from the experts. J Clin Aesthetic Dermatol. 2013;6(Suppl 7):S2–18.

41. Kozel MMA, Sabroe RA. Chronic urticaria: aetiology, management and current and future treatment options. Drugs. 2004;64(22):2515–36.

42. Rombold S, Lobisch K, Katzer K, Grazziotin TC, Ring J, Eberlein B. Efficacy of UVA1 phototherapy in 230 patients with various skin diseases. Photodermatol Photoimmunol Photomed. 2008;24(1):19–23.

43. Hannuksela M, Kokkonen EL. Ultraviolet light therapy in chronic urticaria. Acta Derm Venereol. 1985;65(5):449–50.

44. Maxwell DL, Atkinson BA, Spur BW, Lessof MH, Lee TH. Skin responses to intradermal histamine and leukotrienes C4, D4, and E4 in patients with chronic idiopathic urticaria and in normal subjects. J Allergy Clin Immunol. 1990;86(5):759–65.

45. Sanada S, Tanaka T, Kameyoshi Y, Hide M. The effectiveness of montelukast for the treatment of antihistamine-resistant chronic urticaria. Arch Dermatol Res. 2005;297(3):134–8.

46. Altman K, Chang C. Pathogenic intracellular and autoimmune mechanisms in urticaria and angioedema. Clin Rev Allergy Immunol. 2013;45(1):47–62.

47. Marsland AM, Soundararajan S, Joseph K, Kaplan AP. Effects of calcineurin inhibitors on an in vitro assay for chronic urticaria. Clin Exp Allergy. 2005;35(5):554–9.

48. Wright JD, Chu HM, Huang CH, Ma C, Chang TW, Lim C. Structural and physical basis for anti-IgE therapy. Sci Rep. 2015;5:11581.

49. McCormack PL. Omalizumab: a review of its use in patients with chronic spontaneous urticaria. Drugs. 2014;74(14):1693–9.

50. Aubin F, Avenel-Audran M, Jeanmougin M, Adamski H, Peyron JL, Marguery MC, et al. Omalizumab in patients with severe and refractory solar urticaria: a phase II multicentric study. J Am Acad Dermatol. 2016;74(3):574–5.

51. Metz M, Schütz A, Weller K, Gorczyza M, Zimmer S, Staubach P, et al. Omalizumab is effective in cold urticaria-results of a randomized placebo-controlled trial. J Allergy Clin Immunol. 2017;140:864. https://doi.org/10.1016/j.jaci.2017.01.043.

52. Maurer M, Schütz A, Weller K, Schoepke N, Peveling-Oberhag A, Staubach P, et al. Omalizumab is effective in symptomatic dermographism-results of a randomized placebo-controlled trial. J Allergy Clin Immunol. 2017;140:870. https://doi.org/10.1016/j.jaci.2017.01.042.

53. Cirla AM. Asthma and baker's allergy: experience with health programs. G Ital Med Lav Ergon. 2011;33(1):20–5.

54. Nettis E, Di Leo E, Calogiuri G, Milani M, Delle Donne P, Ferrannini A, et al. The safety of a novel sublingual rush induction phase for latex desensitization. Curr Med Res Opin. 2010;26(8):1855–9.

Management of Contact Urticaria Through Clinical Cases

14

Tabi A. Leslie and David Orton

Introduction

Contact urticaria is the presence of an immediate wheal and flare reaction after direct contact with an external agent, appearing within 30 min and completely clearing, with no residual signs, within hours [1]. The allergic reaction may be caused by a diverse range of substances, from macromolecules (e.g., protein peptides) to simple, low–molecular weight chemicals (haptens), although this is less common [2]. The severity of contact urticaria syndrome can be classified into four stages, with stage 1 as localized contact urticaria reactions and stage IV as anaphylactoid reactions [3]. Contact urticaria can be immunological (sensitization is required to trigger a reaction) or nonimmunological (no sensitization is required). When it is immunological, contact urticaria is a manifestation of type I hypersensitivity and may be missed if the presentation appears as the worsening of a preexisting urticaria or dermatitis. There may be accompanying systemic involvement, including anaphylaxis [4]. If nonimmunological contact urticaria is mild, it may present as erythema or localized pruritus [5].

T. A. Leslie (✉)
Royal Free Hospital, London, UK
e-mail: tabi.leslie@doctors.org.uk

D. Orton
The Hillingdon Hospitals NHS Trust, Uxbridge, UK

Immediate skin reactions are common in dermatological practice but may often be overlooked. These case presentations may alert clinicians to always consider such clinical diagnoses with appropriate investigation and management. The clinical manifestations of immunological contact urticaria reflect the dose and route of exposure to the allergen and can be strictly limited to the contact areas, although ectopic sites may be affected; it can also affect other systems including the gastrointestinal and respiratory tracts.

Protein sources are classically divided into four main groups: group 1 comprises vegetables, fruits, spices, plants, and woods; group 2 includes animal proteins; group 3, grains; and group 4, enzymes [6]. The nature of these causal proteins may affect people in a wide variety of occupations. Food handlers, cooks, caterers, and stay-at-home parents are at risk from fruits, vegetables, and spices. Plants are known to cause immediate skin and mucosal symptoms among gardeners, greenhouse workers, florists, and botanical researchers. Animal proteins constitute the largest group and can cause problems in slaughterhouse workers and butchers, and veterinarians are also at great risk from amniotic or seminal fluid, blood, and saliva. Numerous fish and seafood species, as well as fishing bait maggots, have been reported as causing contact urticaria in fishermen or those who fish as a hobby. Case reports have also been published describing

© Springer International Publishing AG, part of Springer Nature 2018
A. M. Giménez-Arnau, H. I. Maibach (eds.), *Contact Urticaria Syndrome*, Updates in Clinical
Dermatology, https://doi.org/10.1007/978-3-319-89764-6_14

laboratory workers suffering from skin and respiratory symptoms following contact with insects. Different grains and enzymes are known to cause contact urticaria and protein contact dermatitis, and these may be accompanied by respiratory problems in bakers. A variety of low–molecular weight substances (e.g., foodstuffs, preservatives, fragrances) can induce a distinct form of nonimmunological contact urticaria. These agents are frequently encountered in people's surroundings and may produce a reaction without any previous sensitization in most, if not all, exposed persons.

Contact urticaria is diagnosed by taking a detailed history and performing a detailed examination. Identification of the implicated agent may be confirmed by skin prick, scratch, and scratch chamber testing, and measuring the specific IgE may be helpful for some proteins in immunological contact urticaria [7]. Also, a very simple "open test" may be performed on the skin sites suggested by the patient's history to provoke an immediate skin reaction. Management of contact urticaria is based upon avoidance of the suspected agent. Contact urticaria, as other occupational skin diseases, can be prevented by applying the normal hierarchy of preventive measures, that is, elimination, substitution, engineering controls, safe work practices, and personal protective equipment. In a recent Finnish report, almost half the patients (46%) with occupational contact urticaria and protein contact dermatitis had concomitant occupational airway disease. Patients with contact urticaria or protein contact dermatitis should always be asked about respiratory symptoms, and preventive measures at the workplace should include protection of both the skin and the airway [8]. In the case of immunological contact urticaria, there is no pharmacological cure that can reverse sensitization once it has occurred [9]. However, treatments that inhibit mast cell mediator release and effects, or that may control or ameliorate symptoms, may be beneficial. These agents include second-generation non-sedating antihistamines for urticaria, topical calcineurin inhibitors or topical steroids if there is dermatitis, or a short course of oral steroids for rescue treatment of severe symptoms [10]. Nevertheless, the best course of action is to recognize and prevent contact with the eliciting trigger, and therefore correct identification of that substance is vital.

Our collective knowledge of the particular agents that have potential for causing immediate skin reactions is slowly increasing with time, thanks to descriptions of isolated events in case reports. This chapter presents a selection of interesting case reports that demonstrate the wide diversity of clinical presentations by which physicians may be challenged, as well as the appropriate investigations and management. Substances that cause contact urticaria may be classified in a number of ways: by molecular weight, mechanism of action, common use in daily life (e.g., chemicals, cosmetics, plants, foods), or associated occupations. An interesting approach to classifying the causes of contact urticaria could be to consider substances as belonging one to the separate groups of the natural world, for example, animal, vegetable, or mineral.

Clinical Cases

A number of cases where immunological contact urticaria has involved anaphylaxis have been reviewed in case reports. Awareness is important, especially where the use of implicated agents is widespread, but not obviously apparent, as in the following case.

Chlorhexidine is a biguanide topical antiseptic and disinfectant with broad antimicrobial efficacy. It is increasingly being used in instillation gels for urinary catheters, and in contact lens solutions, but also in many cosmetic products in which it may be used as a preservative or an antimicrobial agent at a concentration up to 0.3%, according to the European Cosmetics Regulation. Urticaria following application to intact skin or mucosae in some cases has been accompanied by dyspnea, angioedema, syncope, or anaphylaxis. These reactions have been described via the mucosal route at much lower concentrations than elsewhere, generally as low as 0.05%.

Case 1. From: Anaphylaxis after disinfection with 2% chlorhexidine wand applicator. Bahal S, Sharma S, Garvey, LH, Nagendran V. BMJ Case Rep 2017. [11]

This case report describes a 54-year-old patient who had been attending regular dialysis sessions and taking regular medication (including chlorphenamine 4 mg) with no adverse reactions. He had been feeling well and had not eaten anything unusual on the day of the event. In preparation for the dialysis procedure, the nurse removed his Tesio catheter, and a Chloraprep 3 ml Wand Applicator was used to scrub the insertion area on his chest. Seconds later, the patient developed an urticarial rash accompanied by itching that was widespread and intense. He became dizzy, short of breath, and less responsive with reduced blood pressure. He was treated for anaphylaxis with intramuscular epinephrine 200 µg, intravenous hydrocortisone 200 mg, and chlorphenamine 10 mg, plus high-flow oxygen, nebulized epinephrine 500 µg, and a 750-ml fluid bolus. Over the following 15 min, the patient's symptoms improved and the urticarial rash subsided.

Further management was provided by the hospital immunology team. Although the patient was presumed to be allergic to chlorhexidine, he had been repeatedly exposed to the same product on previous occasions with no reaction or irritation, and had no known drug allergies. The patient had elevated tryptase level 1 h after the reaction. Chlorhexidine IgE levels remained negative over 6 months of repeat testing. Skin prick testing to 0.5% chlorhexidine induced a 10-mm wheal, with appropriate responses from positive and negative control tests. Intradermal testing to 0.0002% chlorhexidine showed a positive result, with a wheal diameter increase from 6 to 15 mm. Both tests were performed with validated concentrations.

Chlorhexidine was identified as the cause by the positive skin prick and intradermal tests, as well as by the evidence apparent from the history. Complete avoidance of products containing chlorhexidine was advised. Disclosure of the allergy upon any interaction with the health service was recommended, to ensure against accidental reexposure in a clinical setting. Furthermore, use of numerous household items was cautioned, such as mouthwashes, toothpastes, creams, lozenges, dressings, disinfectants, and other cleaning solutions. In addition, the patient was equipped with an epinephrine auto-injector for emergency use and a Medic Alert bracelet.

Chlorhexidine may trigger anaphylaxis in patients who have become sensitized by various means of repeated exposure, such as contact with skin wounds, oral mucosa, and catheters. More serious reactions may be preceded by local or generalized urticaria and other mild reactions. In this case, where the allergy developed after many noneventful exposures to chlorhexidine, the authors propose that chlorhexidine applied to inflamed skin may have penetrated the stratum corneum, activating resident antigen-presenting cells, and processing haptenized chlorhexidine. The authors suspect that the use of 2% chlorhexidine in single-application products in the UK may be a factor in increased allergic sensitization to chlorhexidine. In 1997 the U.S. Food and Drug Administration (FDA) issued a warning about chlorhexidine allergic reactions because it was implicated in several cases of anaphylaxis. In February 2017, the FDA released another warning that urged manufacturers of over-the-counter antiseptic products to increase awareness of the risk of serious allergic reactions to chlorhexidine.

Case 2. From: Contact urticaria syndrome and protein contact dermatitis caused by glycerin enema. Suzuki R, Fukuyama K, Yasuhiro M, Namiki T. JAAD Case Reports 2016;2:108–110. [12]

Glycerin is a trihydric alcohol (molecular formula $C_3H_8O_3$). As it has stable nontoxic, nonirritating, and hypoallergenic properties, glycerin is commonly used in medicine, cosmetics, and food. It is also used as a negative control in allergy scratch tests. Although rarely a sensitizer, glycerin may be a cause of contact urticaria syndrome. Suzuki et al. published a case report in

2016 describing an 81-year-old lady who developed a generalized urticarial eruption with a contact urticaria syndrome caused by a glycerin enema. While an inpatient on a medical ward, she was noted to develop eruptions on the days that she received treatment. Symptoms would develop 30 min after the enema containing 50% glycerin was administered and disappear within an hour. These eruptions were associated with a rise in temperature. She was therefore prick tested and scratch prick tested to 50% glycerine and the lubricant used for the enema (dimethylpolysiloxane) as well as the container (polyethylene). All the prick testing results were negative. Scratch-patch testing at the glycerin area revealed an urticarial wheal, in contrast to a slight skin flush with flat exanthemas (with no swelling) at the other two areas. Although scratch tests are less standardized than prick tests, they are useful for investigating a nonstandard allergen.

Contact urticaria syndrome to glycerine was diagnosed and the patient advised to discontinue glycerin enemas. Symptoms did not return after cessation of the enemas. This case was classified by the authors as being stage 2 (generalized urticaria) and immunological, because the patient's symptoms began after repetitive exposure to the enema, and glycerin is a rare sensitizer. It should be noted that the rise in temperature that accompanied the generalized urticaria suggests that the patient had a risk of anaphylaxis.

This case is important because glycerin enemas are commonly used in the hospital setting to control constipation. It has been demonstrated here that glycerin can be a cause of contact urticaria syndrome, which may even lead to anaphylaxis.

Cosmetic Components Causing Contact Urticaria

Adverse reactions to cosmetics include irritant, allergic and photo-allergic contact dermatitis, and contact urticaria.

There are reports of hair dyes causing immediate-type hypersensitivity, some with anaphylaxis or respiratory symptoms: *p*-

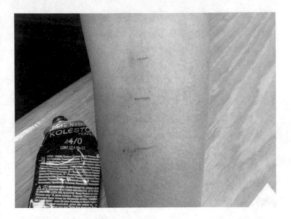

Fig. 14.1 Example of a positive skin prick test to oxidative hair dye whole product. (Courtesy of Dr. Orton)

phenylenediamine (PPD) and its derivatives, such as *p*-aminophenol and *p*-methylaminophenol and toluene-2,5-diamine (Fig. 14.1). The reactions seem to occur only after oxidation by H_2O_2 [13] and are attenuated when the antioxidant sodium sulfite is added to the mix,

Goldberg et al. [14] identified Bandrowski base (CAS no. 20048-27-5), an oxidation product of PPD, as a culprit.

Protein hydrolysates of collagen, keratin, elastin, milk, wheat, almond, and silk are often added to hair conditioners to give the appearance of healthy hair and to add volume. They are also causes of contact urticaria. These substances are capable of producing reactions through a type 1 mechanism, especially in atopic dermatitis patients [15, 16]. Hydrolyzed wheat proteins are also widely used in many other cosmetic products, for which several cases have been reported in the literature, including the induction of wheat-dependent exercise-induced anaphylaxis.

Case 3. From: Fatal latex allergy. Pumphrey RS, Duddridge M, Norton J. J Allergy Clin Immunol 2001;107(3):558. [17]

Pumphrey et al. described the anaphylactic death of a 28-year-old British fashion designer immediately following a hair extension procedure, secondary to exposure to natural rubber latex in the bonding adhesive. The patient had a history of nut allergy and inhalant atopy, and a known strongly positive prick test reaction to natural rubber latex. Moreover, this type of bonding glue may also be used in the application of artificial eyelashes.

There are many cases in the literature illustrating contact urticaria to a wide variety of foodstuffs. Food industry workers are likely candidates for sensitization, with repeated exposure occurring over time, with a response of the immunological contact urticaria type. Occupational groups that are typically at risk include bakers and agricultural and dairy workers, as well as those employed in food-processing factories and restaurants.

Case 4. From: Occupational contact urticaria caused by squid. Ljubojević Hadžavdić S, Marinović Kulišić S, Jurakić Tončić R, Jerković Gulin S, Bradamante M. Contact Dermatitis 2016;74:304–305. [18]

Workers who handle seafood directly are more at risk of developing contact urticaria to fish or crustacea, Sensitization may occur via concentrated skin contact or airway exposure. Occupational allergy to molluscs such as squid has been rarely reported, being much less common than allergy to crustacea (e.g., shrimp). The main allergenic protein in squid is tropomyosin, also found in crustacea and arachnids (house dust mites), and cross-reactive allergens have been identified from squid and octopus. This case report describes a 20-year old restaurant worker who for 2 years experienced recurring localized urticaria within 15 min of contact with squid, with symptoms being more severe during the working week. She had not worn the protective gloves that were provided for her and therefore had frequent direct contact with water and the food to be cooked. Although she was able to handle other shellfish (including oysters and crabs) as well as tolerating eating cooked squid, she suffered from itching and burning when handling octopus.

Prick testing with common food allergens (e.g., fish, cow's milk, egg), as well as with pollen, house dust mites, and pet dander did not reveal any IgE-mediated sensitization. Total serum IgE was elevated slightly, and IgE specific for seafood showed positive results for squid. A clear positive reaction was seen in prick-to-prick testing with squid (12 × 15 mm after 15 min). An open challenge was also performed, wherein fresh squid was applied to the patient's forearm, with contact urticaria being triggered within minutes. Management consisted of advising against further handling of squid and recommending the use of protective gloves while at work, to prevent further reactions.

This case is a rare description of occupational allergy resulting from exposure to squid, which was confirmed by the positive results of prick testing and open skin testing, although an accompanying sensitization to house dust mites, which might have been expected, was not identified.

Case 5. From: Contact urticaria from beer. Koelemij I, van Zuuren EJ. Clin Exp Dermatol 2014;39:407–409. [19]

Two patients with occupational contact urticaria after contact with beer were described in this report. Both patients had a positive medical history of atopic dermatitis and rhinoconjunctivitis. The patients noticed wheals on their hands following direct contact with beer while working in a bar, where one was a bartender and the other was a waitress. The pathomechanism of the development of contact urticaria after contact with beer is not known. The positive prick test result with beer and the presence of IgE antibodies for beer components point to an immunological mechanism in beer-related contact urticaria.

Case 6. From: Contact urticaria from beer. Gutgesell C, Fuchs T. Contact Dermatitis 1995;33:436–437. [20]

A 20-year-old waitress with atopic dermatitis since childhood, rhinoconjunctivitis, and sensitization to numerous inhalant allergens, reported developing urticaria on her hands whenever in contact with beer at work. She maintained that beer did not aggravate her eczema, and that drinking beer did not cause her any problems. Prick and scratch tests were performed, and specific IgE was measured using the radioallergosor-

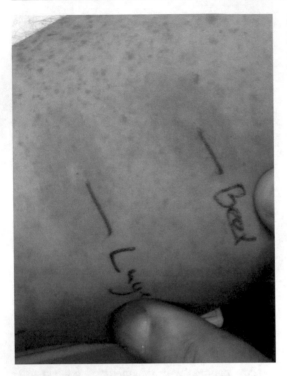

Fig. 14.2 Example of positive skin prick test reactions to beer and lager in a patient reporting contact urticaria. (Courtesy of Dr. Orton)

bent test (RAST) (Fig. 14.2). There were markedly positive scratch test reactions to three different beers and a positive prick test to brewer's yeast, with no eczematous lesions observed at the site after 24 h. The patient's contact urticaria to beer, along with a RAST class 3 result with Budweiser, was suggested by the authors to be caused by an immediate-type reaction to malt (RAST class 3), as well as to brewer's yeast (RAST class 1). The authors concluded that malt allergy is therefore critical to allergy to beer.

Although immunological contact urticaria to proteins is well described in the occupational setting, this case report illustrates the need to consider the diagnosis in other contexts, such as domestic situations.

Case 7 From: Contact urticaria and protein contact dermatitis to chapatti flour. Davies E, Orton DI. Contact Dermatitis 2009;60:113–114. [21]

Chapatti flour is a whole wheat flour used frequently in Asian cookery for the everyday staple

chapattis. They are frequently cooked in Asian households several times a week by combining the flour (often blended with malted barley) with water and then cooking them on a flat heavy hot plate.

Orton et al. described one case of contact urticaria and two cases of protein contact dermatitis to chapatti flour in Asian housewives in their fourth decade. A 36-year-old woman presented with a history of itchy wheals that developed on her hands immediately after handling chapatti flour. She had no personal history of atopy. Prick testing to her chapatti flour as well as to a commercial wheat flour reagent were positive, and a positive weal and flare reaction was also produced by scratch chamber test to chapatti flour. A second 36-year-old woman presented with a 10-year history of fingertip eczema, She would also start sneezing within minutes of exposure to chapatti flour. Patch testing to flour was negative, but positive results were observed with both scratch chamber testing to chapatti flour and prick testing to wheat flour. Both patients were checked for dermographism by abrading an area of normal skin, which also acted as a control for the scratch chamber tests. This test was negative on both occasions. The final patient was a 37-year-old woman with a history of lifelong atopic dermatitis, presenting with a 3-year history of persistent hand eczema, which affected fingertips and the palmar surface of both hands. On further questioning, the patient disclosed that immediately after handling chapatti flour, she experienced itching and burning of her hands. Skin prick tests to chapatti and wheat flour were both positive. Management of all three patients was based on advice to avoid direct contact with chapatti flour while preparing and cooking the chapattis by wearing latex-free gloves. The eczema improved considerably in two of the cases. However, the third patient reported difficulty in handling the dough wearing gloves, and her eczema persists.

The authors concluded that the diagnoses of contact urticaria and protein contact dermatitis should also be considered in the domestic as well as an occupational setting. All patients presenting with hand eczema, particularly Asian housewives, should be examined for clinical features of contact urticaria.

**Case 8. From: Silk contact anaphy-
laxis.** Makatsori M, Scadding GW, Skypala I,
Durham SR. Contact Dermatitis 2014;71:314–
315. [22]

Silk, gathered from the cocoon of the silkworm, is a common cause of occupational asthma
among workers in the industry. The two major
types are cultivated mulberry silk and wild silk,
produced by different species of silkworm. The
silk used in clothing is stripped of allergenic proteins, and because the structural protein of silk
(fibroin) has low allergenic potential, allergy to
silk in clothing is rare. Makatsori et al. present
the case of a 23-year-old female with a past history of mild eczema, asthma, and allergic rhinitis.
She had already been diagnosed as sensitized to
house dust mites, tree pollens, and grass, confirmed by specific IgE and prick tests, and had a
history of anaphylactic reactions to tree nuts,
peanuts, and lemon seeds. The patient then experienced anaphylaxis without having been exposed
to these foods, although she had eaten a bread roll
with sunflower seeds 2 h before the reaction. This
event had led her to believe that sunflower seeds
may have been the cause, and she proceeded to
strictly avoid these, along with all other seeds.
However, upon comprehensive questioning after
further referral, a detail emerged that implicated
silk as the suspect agent. The patient had gone
shopping on the day of the reaction, and tried on
a silk blouse and silk dress. An urticarial rash
developed within 5 min, followed closely by difficulty breathing and faintness, consistent with
anaphylaxis criteria. The patient was treated with
intramuscular adrenaline by attending paramed-
ics and she recovered fully. Through taking a
detailed history, it was also revealed that several
months after the anaphylactic reaction, the patient
had developed generalized urticaria subsequent
to putting on a silk dress at home.

Investigations were performed to test both
sunflower seeds and silk. The patient's total IgE
level was 725 IU/ml, with the level of specific
IgE against sunflower seeds 8.50 IU/ml. Prick-
prick testing with whole sunflower seed induced
a 2-mm wheal. A positive prick test is defined as

a wheal with diameter ≥ 3 mm; therefore, further
graded challenges to sunflower seeds were made,
with no adverse reaction. Prick testing was then
performed with the same silk fabric that had previously caused urticaria in the patient. With dry
silk, the prick testing caused a wheal of 2 mm,
but with damp silk, a wheal of 22 mm was provoked. The same damp silk fabric gave negative
results from prick testing with two control subjects. Next, a modified patch test was implemented with a piece of the silk fabric applied to
the forearm and left for 15 min in contact with the
skin. After 15 min the damp silk gave multiple
wheals, which spread for several centimeters
away from the region of direct contact. Last, the
level of specific IgE against mulberry silk was
tested and found to be 1.00 IU/ml, although specific IgE against wild silk waste matter was negative (<0.35 IU/ml).

Along with the detailed history that was even-
tually obtained, the results of the investigations
confirmed the diagnosis of contact allergy to silk.
The patient was advised to avoid silk clothing.

This is thought to be the first reported case of
anaphylaxis requiring epinephrine treatment
caused by skin contact with silk. Fibroin is considered to be of low allergenic potential but is
held together by sericin, a sticky water-soluble
glycoprotein. Given that the patient had a positive skin test reaction to damp but not to dry silk
fabric, the authors of this case report hypothesize
that prolonged skin contact in conjunction with a
sufficient amount of surface sweat was required
to provoke the anaphylactic reaction. Silk is promoted as being a hypoallergenic fabric and is
often recommended for people with atopic dermatitis. Therefore, this case makes an important
contribution to the literature in highlighting the
potential of silk to act as an IgE-mediated contact
allergen, which may cause anaphylaxis.

Human Seminal Plasma

*Human seminal plasma (HSP) hypersensitivity is
defined as a spectrum of systemic and/or localized
symptoms after exposure to specific protein components in seminal plasma.*

HSP allergy was first reported in 1958 by Specken [23], who described the case of a 65-year-old woman who, after coitus, would have a generalized urticarial skin reaction, sometimes accompanied by asthma attacks, which would disappear after some 3 h. It is rarely diagnosed, as in most cases, only vulvovaginal symptoms are elicited, which are often chronic and for which no cause is readily apparent [24]. The major antigen is believed to be prostate-specific antigen, although this heterogeneous disorder is likely to involve other proteins. Although there are no known risk factors for developing HSP hypersensitivity, women who develop systemic symptoms are more often also atopic. Symptoms can appear after first time intercourse in up to 50% of cases, in both systemic and localized forms [25]. The development of systemic reactions may be preceded by mild local reactions for many months or years. This diagnosis should also be considered in cases of vulvovaginitis.

Diagnosis requires a careful history, with the gold standard for diagnosing HSP hypersensitivity being that symptoms completely subside when a condom prophylactic is habitually used. Patients with HSP hypersensitivity often elicit positive skin prick testing and/or serum-specific immunoglobulin E to whole seminal fluid or fractionated seminal plasma proteins (Fig. 14.3). Infertility has not been demonstrated to be related

to HSP hypersensitivity. However, it is often difficult for women with HSP hypersensitivity to conceive because they are unwilling to have unprotected sex, and because treatment often involves the use of condoms. Other treatments which may facilitate conception involve local desensitization, which may be achieved by intravaginal administrations of the partner's seminal plasma in serial dilutions [26]. Alternatively, subcutaneous desensitization to relevant fractionated seminal plasma proteins obtained from the woman's sexual partner may achieve systemic tolerance in patients with anaphylactic sensitivity [27]. In most cases, HSP hypersensitivity is successfully managed using a combination of these approaches.

Case 9. From: Allergy to human seminal plasma and latex: case report and review of the literature. Kint B, Degreef H, Dooms-Goossens A. Contact Dermatitis 1994;30(1):7–11. [24]

The case is reported of a 32-year-old atopic woman with combined type I and possible type IV allergy to human seminal plasma, as well as type I allergy to latex. Clinical symptoms were swelling and a burning sensation on the vulva and in the vulvovaginal area during or after coitus, followed by vesiculation, lichenification, and the development of generalized eczema. Diagnosis was confirmed by investigation with positive prick tests to seminal fluid and natural rubber latex.

Conclusion

The management of contact urticaria can be straightforward, but many cases may present diagnostic challenges. This chapter has highlighted some interesting cases to provide clinicians with a range of possibilities to bear in mind when assessing their next patient presenting with a complicated or unexpected presentation or clinical history.

It will be helpful for diagnosis if in vivo tests can be replaced by effective in vitro tests. Presently there are only a small number of in

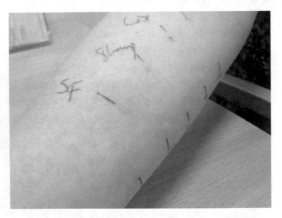

Fig. 14.3 Example of a positive skin prick test to seminal fluid (SF) in a lady reporting severe vulval itching after coitus and resolution when the partner wore condoms. (Courtesy of Dr. Orton)

vitro tests available for a few immunological allergens, including natural rubber latex [10].

Once the agent has been identified and the symptoms controlled, the current mainstay of treatment for contact urticaria remains to be trigger avoidance and use of personal protective equipment. Additional treatments may be considered, with the intention of suppressing or improving symptoms. Second-generation non-sedating antihistamines are the recommended first-line treatment for urticaria, although a pulse of oral prednisolone or the addition of other medications may be necessary.

Further research will aid the better understanding and prevention of contact urticaria, with the aim of developing a global approach to its management.

References

1. Fisher AA. Contact dermatitis. Philadelphia: Lea & Febiger; 1973.
2. Wilkinson M, Orton D. Allergic contact dermatitis. In: Griffith's C, Barker J, Chalmers R, Bleiker T, Creamer D, editors. Rook's textbook of dermatology. 9th ed. Oxford: Wiley; 2016.
3. von Krogh G, Maibach HI. The contact urticaria syndrome – an updated review. J Am Acad Dermatol. 1981;5(3):328–42.
4. McFadden J. Immunologic contact urticaria. Immunol Allergy Clin N Am. 2014;34(1):157–67.
5. Wakelin SH. Contact urticaria. Clin Exp Dermatol. 2001;26(2):132–6.
6. Amaro C, Goossens A. Immunological occupational contact urticaria and contact dermatitis from proteins: a review. Contact Dermatitis. 2008;58(2):67–75.
7. Gimenez-Arnau A. Contact urticaria and the environment. Rev Environ Health. 2014;29(3):207–15.
8. Helaskoski E, Suojalehto H, Kuuliala O, Aalto-Korte K. Occupational contact urticaria and protein contact dermatitis: causes and concomitant airway diseases. Contact Dermatitis. 2017;77:390.
9. Wang CY, Maibach HI. Immunologic contact urticaria – the human touch. Cutan Ocul Toxicol. 2013;32(2):154–60.
10. Gimenez-Arnau A, Maurer M, De La Cuadra J, Maibach H. Immediate contact skin reactions, an update of Contact Urticaria, Contact Urticaria Syndrome and Protein Contact Dermatitis – "A Never Ending Story". Eur J Dermatol. 2010;20(5):552–62.
11. Anaphylaxis after disinfection with 2% chlorhexidine wand applicator. Sameer Bahal, Samriti Sharma, Lene Heise Garvey, Vasantha Nagendran. BMJ Case Reports 2017:published online 8 August 2017, doi:10.1136/bcr-2017-219794
12. Suzuki R, Fukuyama K, Miyazaki Y, Namiki T. Contact urticaria syndrome and protein contact dermatitis caused by glycerin enema. JAAD Case Rep. 2016;2(2):108–10.
13. Pasche-Koo F, French L, Piletta-Zanin PA, Hauser C. Contact urticaria and shock to hair dye. Allergy. 1998;53(9):904–5.
14. Goldberg BJ, Herman FF, Hirata I. Systemic anaphylaxis due to an oxidation product of p-phenylenediamine in a hair dye. Ann Allergy. 1987;58(3):205–8.
15. Niinimaki A, Niinimaki M, Makinen-Kiljunen S, Hannuksela M. Contact urticaria from protein hydrolysates in hair conditioners. Allergy. 1998;53(11):1078–82.
16. Verhulst L, Goossens A. Cosmetic components causing contact urticaria syndrome: an update. In: Gimenez Arnau A, Maibach H, editors. Contact urticaria syndrome. Boca Raton: CRC Press; 2014. p. 203–18.
17. Pumphrey RS, Duddridge M, Norton J. Fatal latex allergy. J Allergy Clin Immunol. 2001;107(3):558.
18. Ljubojevic Hadzavdic S, Marinovic Kulisic S, Jurakic Toncic R, Jerkovic Gulin S, Bradamante M. Occupational contact urticaria caused by squid. Contact Dermatitis. 2016;74(5):304–5.
19. Koelemij I, van Zuuren EJ. Contact urticaria from beer. Clin Exp Dermatol. 2014;39(3):407–9.
20. Gutgesell C, Fuchs T. Contact urticaria from beer. Contact Dermatitis. 1995;33(6):436–7.
21. Davies E, Orton D. Contact urticaria and protein contact dermatitis to chapatti flour. Contact Dermatitis. 2009;60(2):113–4.
22. Makatsori M, Scadding GW, Skypala I, Durham SR. Silk contact anaphylaxis. Contact Dermatitis. 2014;71(5):314–5.
23. Specken. A strange case of allergy in gynecology. Ned Tijdschr Verloskd Gynaecol. 1958;58(5):314–8; discussion 8–21.
24. Kint B, Degreef H, Dooms-Goossens A. Combined allergy to human seminal plasma and latex: case report and review of the literature. Contact Dermatitis. 1994;30(1):7–11.
25. Bernstein JA. Human seminal plasma hypersensitivity: an under-recognized women's health issue. Postgrad Med. 2011;123(1):120–5.
26. Lee J, Kim S, Kim M, Chung YB, Huh JS, Park CM, et al. Anaphylaxis to husband's seminal plasma and treatment by local desensitization. Clin Mol Allergy. 2008;6:13.
27. Mittman RJ, Bernstein DI, Adler TR, Korbee L, Nath V, Gallagher JS, et al. Selective desensitization to seminal plasma protein fractions after immunotherapy for postcoital anaphylaxis. J Allergy Clin Immunol. 1990;86(6 Pt 1):954–60.

Index

© Springer International Publishing AG, part of Springer Nature 2018
A. M. Giménez-Arnau, H. I. Maibach (eds.), *Contact Urticaria Syndrome*, Updates in Clinical
Dermatology, https://doi.org/10.1007/978-3-319-89764-6

Printed in the United States
By Bookmasters